Statistical Methods in Psychiatry and Related Fields

Longitudinal, Clustered, and Other Repeated Measures Data

CHAPMAN & HALL/CRC

Interdisciplinary Statistics Series

Series editors: N. Keiding, B.J.T. Morgan, C.K. Wikle, P. van der Heijden

Published titles

AGE-PERIOD-COHORT ANALYSIS: NEW MODELS, METHODS, AND EMPIRICAL APPLICATIONS Y. Yang and K. C. Land

ANALYSIS OF CAPTURE-RECAPTURE DATA R. S. McCrea and B. J. T. Morgan

AN INVARIANT APPROACH TO STATISTICAL ANALYSIS OF SHAPES S. Lele and J. Richtsmeier

ASTROSTATISTICS G. Babu and E. Feigelson

BAYESIAN ANALYSIS FOR POPULATION ECOLOGY R. King, B. J. T. Morgan, O. Gimenez, and S. P. Brooks

BAYESIAN DISEASE MAPPING: HIERARCHICAL MODELING IN SPATIAL EPIDEMIOLOGY, SECOND EDITION A. B. Lawson

BIOEQUIVALENCE AND STATISTICS IN CLINICAL PHARMACOLOGY S. Patterson and B. Jones

CAPTURE-RECAPTURE METHODS FOR THE SOCIAL AND MEDICAL SCIENCES D. Böhning, P. G. M. van der Heijden, and J. Bunge

CLINICAL TRIALS IN ONCOLOGY, THIRD EDITION S. Green, J. Benedetti, A. Smith, and J. Crowley

CLUSTER RANDOMISED TRIALS R.J. Hayes and L.H. Moulton

CORRESPONDENCE ANALYSIS IN PRACTICE, THIRD EDITION M. Greenacre

THE DATA BOOK: COLLECTION AND MANAGEMENT OF RESEARCH DATA M. Zozus

DESIGN AND ANALYSIS OF QUALITY OF LIFE STUDIES IN CLINICAL TRIALS, SECOND EDITION D.L. Fairclough

DYNAMICAL SEARCH L. Pronzato, H. Wynn, and A. Zhigljavsky

FLEXIBLE IMPUTATION OF MISSING DATA S. van Buuren

GENERALIZED LATENT VARIABLE MODELING: MULTILEVEL, LONGITUDINAL, AND STRUCTURAL EQUATION MODELS A. Skrondal and S. Rabe-Hesketh

GRAPHICAL ANALYSIS OF MULTI-RESPONSE DATA K. Basford and J. Tukey

INTRODUCTION TO COMPUTATIONAL BIOLOGY: MAPS, SEQUENCES, AND GENOMES M. Waterman

MARKOV CHAIN MONTE CARLO IN PRACTICE W. Gilks, S. Richardson, and D. Spiegelhalter

Published titles

MEASUREMENT ERROR ANDMISCLASSIFICATION IN STATISTICS AND EPIDEMIOLOGY: IMPACTS AND BAYESIAN ADJUSTMENTS P. Gustafson

MEASUREMENT ERROR: MODELS, METHODS, AND APPLICATIONS
J. P. Buonaccorsi

MEASUREMENT ERROR: MODELS, METHODS, AND APPLICATIONS
J. P. Buonaccorsi

MENDELIAN RANDOMIZATION: METHODS FOR USING GENETIC VARIANTS IN CAUSAL ESTIMATION S.Burgess and S.G. Thompson

META-ANALYSIS OF BINARY DATA USINGPROFILE LIKELIHOOD D. Böhning, R. Kuhnert, and S. Rattanasiri

MISSING DATA ANALYSIS IN PRACTICE T. Raghunathan

MODERN DIRECTIONAL STATISTICS C. Ley and T. Verdebout

POWER ANALYSIS OF TRIALS WITH MULTILEVEL DATA M. Moerbeek and S. Teerenstra

SPATIAL POINT PATTERNS: METHODOLOGY AND APPLICATIONS WITH R
A. Baddeley, E Rubak, and R. Turner

STATISTICAL ANALYSIS OF GENE EXPRESSION MICROARRAY DATA T. Speed

STATISTICAL ANALYSIS OF QUESTIONNAIRES: A UNIFIED APPROACH BASED ON R AND STATA F. Bartolucci, S. Bacci, and M. Gnaldi

STATISTICAL AND COMPUTATIONAL PHARMACOGENOMICS R. Wu and M. Lin

STATISTICS IN MUSICOLOGY J. Beran

STATISTICS OF MEDICAL IMAGING T. Lei

STATISTICAL CONCEPTS AND APPLICATIONS IN CLINICAL MEDICINE
J. Aitchison, J.W. Kay, and I.J. Lauder

STATISTICAL AND PROBABILISTIC METHODS IN ACTUARIAL SCIENCE
P.J. Boland

STATISTICAL DETECTION AND SURVEILLANCE OF GEOGRAPHIC CLUSTERS
P. Rogerson and I. Yamada

STATISTICAL METHODS IN PSYCHIATRY AND RELATED FIELDS: LONGITUDINAL, CLUSTERED, AND OTHER REPEATED MEASURES DATA
R. Gueorguieva

STATISTICS FOR ENVIRONMENTAL BIOLOGY AND TOXICOLOGY A. Bailer and W. Piegorsch

STATISTICS FOR FISSION TRACK ANALYSIS R.F. Galbraith

VISUALIZING DATA PATTERNS WITH MICROMAPS D.B. Carr and L.W. Pickle

Statistical Methods in Psychiatry and Related Fields

Longitudinal, Clustered, and Other Repeated Measures Data

Ralitza Gueorguieva

CRC Press
Taylor & Francis Group
Boca Raton London New York

CRC Press is an imprint of the
Taylor & Francis Group, an **informa** business
A CHAPMAN & HALL BOOK

CRC Press
Taylor & Francis Group
6000 Broken Sound Parkway NW, Suite 300
Boca Raton, FL 33487-2742

CRC Press is an imprint of Taylor & Francis Group, an Informa business

Printed on acid-free paper

International Standard Book Number-13: 978-1-4987-4076-0 (Hardback)

Library of Congress Cataloging-in-Publication Data

Names: Gueorguieva, Ralitza, author.
Title: Statistical methods in psychiatry and related fields : longitudinal, clustered, and other repeated measures data / by Ralitza Gueorguieva.
Description: Boca Raton, Florida : CRC Press, [2018] | Includes bibliographical references and index.
Identifiers: LCCN 2017029497| ISBN 9781498740760 (hardback) | ISBN 9781315151526 (e-book) | ISBN 9781498740777 (e-book) | ISBN 9781351647564 (e-book) | ISBN 9781351638043 (e-book)
Subjects: LCSH: Psychiatry--Research--Statistical methods.
Classification: LCC RC337 .G87 2018 | DDC 616.890072/7--dc23
LC record available at https://lccn.loc.gov/2017029497

Visit the Taylor & Francis Web site at
http://www.taylorandfrancis.com

and the CRC Press Web site at
http://www.crcpress.com

To my mother, Vesela, who was my strongest supporter

and greatest influence.

Contents

Preface

Clinical trials and epidemiological studies in the area of psychiatry and related fields present unique challenges to study design and data analysis. Often, outcomes are imprecisely ascertained, repeatedly measured over time or in related individuals, and may represent heterogeneous populations. This requires proper statistical methods for data analysis to be used in order to take into account the inherent variability in the data, correlations between repeated observations, and underlying traits or processes. However, a large number of studies in the area still use standard statistical techniques with oversimplified assumptions (e.g., endpoint analysis with last observation carried forward imputation, repeated measures analysis of variance models on complete data) that may lead to biased conclusions. Features of the data, such as floor or ceiling effects, and strength of correlation depending on the closeness of the repeated observations, are also often ignored.

Multiple statistical developments in recent years have revolutionized our ability to analyze data from clinical trials and epidemiological studies. First, mixed models use all data on subjects without the need for imputation, properly account for correlations of the repeated measures within individuals, minimize bias in estimates, and are appropriate for a wide range of applications from longitudinal to brain imaging data. Second, mixture models allow for data-driven estimation of underlying latent classes of trajectories over time and are suitable when individuals are expected to demonstrate categorically different patterns of change over time. Third, non-parametric methods are useful when there are excess observations at the lower or upper end of the measurement scales (i.e., floor or ceiling effects) or data distributions are otherwise unwieldy. In recent years, methods for dealing with missing data, such as multiple imputation, inverse probability weighting, and different types of models for incorporating the reasons for dropout in the analyses, have been proposed in the statistical literature.

Whereas some novel statistical methods have been used to plan studies and analyze data in psychiatry and related fields, bridging the gap between methodological developments in statistics and analyses of clinical trials and epidemiological studies has not been achieved. This is partly due to difficulties in "translating" statistical methods so that their assumptions, applicability, model fitting, and interpretation are understandable to quantitatively oriented non-statisticians. Statistical methodological papers are often full of statistical notation and jargon that make them hard to follow by applied researchers. Many other published works have aimed to explain statistical methods to nonstatistical audiences, but they are spread over many different specialized journals and often focus on just a particular aspect of statistical methods or only on a particular area of application. The current book summarizes recent statistical developments to a nonstatistical audience of quantitatively oriented researchers in psychiatry and related fields and is expected to be a valuable resource, aimed at promoting the use of appropriate statistical methods for analysis of complex data sets.

The book starts with an introductory chapter (Chapter 1) describing the notions of repeated observations, within-subject correlation, longitudinal data, and clustering. The advantages of collecting and analyzing repeatedly measured data are outlined together with the most commonly used statistical designs. The chapter also includes a review of the challenges in formulating appropriate models, basic statistical terminology and notation, and introduces the data sets that are used for illustration throughout the book.

Several of the following chapters (Chapters 2 through 5 and 10) present, at a non-technical level, approaches for the analysis of correlated data. Chapter 2 reviews traditional methods such as endpoint analysis, analysis of summary measures, and ANOVA-based approaches (rANOVA, rMANOVA), and discusses the limitations of these approaches in addressing the complexity of modern longitudinal and clustered data sets.

Linear mixed models (LMM) for continuous outcomes with bell-shaped distributions are presented in Chapter 3, with emphasis on how correlations within individuals (or clusters) and data variability are taken into account by random effects, structured variance–covariance matrices, or combinations of the two. The chapter also includes a presentation of the most commonly used linear mixed models, graphical methods for visualizing results and checking model assumptions, several data examples, and a detailed description of the advantages of linear mixed models over traditional methods.

Chapter 4 is devoted to two generalizations of linear mixed models for repeatedly measured categorical or count outcomes, or outcomes with skewed distributions. Generalized linear mixed models (GLMM) take into account the correlation among repeatedly measured observations via random effects whereas generalized estimating equations (GEE) use a working correlation structure to directly define the nature of interdependence among repeated observations. The two approaches are contrasted at a conceptual level, and emphasis is placed on model formulation and interpretation, with technical details kept to a minimum.

Chapter 5 introduces non-parametric methods for repeated measures that are useful for data distributions that are not well described by the standard choices from Chapters 3 and 4. The process of ranking the observations and then analyzing the ranks using LMM with special choices for the estimation procedures is illustrated on data examples, and the advantages and disadvantages of this approach are discussed.

Finally, two types of models aimed at identifying distinct classes of trajectories over time are described in Chapter 10: latent class growth models (LCGM) and the more general growth mixture models (GMM). The discussion focuses on the assumptions of both approaches and on result interpretation. Common computational and model identifiability problems are also presented and data examples are used for illustration.

Chapter 2 can be skipped by readers who are familiar with or not interested in learning about traditional methods for the analysis of repeated measures. Chapter 3 is key and should be read before Chapters 4, 5, and 10. Chapters 5 through 12 rely on information presented in Chapters 3 and 4 but are otherwise free-standing.

Chapter 6 discusses the need and techniques for multiple comparison correction when multiple outcomes or post hoc tests or estimations are performed. Procedures for control of the familywise error rate and the false discovery rate are presented at a non-technical level. General guidelines are provided, with special attention paid to the selection of the family of comparisons and the type of adjustment needed.

Chapter 7 is devoted to missing data and techniques for proper analysis in the presence of dropout. The three missing data mechanisms (missing completely at random, missing at random, and not missing at random) are defined, and models are contrasted in terms of their ability to handle data under these different mechanisms. State-of-the-art methods such as multiple imputation, full information maximum likelihood, and inverse probability weighting are presented together with methods for sensitivity analysis.

Chapter 8 is devoted to the issue of adjustment for covariates in statistical models. Common misuses of analysis of covariate as a bias-correction method (rather than as a method to enhance efficiency or power) are discussed together with explanations of the utility and the goals of adjustment in experimental and observational studies. Propensity score adjustments for multiple covariates are presented and their advantages discussed.

Chapter 9 focuses on two special types of variables that affect the relationship between a predictor of interest and an outcome, namely moderators and mediators. The causal inference framework is described and careful attention is paid to the assumptions under which causality can be claimed in assessing mediated relationships. Assessment of moderator and mediator effects is considered in the context of randomized and observational studies.

Chapter 11 reviews design considerations for studies with correlated data and focuses specifically on power calculations. Sample size estimation for traditional methods, mixed-effects models, and generalized estimating equations is considered. Common randomization approaches for experimental studies are also reviewed.

The book concludes with a summary and additional topics for interested readers (Chapter 12). In particular, references for models for multiple outcomes, spline modeling of time effects, transition models, survival analysis, analysis of intensive longitudinal data, models for spatial data, and Bayesian estimation approaches are included. An overview of commonly used software for the analysis of correlated data is also provided.

The target audience are researchers in psychiatry and related areas with minimal statistical knowledge. The book is intended to be used primarily as a guide to understand the different methods. It could also be used to teach modern statistical methods to doctoral students and post-doctoral researchers, medical residents, and faculty who are interested in improving their knowledge of statistical methods. Applied statisticians collaborating in psychiatry and related fields should also find it useful.

Online materials are provided at **http://medicine.yale.edu/lab/statmethods/** and include data sets or links to locations of data sets, programs, and output for the data examples in the book. The book, together with the online materials, allows readers to work through a variety of examples and aims to promote the use of appropriate statistical methods for the analysis of repeated measures data.

The book is partially based on a series of my lectures in modern statistical methods for the analysis of psychiatric data presented to researchers in the Department of Psychiatry at Yale School of Medicine, and on several of my manuscripts intended to popularize statistical methods in the psychiatry literature. As a Senior Research Scientist at the Department of Biostatistics at Yale School of Public Health, I have greatly benefited from discussions and collaborative work with my colleagues in biostatistics and psychiatry. I very much appreciate the flexibility of the Yale environment that has allowed me to work on this book project. I would also like to acknowledge the support of the Institute of Mathematics and Informatics at the Bulgarian Academy of Sciences that has allowed me to be an active member of the Bulgarian statistical community.

I would like to thank all individuals who provided feedback on the book, the researchers who allowed me to use their data for illustration, and all my statistical and subject-matter collaborators from whom I have learned so much over the years. I am especially grateful to Brian Pittman, Eugenia Buta, and several anonymous reviewers who read a number of chapters of the book and provided excellent feedback, as well as to Alan Agresti, not only for his thoughtful comments, but also for giving me the confidence to attempt this book project. I also appreciate the helpful discussions with Ran Wu. Special thanks go to my collaborators and mentors John Krystal and Stephanie O'Malley who have been instrumental in my career and development as an independent scientist. I am also grateful to Neill Epperson, Gerard Sanacora, Mehmet Sofuoglu, Naomi Driesen, Peter Morgan, and Scott Woods for allowing me to use their data sets. I would also like to acknowledge my editor, Rob Calver, and his assistant, Lara Spieker, for their guidance and support, and

Denise Meyer for her work on the book website with online materials. Last but not least, I would like to thank my immediate and extended family who put up with my physical and/or mental absence in the many days I devoted to work on this book. In particular, I appreciate the patience of my husband Velizar and my children Alex and Lili, the support of my father Vladislav, sister Annie, brother-in-law Nathan, and mother-in-law Lili.

1

Introduction

Repeatedly measured data are paramount in medicine, epidemiology, public health, psychology, sociology, and many other fields. The simplest case of such data is when a single measurement is collected repeatedly on the same individual or experimental unit. Each repeated measurement is called an *observation* and observations can be obtained over time, over a spatial map, or can be unordered temporally or spatially but nested (clustered) within larger experimental units.

Clustered data occur when repeated measures are not ordered and can be considered symmetrical within the larger experimental unit (cluster). For example, members of the same household can be interviewed, and in this case, their responses are repeated measures within the family. The family, rather than the individual, is the experimental unit and serves as the cluster. Observations on different individuals within the cluster are likely to be related to one another because individuals share the same environment and/or genetic predisposition. Similarly, patients may be clustered (or nested) within the same therapy group or clinic. Their treatment responses are also expected to be related because of the common influence of group or clinic, and can be considered repeated measures within the group or clinic. Several layers of clustering can be present in a data set. For example, the individual can be nested within family and the family can be nested within the neighborhood.

Longitudinal data occur when repeated measures are collected over time. In clinical trials in psychiatry and related fields, often the same rating instrument is administered to each individual at baseline, at intermediate time points, at the end of the randomized phase, and at follow-up. For example, depression severity can be measured weekly, biweekly, or monthly, in order to assess treatment effects over time. Similarly, in observational studies, the natural progression of a disease or other measures is ascertained repeatedly over time. In animal or human laboratory experiments, often responses from the same individual to different randomly ordered experimental conditions are recorded and compared.

Spatial data occur when repeated measures are spatially related. In imaging data sets, voxels are arranged in three-dimensional space where an observed value in a particular voxel is likely related to the observed values in neighboring voxels. In functional imaging studies, brain activation maps are created and often averaged region of interest signals are analyzed in order to measure and compare responses to different stimuli. In epidemiological studies, disease maps over geographical areas are created and analyzed. Methods for voxel-based data analysis of imaging studies and geographic and information systems are beyond the scope of this book, but we consider region of interest analyses of imaging data.

In all these situations, repeated observations within the same individual or cluster are related. Failure to take this interrelationship into account in statistical analyses, can lead to flawed conclusions. In this chapter, we review some terminology relevant to repeated measures data, such as mean response and measures of variability and correlation, present types of studies with longitudinal and clustered data, discuss advantages and challenges of collecting and analyzing repeatedly measured data, describe data sets that are used for illustration throughout the book, and provide a brief historical overview of approaches for the analysis of correlated data. We focus on continuous (quantitative, dimensional) measures. Later chapters deal specifically with categorical measures which can be dichotomous, ordinal with few ordered levels, and nominal (unordered). Some statistical terminology and basic notation is presented in Section 1.7 and can be skipped by readers who are confident of their statistical knowledge of basic concepts. Statistical Analysis System (SAS) code for the graphs in this chapter and for all models considered in further chapters, together with actual output and available data sets, is available on the book website.

1.1 Aspects of Repeated Measures Data

1.1.1 Average (Mean) Response

The goals of many studies with repeatedly measured data are to estimate the average response in a population of interest and see whether it changes significantly as a result of treatment, exposure, covariates, and/or time. Herein, *response* is used in the sense of an outcome (outcome variable, dependent variable) that measures the main characteristic in the population of interest. *Population* is the target group of individuals for whom statistical inference should be generalizable and from where the study *sample* is obtained. For example, in depression studies, the response can be depression severity measured by a standard depression rating scale, such as the Hamilton Depression Rating Scale (HDRS), or a dichotomous measure of improvement defined as at least 50% decrease from baseline on the HDRS, and the population can be all individuals with major depression. In substance abuse studies, the response can be the percentage of days without substance use in a particular time period, and the population can be all individuals with alcohol dependence. In functional imaging studies, the response can be activation change in a brain region and the population can be all individuals, healthy or otherwise. The sample should be randomly obtained from the population if it is to be representative of the population of interest.

Average response refers to the mean of the individual responses in the sample or the population. In the simplest case of a single random sample from a population without repeated measures, the sample average response is just the arithmetic mean of all response values for the individuals in the sample (see Section 1.7 for exact formula). The population-average response is the mean response of all individuals in the population and, since it is usually not possible to measure, we use the sample mean to make inferences about the population mean. In longitudinal or clustered data, response is measured repeatedly within the individual over time or within the cluster, and the average response is usually a sequence or collection of numbers that correspond to each repeated measurement occasion. For example, the average response in a depression clinical trial that takes 8 weeks may be a sequence of eight averages of the individual responses (one for each week of the study). The average response in an imaging study may be a collection of several average responses, each corresponding to a different brain region.

Average response usually depends on a number of *predictors*. In clinical trials, we always have treatment as the main predictor of interest while participant characteristics such as age, gender, and disease severity are additional predictors that can also affect the response. Such additional predictors are usually called *covariates*. In observational studies, we might be interested in the effect of exposures, such as smoking or drinking, on the response. In imaging studies, we may want to measure brain activation while individuals perform different tasks. In all these situations, estimation of the average response and how it depends on different predictors is of primary interest.

1.1.2 Variance and Correlation

The variability and interdependence of repeated measures within the individual or cluster are usually of secondary interest, although there are situations where they may be of equal or even higher interest than the estimation of the average response. For example, in clinical trials, the main goal may be to test whether an experimental treatment is on average better than a standard treatment or a placebo in terms of improvement in response over time. The variability in the responses of individuals needs to be taken into account but it is usually not of primary interest. However, it is possible that the experimental treatment may have a very similar average response to the standard treatment, but inter-individual variability in response may be lower (i.e., individuals may respond to treatment more consistently and similarly to one another). In this situation, the new treatment may be preferable and estimation of the variability of response is of interest too.

Variability of observations around the mean from a simple random sample is described by the *variance* or *standard deviation* of the observations (see Section 1.7). The sample standard deviation is often preferable as it provides a measure of variability that is evaluated in the same units as the mean. In repeated measures situations with longitudinal data, often the variability of the response at one particular time point differs from the variability at another, in which case it makes sense to estimate separate variances in order to assess data spread at individual time points. However, in some situations it may be reasonable to assume that the variances on all repeated occasions are the same. In this case, a better statistical estimate of the common variance can be obtained by pooling information from all occasions. Examples of both scenarios are considered in Chapter 2.

Repeated measures within individuals or clusters are often correlated. *Correlation* reflects the degree of linear dependence between two variables and varies between –1 and 1. It is important to emphasize that the definition includes the word "linear." Two variables may be perfectly related in a curvilinear fashion and have a correlation of zero. Correlation values of 1 or –1 correspond to perfect linear dependence between two variables. In these cases, knowing the values of one of the variables exactly predicts the values of the other variable, but does not imply that the two variables take the same value. Correlations are positive when larger values on one of the variables correspond to larger values on the other variable. Correlations are negative when larger values on one of the variables correspond to smaller values on the other variable. Please note that the proper statistical term for the latter case is "negative correlation," not "inverse correlation," as is often erroneously used. Section 1.7 shows how correlations are calculated and illustrates different scenarios.

Repeated measures within individuals, especially in longitudinal studies, are usually positively correlated although, in some situations, it is possible for observations to be negatively correlated. Individual responses tend to be systematically higher or lower than the mean response, which is reflected in a positive correlation. For example, if individuals start a study with higher illness severity than most other individuals, their repeated severity measures are likely to stay above average, at least for a while. Thus, repeated observations on the same individual are positively correlated with stronger correlation the closer the observations are to each other in time. This is very typical of longitudinal studies.

Some situations where negative correlation is more likely to be present are as follows: clustered data where individuals within a cluster may be competing for resources (e.g., individual weights of fetuses within a litter may be negatively correlated), longitudinal data where a positive response on one occasion makes a positive response less likely in another situation (e.g., immunity built after a viral illness may prevent a person from getting sick with the same or similar virus in the future), and clustered imaging data where a positive response in one brain region may occur simultaneously with a negative response in another region. Different types of statistical models provide varied levels of flexibility in specifying the structure of the correlations and variances within a data set. Subsequent chapters deal with this issue in detail.

1.2 Types of Studies with Repeatedly Measured Outcomes

Repeated measures can be collected on the same individual over time, on different parts of the body of the same individual, on members of the same family, or on individuals in clusters where measurements are expected to be related to one another, for example, students in schools or patients in clinics. The variability of the individual measures and interdependence between repeated measures can follow different patterns and needs to be properly taken into consideration in the statistical analysis of the data. Herein, we consider different types of studies with repeated measures data and discuss the implications of the patterns of variability in each of these situations for statistical modeling.

In *longitudinal studies* repeated measures are collected on the same individuals over time. Longitudinal studies are often prospective (i.e., individuals are recruited at a particular moment in time and followed up) and most often their focus is on assessing the effect of an intervention or an exposure over an extended period of time. They can also be used to ascertain trajectories of change and to compare temporal patterns of response of different groups of individuals. In some cases, subjects are assessed over time under experimental conditions (i.e., individuals are randomized to receive a particular treatment), whereas other times subjects are simply observed (i.e., when it might be unethical or too expensive to randomize individuals, for example, in studies investigating the effects of smoking or when analyzing the progression of a rare disease). These two types of studies are known as *experimental* and *observational*, respectively.

Clinical trials are the most common type of experimental longitudinal studies. Even though the primary endpoint of a clinical trial may be a single measure (e.g., time to remission, relapse, or outcome measured at the end of the trial), data are collected repeatedly on the same individuals over time. Double-blind randomized clinical trials, in which both the patient and the clinician are blind to treatment assignment, are considered the gold standard of evaluating intervention effects and are the only studies where direct causal interpretation is possible because randomization balances the study groups at baseline on potentially confounding variables for the relationship of the main predictor of interest and the outcome.

The simplest and most frequently used clinical trial design is the *parallel group design* where each individual is randomly assigned to an intervention and individuals receiving different interventions are followed in parallel. Participants do not switch treatments in this design unless necessitated for safety or other reasons. Figure 1.1 presents an example of such a design with three groups and four equally spaced assessment points over time.

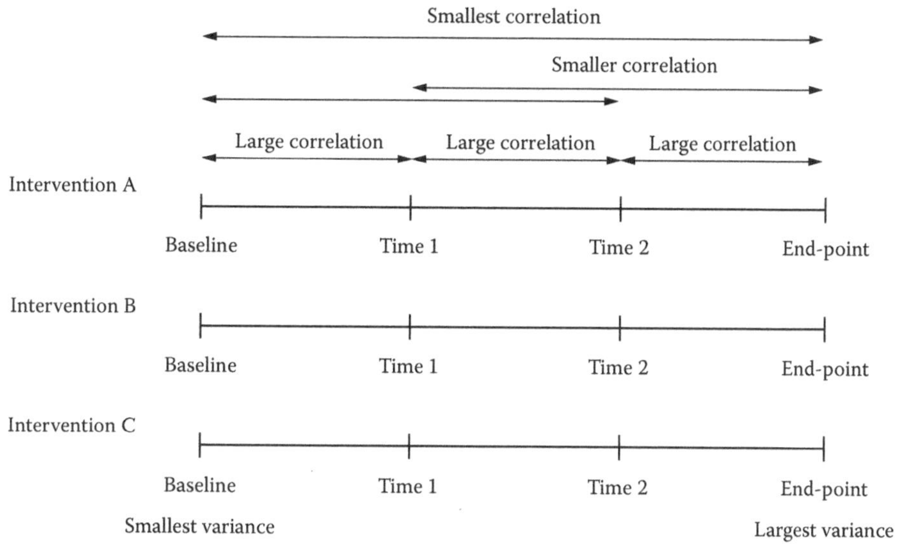

FIGURE 1.1
Parallel group clinical trial with three interventions and four repeated measures.

In the data example subsection of this chapter (Section 1.5), we present parallel group clinical trials in depression and alcohol dependence. In these studies, individuals are randomly assigned to different interventions and the outcomes (depression severity in the depression trials and drinking in the alcohol dependence trial) are repeatedly measured on individuals during treatment.

In such parallel group trials, the variability of repeated measures on the same outcome often increases over time because individuals are most comparable at baseline as they need to satisfy a strict set of inclusion/exclusion criteria. With time, differences emerge as some individuals respond more favorably to treatment than others. This leads to an increase in variability of the measurements toward the end of the trial. This increase is sometimes small and can be ignored, but occasionally the increase may be quite dramatic and needs to be taken into account in the data analysis. Furthermore, measurements within the same individual that are closer in time tend to be more highly correlated than measurements that are further apart in time. This is almost always the case and needs to be properly modeled so that statistical inferences are valid. Different ways to take into account the pattern of correlations in the statistical model are discussed in Chapter 3.

Another frequently used clinical trial design, is the *cross-over design*, which is popular in both human and animal laboratory studies. In this design, individuals are assigned several treatments in randomized order, that is, they are randomized to a particular sequence of treatment assignments. Figure 1.2 shows an example of a cross-over design with three treatments. In Section 1.5, we present a human laboratory study in which smokers received different doses of nicotine and menthol in randomized order. The outcome was nicotine reinforcement and was measured for each menthol and nicotine dose combination. The study focused on assessment of the independent and interactive effects of nicotine and menthol.

The cross-over design can be particularly useful when individuals vary considerably in their response from one another, repeated measures on the same individual are substantially correlated, when interventions are relatively short in duration, and when there is no or low possibility of carry-over effects from one treatment to another. Carry-over

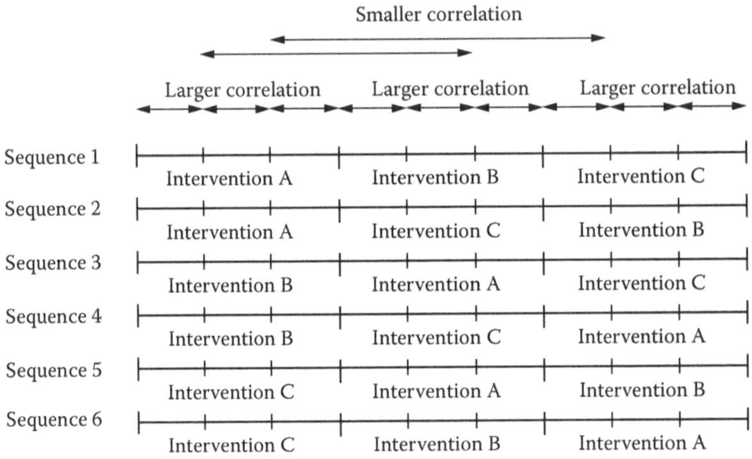

FIGURE 1.2
Cross-over trial with three interventions and three repeated measures within intervention period.

effects are minimized when a sufficient washout period is allowed in between treatments. This design is more efficient (i.e., can detect differences between treatments with greater power or with fewer individuals) than the parallel group design when there is large between-subject variability because it allows a direct comparison of the treatment effects within each individual, i.e., each subject serves as their own control. However, this design may also be associated with higher probability of dropout and order effects must be controlled. It is also difficult to implement in scenarios when there are carry-over effects and treatment effects take long to manifest. In cross-over designs, correlations between repeated measures on the same individual within the same treatment period are usually higher than correlations between repeated measures on the same individual from different treatment periods. Within each period, correlations can be modeled using the same approach as correlations from a parallel group clinical trial.

Observational longitudinal studies usually follow groups of individuals over time. For example, in the Health and Retirement Study, presented in Section 1.5, individuals aged 55 and older were followed more than 10 years with interviews every 2 years. Participants in the study of association between unemployment and depression were interviewed up to three times in a period of up to 16 months after job loss.

Observational longitudinal studies are used when it is not possible or ethical to randomize individuals, or when it may be too expensive to perform an experimental study. For example, assessing the effect of smoking, or of genetic factors, on the emergence or progression of some disease over time can only be performed using observational studies. In these studies, the same issues about modeling variability and correlations between repeated measures on the same individual as in randomized clinical trials apply.

In studies where the same outcome is measured on related individuals (e.g., twins, sibling pairs, or members of the same family) or in clustered settings (e.g., individuals within the same clinic or treated by the same doctor), correlations are also expected to be present. For example, in the Health and Retirement Study, data were collected on married individuals. In the mother–infant study presented in Section 1.5, there are positive correlations between mothers and their infants. Correlations may be naturally occurring (e.g., individuals living together or genetically related are expected to exhibit some level of correlation on some responses) or may be introduced by the researcher via the study design. For example, in cluster-*randomized clinical trials,* the units receiving a particular intervention are clinics, not individual patients. However, the responses to the intervention are usually measured on the individual patients within clinics. Failure to take into account the correlation between the observations on different patients within the same clinic can result in erroneous conclusions. Regardless of the reason for correlations between the observations in clustered settings, statistical methods need to appropriately model this correlation in order to provide valid results.

Unlike in situations with longitudinal data, where correlations are stronger or weaker depending on the time lag between observations on the same individual, in clustered settings with only one level of clustering it is likely that observations within clusters are equally correlated while observations from different clusters are uncorrelated. For example, observations on individuals within the same clinic may be correlated but observations on individuals from different clinics should be uncorrelated. Additionally, the variances of the observations on individuals in the same cluster are expected to be the same. This structure of variances and correlations is the simplest possible structure in repeated measures scenarios and is called *compound symmetry structure.* This structure will be presented in more detail in Chapters 2 and 3.

Different levels of clustering are also possible. For example, individuals can be nested within families and families can be nested within neighborhoods, which leads to different levels of correlations within the family and within the neighborhood. In this case, a multilevel version of the compound symmetry structure may arise, such that observations on members of the same family are strongly correlated, observations on members of different families but living in the same neighborhood may be weakly correlated, and observations on members of different families in different neighborhoods are uncorrelated. The variance of each observation in this case can be represented as the sum of the variance due to neighborhood, the variance due to family, and the variance due to the individual. Figure 1.3 illustrates the situation with two different levels of clustering: individuals are

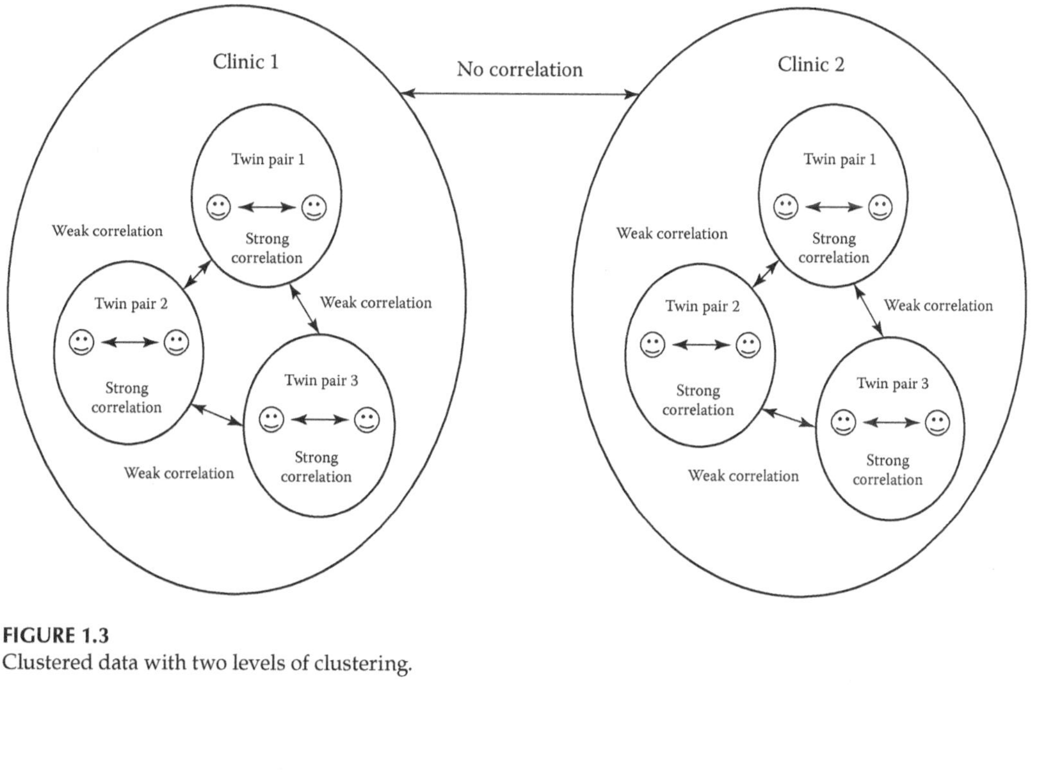

FIGURE 1.3
Clustered data with two levels of clustering.

nested within twin pairs and twin pairs are nested within clinics where they might be undergoing a particular treatment together with other twin pairs. More than two levels of clustering may also be present and need to be taken into account for proper statistical inference.

It is also possible to have correlations in a data set due to both clustering and to repeated observations on the same individual over time. For example, some interventions in psychiatry and related fields (e.g., some behavioral interventions) are administered in a group setting (e.g., therapy group) and then participants' responses are repeatedly assessed over time. Since the same therapist is providing treatment to a group of individuals at the same time, correlations may arise between measurements on individuals in the same group. These correlations are in addition to the correlations that exist between repeated measures on the same individual over time. This leads to layers of correlation in the data. In particular, measurements on the same individual at two adjacent time points are usually strongly correlated and measurements on the same individual further apart in time are weakly correlated. Furthermore, measurements on different individuals within the same therapy group are correlated, with the strongest correlation observed for pairs of observations at the same time point and correlations decreasing with time lag between observations. The models considered in Chapters 3 and 4 demonstrate how such fairly complicated situations can be seamlessly and appropriately handled and illustrate the methods on data introduced in Section 1.5.

Imaging data present their own set of challenges in accounting for correlations between observations because of the spatial relationship between units of analysis. Different imaging techniques (e.g., magnetic resonance imaging [MRI], functional magnetic resonance imaging [fMRI], and diffusion tensor imaging [DTI]) and different resolution levels may require different techniques for the handling of correlated measures. At the highest resolution level of MRI or fMRI analyses, signal intensities at adjacent voxels (points in three-dimensional space) are expected to be more highly correlated than observations at voxels that are more distant. Also, variability of signals measured at individual voxels do not in general vary considerably. However, at the level of region of interest (ROI), where sets of voxels have been combined into anatomically or functionally defined areas and overall measures have been calculated over the entire ROI, distance between regions is no longer of utmost importance and measures in regions closer in space are not necessarily more highly correlated than measures from regions that are further apart. Moreover, variances of measures in different regions may be vastly different from one another due to the size of the region or other factors. In-depth consideration of issues and techniques of analysis of different types of imaging data are beyond the scope of this book. However, in Chapter 3, we discuss techniques for analysis of ROI data and illustrate with the data from the fMRI study of working memory in schizophrenia, introduced in Section 1.5. For details on issues in brain imaging analysis the interested reader is referred to Chung (2014). Friston (2007) provides a detailed overview of statistical parametric mapping for functional brain images.

1.3 Advantages of Collecting and Analyzing Repeatedly Measured Data

The main advantage of collecting repeatedly measured data is that each individual or experimental unit serves as their own control. When an intervention or exposure can be varied within an individual, repeated measures allow one to assess or compare the effects within the subject. This means that the effects of potentially confounding variables that vary between subjects can be controlled and, as a result, the variability of estimating effects of an intervention or exposure is reduced, compared to studies at a single time point (*cross-sectional studies*). This is reflected in increased power for within-individual or within-cluster comparisons, that is, there is higher probability of finding differences in response within clusters or individuals when true differences exist.

Furthermore, patterns of change over time can be assessed when longitudinal data are collected. Prospective studies collect information over a period of time, starting at study entry. Clinical trials and cohort studies are examples of prospective studies. In such investigations, repeated measures on a number of variables can be collected on the same individuals. This allows one to estimate trajectories over time, to test between-group differences on trajectories over time, and to assess variability of measurements both within and between subjects. Such studies have greater *statistical power* for testing time effects and differences between groups over time than corresponding cross-sectional methods. Additionally, such analyses that take into account the variability and correlation of repeated measurements can better control the probability of finding differences where true differences do not exist (i.e., better control of *type I error* in statistical testing).

1.4 Challenges in the Analysis of Correlated Data

To analyze a data set with correlated data, proper statistical models need to be constructed. In this section, we consider parametric models in which all aspects of the models need to be specified. *Non-parametric models* that do not make specific assumptions about the distribution of the response variable are considered in Chapter 5. *Semi-parametric models* that make assumptions about some aspects of the response distribution and leave others unspecified, such as *generalized estimating equations* (GEE), are considered in Chapter 4.

The first aspect of the statistical model, is the specification of the patterns of the means of the response variable within a cluster or over time. The means are usually assumed to depend on individual or cluster characteristics, on predictors that may vary within a cluster or over time, and very often on time and treatment. The model should provide a good smoothing of the unknown true relationship between predictors and the response that is useful for a relatively simple description of reality. In the model definition, the relationship is described by a mathematical equation, which is usually a linear function of the predictors and hence is called a *linear predictor* (see Section 1.7 for model definition). Some statistical models are more general and assume non-linear relationships. But in all cases, the equation that describes how the mean response varies as a function of the predictors needs to be matching reality reasonably well. This requires that measured predictors that affect the mean be included in the equation and that the form of the equation corresponds to the relationship between the predictors and the mean outcome. An example of poor correspondence between model and reality is when the model assumes that the response varies linearly with the predictor but in fact the relationship is curvilinear. If the mean response is not correctly specified, other aspects of the model definition can be affected and statistical inferences may be misleading.

The second aspect of the statistical model is the *distribution of the response variable.* When the response variable is continuous or approximately continuous (e.g., scores on instruments assessing symptoms of depression or schizophrenia), the natural and mathematically most convenient distribution that is considered first is the normal distribution. However, if a histogram of the response distribution does not appear approximately bell-shaped (with most observations in the middle and a few large and small observations in the tail of the distribution), then directly assuming normal distribution can lead to problems with the conclusions from the statistical analysis, especially in small samples. One possible solution to this issue is to apply a transformation to the response variable prior to analysis, in order to have the distribution of the transformed variable more closely resemble the normal distribution, and then use models for normally distributed data. This is mathematically most convenient but is not straightforward to interpret as all statistical estimates are on the transformed scale and in general can't be directly transformed back. Chapter 3 is devoted to models for repeated measures with a normal response. Alternative distributions can be considered for continuous response variables and some of these models are considered in Chapter 4. Chapter 4 also covers models for dichotomous (binary) and count data.

The third aspect of the model formulation is describing the variances of repeated observations and the correlations between repeated measures within clusters and/or over time. In Chapters 3 and 4, we consider different approaches for accounting for the variance and covariance, based on mixed-effects models and estimating equations.

In summary, due to the complexity of the variances and correlations between repeatedly measured observations, formulating an appropriate statistical model is challenging and should be done in steps with proper checks of each aspect of the model formulation. Descriptive statistics and data visualization techniques are used to inform decisions about model formulation. Such techniques are illustrated using the data sets in the next section.

1.5 Data Sets

Several data sets are considered for illustration of the methods described throughout the book. We consider data sets from both clinical trials and observational studies, with longitudinal and clustered data, with balanced and unbalanced designs. Most data sets have missing data which can present problems for analysis. Specific features of the different data sets are emphasized and graphical and tabular methods for data exploration are presented.

1.5.1 Augmentation Treatment for Depression

The first data set is from a parallel group clinical trial of an *augmentation treatment for depression* (Sanacora et al., 2004). In this study, 50 patients were randomly assigned to either fluoxetine + yohimbine (augmentation treatment) or fluoxetine+placebo (control treatment) for six weeks. The main study hypothesis was that the augmentation treatment group would show faster improvement than the control group on the HDRS total score, which measures severity of depression symptoms. The primary analysis of these data reported in Sanacora et al. (2004) showed that patients in the augmentation group achieved responder status (HDRS score of 10 or less) faster than the control group. In subsequent chapters (e.g., Chapters 3, 6, and 7) we use this data set to illustrate model fitting that allows for comparison of the treatment response profiles of the two groups over time.

But before we proceed with consideration of the statistical models, we explore the data with some graphical representations. Figure 1.4 shows two *profile plots* of the HDRS scores of all patients in the study by treatment group. This type of plot (also known as a *spaghetti plot*) is useful for visualizing longitudinal data in small- to medium-sized data sets, as it shows the individual trajectories of observed responses over time. It provides a visual impression of the mean trend over time, the variability of observations, and the strength of correlation between adjacent observations of individuals over time. From Figure 1.4 we see that the individuals in the two treatment groups appear to have similar baseline scores, although the scores in the control group are slightly higher. We also see that most patients have substantial decrease in depression severity over time and that variances appear to slightly increase from baseline, especially for the control group in the middle of

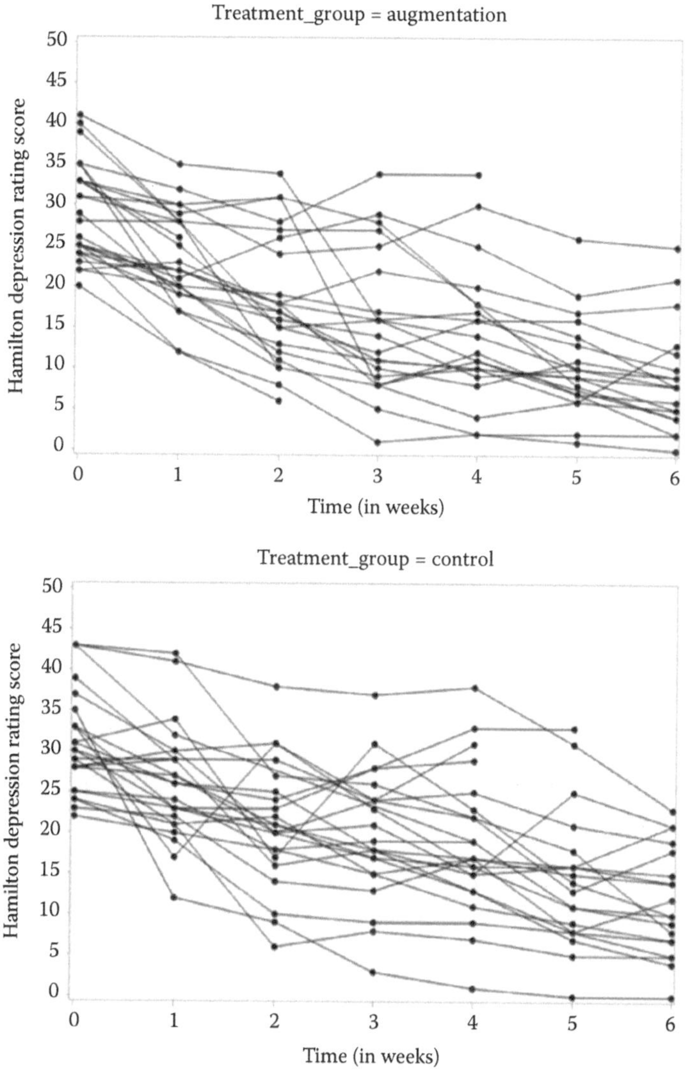

FIGURE 1.4
Profile plots of Hamilton Depression Rating Scale scores of all subjects in the augmentation depression data set by treatment group.

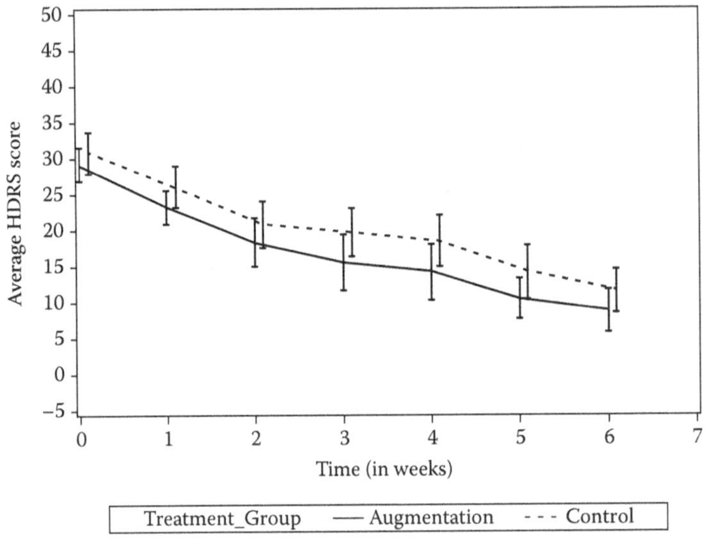

FIGURE 1.5
Means and standards error of the Hamilton Depression Rating Scale scores over time by treatments group in the augmentation depression data set.

the observation period. Furthermore, most patients' responses tend to stay either above or below the corresponding average scores of their respective treatment group which suggests that correlations between repeated observations within the individual are positive.

Figure 1.5 presents a plot of the means and standard errors of the means over time for each treatment group, based on all available observations at each time point. This plot confirms our observations from Figure 1.4 concerning the average trend and the variability over time. However, it does not provide any information about the correlation of observations within individuals. Also, in the presence of missing data, it may present a distorted picture of the average trends over time. For example, if subjects in the control group selectively drop out due to inefficacy of the treatment and subjects in the active group drop out due to side effects, the between-group differences shown in the figure at later time points may be smaller than the real differences. Analysis in the presence of missing data is considered in detail in Chapter 7 and these data are used for illustration.

Despite the limitation of the mean plot, it is quite useful for spotting changes in average treatment response between groups over time and can be used with a data set of any size. Since standard errors of the means decrease with increasing sample size and the corresponding error bars get tighter around the means, sometimes the same type of plot is created with bars corresponding to standard deviations, rather than standard errors of the mean. Standard deviation estimates do not in general decrease with increasing sample size and provide an estimate of the variation of individual observations in the sample, rather than of the means.

1.5.2 Sequenced Treatment Alternatives to Relieve Depression (STAR*D)

The second data set is from the Sequenced Treatment Alternatives to Relieve Depression (STAR*D) clinical trial (Gaynes et al., 2008; Trivedi et al., 2006). STAR*D is the largest randomized prospective study of outpatients with major depression to date. The first stage of this study was a 12-week course of citalopram, a selective serotonin reuptake inhibitor

(SSRI) antidepressant and the outcome of interest was improvement in the total score from the Quick Inventory of Depression Symptomatology (QIDS) (Rush et al., 2006) questionnaire. Four thousand and nineteen subjects provided data on QIDS in the first phase. The total QIDS score is similar to the total HDRS score considered in the previous example and reflects total depression severity.

Prediction of initial response to antidepressant treatment in STAR*D was recently considered by Chekroud et al. (2016) with responder status over the entire 12 weeks defined, based on the improvement in total QIDS score. Subsequent analyses identified three different clusters of depression symptoms (core depression symptoms, sleep symptoms, and atypical symptoms) in this study and in two other large clinical trials in depression, and showed that treatments are not equally effective for the three clusters (Chekroud et al., 2017) across trials. In this book, we focus on the effects of citalopram treatment in the first phase of the STAR*D trial on the three clusters and illustrate how the models introduced in Chapter 3 can be used to model the three aspects of depression severity simultaneously.

The design of the study was intended to be balanced with subjects scheduled for visits at weeks 0, 2, 4, 6, 9, and 12. However, participants were sometimes seen in intermediate weeks and occasionally had repeat visits during the same week. Thus, the measurement times of subjects were somewhat different and the design was actually unbalanced. This limits the set of possible approaches that could be used for such data and requires that one makes the assumption that the time points are independent of the outcome and of the other effects in the model. This assumption is considered in more detail in Chapter 3.

Figure 1.6 shows a *panel plot* of the observed symptom cluster scores over time of three participants in the study. The rows correspond to different individuals and the columns correspond to different clusters. Each dot in the graph is the average of the scores on the individual items for the participant in the cluster of symptoms. The observation times are different for the three individuals but are all within the 12-week period. The superimposed regression lines are based only on the observations in the graph and are used to illustrate visually the linear trend in change over time. Note that the linear trend does not necessarily fit the data well. In particular, the trends of change in the sleep cluster appear curvilinear for these three individuals, but since these are only a few of the participants, we can't make any conclusions about the pattern of change over time for the entire sample.

The panel plot is an alternative way of presenting individual change over time to the spaghetti plot, but it is limited to showing only a few individuals at a time. We consider these data in more detail in Chapters 3 and 10.

1.5.3 Combined Pharmacotherapies and Behavioral Interventions for Alcohol Dependence (COMBINE) Study

The Combined Pharmacotherapies and Behavioral Interventions for Alcohol Dependence (COMBINE) Study (Anton et al., 2006) represents the largest study of pharmacotherapy for alcoholism in the United States to date. This parallel group clinical trial was designed to answer questions about the benefits of combining behavioral and pharmacological interventions on drinking outcomes in individuals with alcohol dependence. Eight groups (1226 participants in total) received medication management and a combination of active or placebo naltrexone, active or placebo acamprosate, and combined behavioral intervention (CBI), or no CBI in a $2 \times 2 \times 2$ factorial design (Figure 1.7). A ninth group received only CBI without medication management and is not considered herein. Double-blind medication treatment (naltrexone and acamprosate) and CBI were provided for approximately four months and participants were followed for up to one year after randomization.

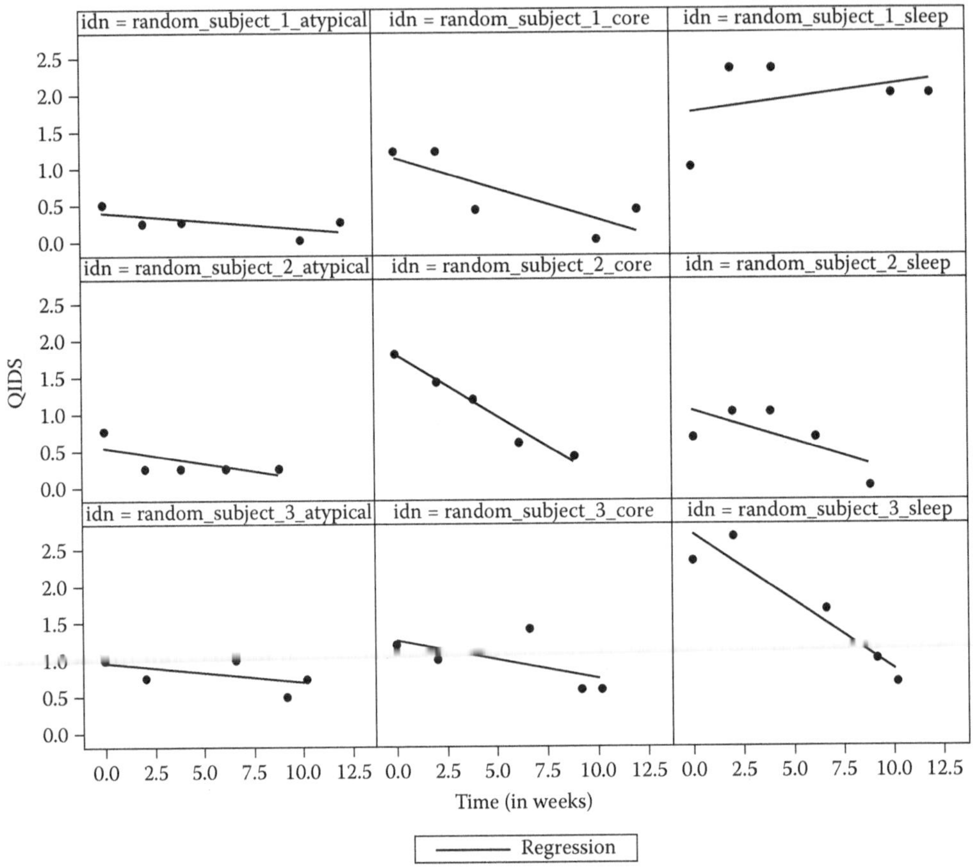

FIGURE 1.6
Cluster symptom scores of three individuals from the STAR*D trial in depression.

Combined behavioral intervention
+
Medication management

Placebo acamprosate + Placebo naltrexone	Placebo acamprosate + Active naltrexone
Active acamprosate + Placebo naltrexone	Active acamprosate + Active naltrexone

Medication management only

Placebo acamprosate + Placebo naltrexone	Placebo acamprosate + Active naltrexone
Active acamprosate + Placebo naltrexone	Active acamprosate + Active naltrexone

FIGURE 1.7
Design of the COMBINE study.

Participants were required to abstain from drinking for at least four days prior to randomization and the main outcomes in the primary analyses were: time to first heavy drinking days and percent days abstinent over the entire treatment period. The primary analyses found significant benefit of naltrexone and CBI on drinking outcomes, but the combination of naltrexone and CBI was not better than the monotherapies. The effects of acamprosate were not significant.

Drinking data in this study were collected daily using the timeline follow-back method (TLFB). This method was also used to collect daily drinking data for the 90 days prior to the baseline assessment and during follow-up. Since daily drinking data are available, it is possible to look at changes in drinking patterns over time pre-treatment, during treatment, and during follow-up. In this book, we use monthly summaries of drinking data for illustration, which allow estimation of trajectories of treatment response over time and allow us to ignore variability in the daily measures due to the day of the week. Depending on the model that we are illustrating, we focus on several different measures: average number of drinks per day, average number of drinks per drinking day (day on which drinking occurred), and number of drinking days.

Figure 1.8 shows the average number of drinks per drinking day in four treatment arms during the treatment period. Note that this measure is calculated only for the drinking days and thus reflects only one aspect of drinking behavior (i.e., intensity of drinking). Additional outcomes, such as percent of drinking days, need to be considered in order to describe other aspects of drinking (i.e., frequency of drinking). We consider these aspects separately in subsequent chapters. Joint analysis of the different aspects is also possible but requires more sophisticated statistical models and is beyond the scope of this book. Interested readers are referred to Liu et al. (2008) and Liu et al. (2012) for more details.

In Figure 1.8, we omit the standard errors of the means from the graph and also ignore acamprosate assignment in order to have a less cluttered figure. This type of figure shows

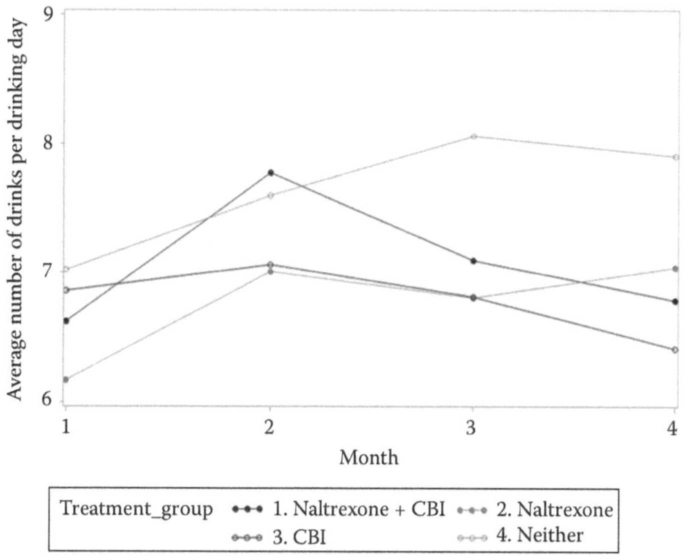

FIGURE 1.8
Average number of drinks per drinking day by treatment group in the COMBINE data set.

the average trends over time but does not provide information about the data distribution at each time point. Profile plots will not be very useful for data visualization in this study because there are several hundred participants within each group and it will be difficult to distinguish the individual trajectories. Standard error or standard deviation bars will also be hard to distinguish if added to Figure 1.8 because there are several groups and many time points. Instead, histograms or box plots can be used to visualize the data distribution at each time point. Figure 1.9 shows *box plots* of the outcome (average number of drinks per

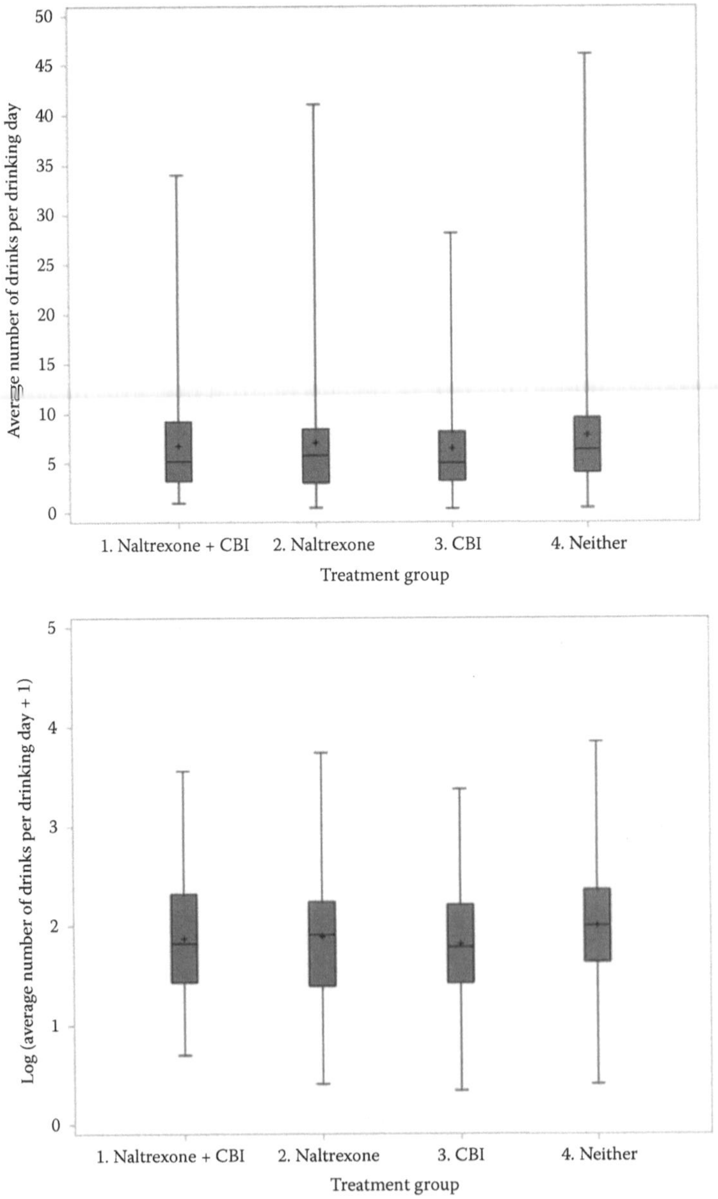

FIGURE 1.9
Box plots of average number of drinks per drinking day by treatment group at month four in the COMBINE study.

drinking day) at month four by treatment group. In the top panel of the figure are four box plots of the original response variable. In each box plot, the middle line shows the median of the data (i.e., the value below which 50% of the observations lie), the lower and upper ends of the box show the 25th and the 75th percentile, respectively (i.e., the values below which we have 25% and 75% of the observations, respectively), the plus (+) sign shows the mean of the data and the whiskers of the box plot show the minimum and maximum value in the corresponding treatment group. From this set of box plots, we see that drinking data are right-skewed (i.e., there are a few large observations whereas the majority of the observations are clustered together at the lower end of the scale). When data are right-skewed, usually a transformation is applied prior to statistical analysis and the log transformation is most commonly used. The bottom panel of Figure 1.8 shows the box plots of the data after the data have been transformed using the log transformation. We add 1 to each observation prior to transformation in order to avoid problems with taking log of values that are equal or close to 0. The box plots of the transformed data show that the transformation makes the data more symmetric and the medians and the means are much closer to one another than before the transformation.

In subsequent chapters, we show how to fit different statistical models to the COMBINE data to assess changes over time and the effect of baseline covariates on trajectories over time. We use these data to illustrate models for longitudinal data with continuous and categorical responses, mixture models for empirical derivation of heterogeneous trajectories over time, and assessment of moderating and mediating effects. We also demonstrate how to interpret significant interactions and main effects via appropriate post hoc comparisons.

1.5.4 The Health and Retirement Study

The Health and Retirement Study (HRS, http://hrsonline.isr.umich.edu/) is a longitudinal survey among American citizens born between 1931 and 1941 and their spouses that assesses changes in labor force participation and health status over the transition period from working to retirement, and the years after. The initial HRS panel (N=12,652) was first interviewed in 1992 with subsequent interviews taken every two years. This survey is an observational longitudinal study that provides a wealth of information to address important questions about aging and the transition from working to retirement. In this book, we focus on changes in self-rated health (SHLT) and body-mass index (BMI), and the effects of covariates on these changes. Body-mass index is calculated as weight, in kilograms, divided by the square of height, in meters, and is considered a continuous measure. Self-reported health is an ordinal measure that takes the following possible values: excellent (coded as 1), very good (2), good (3), fair (4), and poor (5). BMI increases on average over time while SHLT deteriorates on average over the first seven waves of data. Mean plots with or without variance estimates could be created to illustrate this, as shown for the previous data sets.

Within this data set, correlations are present between repeated measures on the same variable within individuals and on different variables within individuals. Figure 1.10 is a scatterplot matrix that shows the distributions of BMI and SHLT at the first wave and at the seventh wave, and gives visual clues as to whether the measurements are correlated and in what direction the correlation is. For this plot, we chose a subset of 250 individuals since plotting the entire data set of several thousand individuals would have made the graphs hard to read. Each of the individual plots in the scatterplot matrix illustrates the relationship between two variables and to a certain extent the distribution of each variable.

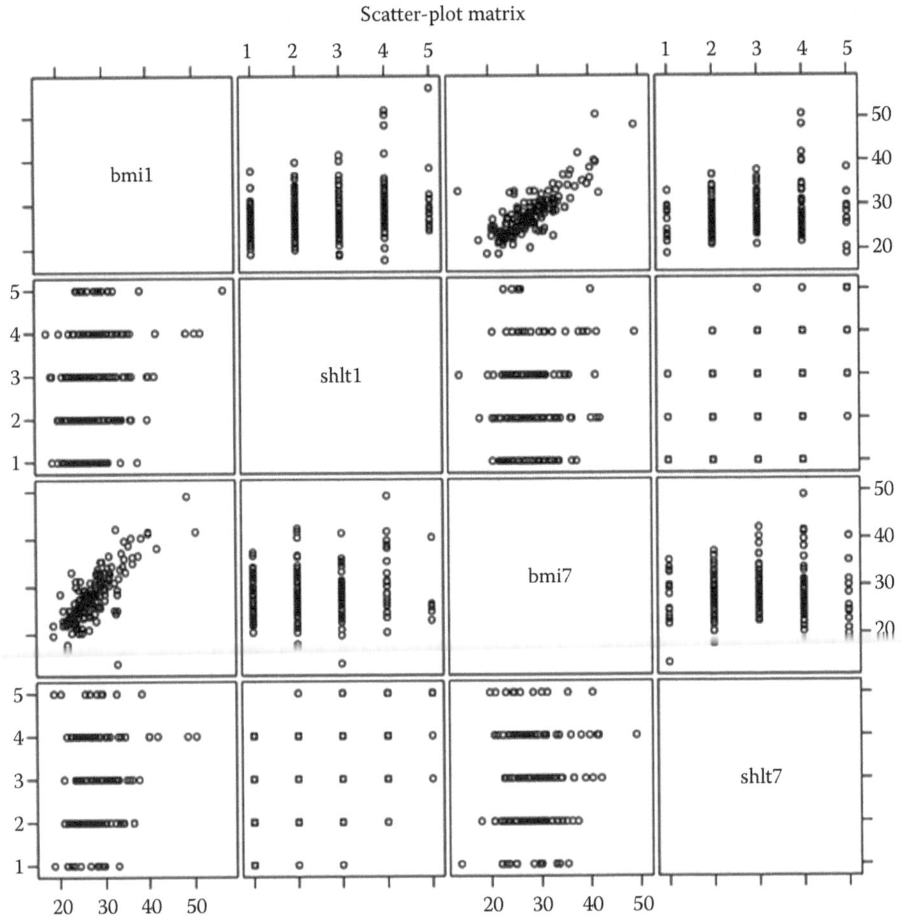

FIGURE 1.10
Scatterplot matrix of body-mass index (BMI) and self-rated health (shlt) measures in wave 1 and wave 7 of the Health and Retirement Study.

For example, the plot in the first row and second column is a scatterplot for the relationship between BMI at wave 1 (bmi1) and self-rated health at wave 1 (shlt1). Since SHLT takes only five possible values, the observations are concentrated in five columns of individual circles, each circle corresponding to an individual in the sample. The increasing height of the columns from left to right indicates that participants with higher BMI tend to have worse self-reported health (i.e., higher scores on the self-rated health variable). Also, some outliers in terms of BMI are noted in the upper right corner of this plot.

Similarly, the plot in the first row and third column visualizes the relationship between BMI at wave 1 (bmi1) and BMI at wave 7 (bmi7). As expected BMI measures are strongly positively correlated even though the observations are 14 years apart. The plot in the second row and the fourth column visualizes the relationship between self-rated health during wave 1 (shlt1) and wave 7 (shlt7). Self-rated health measures are also positively correlated but this is harder to see since this variable is ordinal with five levels and the dots representing individuals are on top of each other. We notice that there is nobody in this sample with poor (5) or fair (4) self-rated health at wave 1 who is with excellent health (1) at wave 7. Participants with poor (5) self-rated health at wave 1 also do not have very good (2) health at wave 7 and participants with excellent health (1) at wave 1 do not have poor health (5) at wave 7.

Note that the plots in the lower left part of this scatterplot matrix are flipped images of the plots in the upper right part of the matrix. For example, the plot in the second row and first column represents the same information concerning the relationship between BMI and SHLT at wave 1 as the plot in the first row and second column but with the vertical and horizontal axes switched. Choosing which of the two plots to focus on is a matter of convenience and depends on the application.

Scatterplot matrices are very useful for visualization of relationships between variables since they allow simultaneous consideration of multiple variables. However, scatterplot matrices that are too large should be avoided since detail may be hard to see. The HRS data set will be used in subsequent chapters for illustration of models for correlated data and also for the effects of different types of missing data on inferences.

1.5.5 Serotonin Transport Study in Mother–Infant Pairs

This study evaluates the effects of maternal treatment with an antidepressant (sertraline) for post-partum depression on serotonin transport in breastfeeding mother–infant pairs (Epperson et al., 2001). Treatment with selective serotonin reuptake inhibitors (SSRIs) is associated with significant blockade of serotonin reuptake in patients. Infants of breastfeeding mothers are exposed to sertraline through maternal breast milk. The critical question is whether SSRI exposure is safe for infants. One aspect of this assessment is to test whether sertraline exposure is associated with significant blockade of serotonin reuptake in infants and to compare magnitude of blockade between mothers and infants. The data set consists of 14 mother–infant pairs with serotonin measurements in both mothers and infants before and after exposure to sertraline. Figure 1.11 shows serotonin levels in mothers and infants before and after antidepressant treatment. The plot clearly shows a decrease in mothers after treatment and no change in their infants.

There are two types of correlations in these data: between measurements on mothers and infants within the same pair, and between pre- and post-measurements for each infant or mother. These correlations are shown in a table form in Table 1.1. In this table *mpre* is the variable "serotonin level in mother before the intervention," *mpost* is "serotonin level in mother after the intervention," *cpre* is "serotonin level in child before the intervention," and *cpost* is "serotonin level in child after the intervention." All correlations are positive and most are fairly strong. The only two that are not statistically significantly different from zero are between mothers' and children's measures after treatment, and between mothers' measures after the treatment and children's measures before the treatment. The correlations, as well as the apparent differences in variability of the measurements of mothers before and after the intervention, need to be taken into account for proper statistical analysis. We use these data to illustrate how mixed models can be fitted to analyze clustered correlated data.

1.5.6 Meta-Analysis of Clinical Trials in Schizophrenia

This study (Woods et al., 2005) assessed whether the degree of improvement with antipsychotic medication in clinical trials differed depending on control group choice. The meta-analysis evaluated 66 treatment arms from 32 studies of four medications (risperidone, olanzapine, quetiapine, and ziprasidone) for the treatment of schizophrenia symptoms

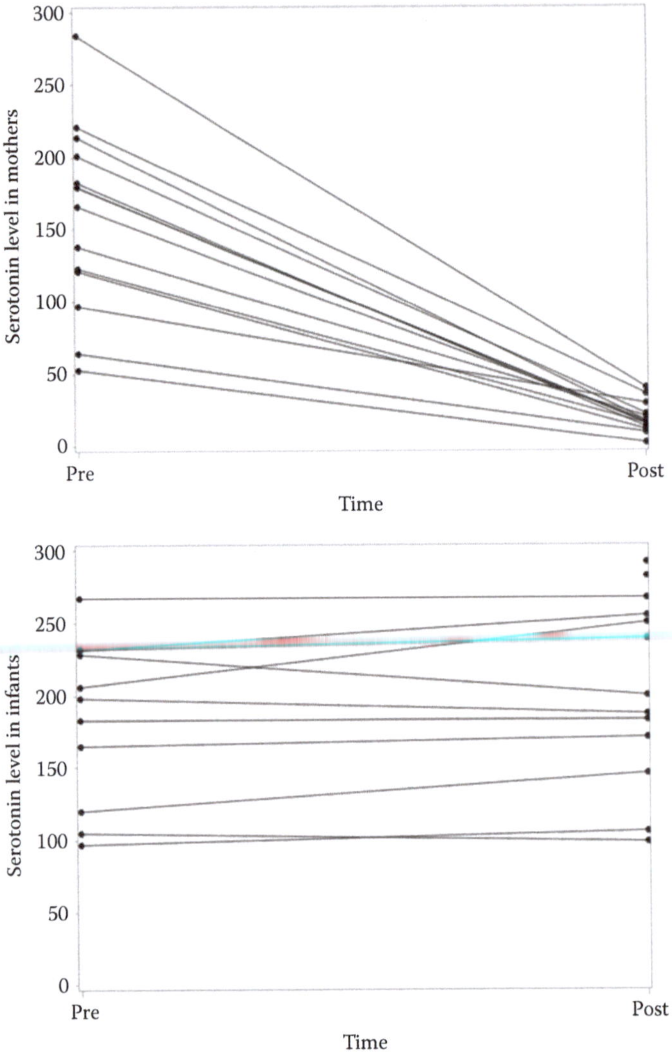

FIGURE 1.11
Serotonin levels in mothers (on the left) and their infants (on the right) before and after antidepressant treatment in the serotonin transport study in mother–infant pairs.

TABLE 1.1

Correlations between Serotonin Level Measurements on Mothers and Infants before and after Antidepressant Treatment

	mpre	mpost	cpre	cpost
mpre	1.00	0.70	0.71	0.56
mpost		1.00	0.48	0.34
cpre			1.00	0.91
cpost				1.00

TABLE 1.2

Average Change in BPRS Scores from Baseline to Endpoint and Standard Deviations by Dose and Type of Design in Antipsychotic Clinical Trials

Type of Design Dose	Placebo-Controlled Mean (SD)	Low Dose-Controlled Mean (SD)	Active Control Mean (SD)
Effective dose	9.0 (2.9)	11.2 (2.7)	14.7 (4.0)
Intermediate dose	6.3 (2.7)	9.8 (3.9)	—
Ineffective dose	2.8 (0.8)	6.7 (2.2)	—

with a total of 7264 patients. Average improvements and corresponding standard deviations by dose and type of design are shown in Table 1.2. Based on this table, the largest improvement from baseline occurs in studies with active control at effective medication doses. The average improvement in this type of design is by about 50% more than the average improvement at the same dose level in placebo-controlled trials (14.8 compared to 9.0). This corresponds to more than one standard deviation difference, which is considered a substantial effect. The original study (which applied mixed models to these data) concluded that the degree of improvement with antipsychotic medication in clinical trials differed significantly depending on control group choice. The modeling took into account the correlations between measurements on different treatment arms within the same study that are due to sampling individuals from the same population and the common effect of the environment in which the treatments within the same study were offered. In Chapter 3, we describe how an appropriate model is constructed and show the results from the analysis.

1.5.7 Human Laboratory Study of Menthol's Effects on Nicotine Reinforcement in Smokers

Menthol is a common ingredient in e-cigarettes and in other modified tobacco products that may facilitate the development and maintenance of addiction, especially in young adults who increasingly use e-cigarettes. This study (Valentine et al., under review) used a two-level cross-over experimental design to examine whether menthol at different doses, compared to placebo, altered nicotine reinforcement in young adult smokers. Smokers of mentholated and smokers of non-mentholated cigarettes were randomized to receive the three doses of menthol (high dose, low dose, and no menthol) by an e-cigarette in random order and in a double-blind fashion. Each menthol dose was given on a separate test day. On each of these days, all three nicotine doses (saline, 5, 10 μg/kg) were infused in random order. The design is illustrated with the schematic in Figure 1.12. This type of design leads to increased power for testing the main and interactive effects of the two factors (nicotine and menthol) compared to a parallel group design. The main outcome of interest in this study is the rewarding effect of nicotine measured by the Drug Effects Questionnaire. The hypothesis is that concurrent menthol and nicotine administration, as compared to nicotine and control flavor, or saline and control flavor, enhances the rewarding effects of nicotine. We use these data to illustrate how to model correlations within subjects between repeated observations on the same test day and on different test days.

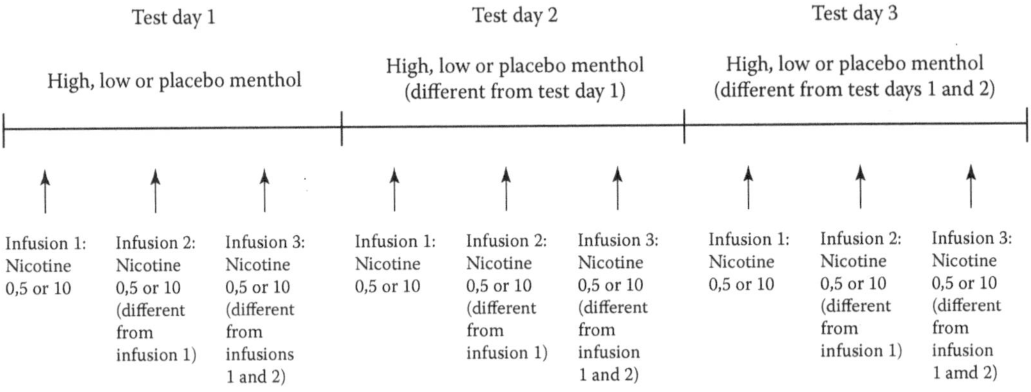

FIGURE 1.12
Double cross-over design of the human laboratory study of menthol's effects on nicotine reinforcement in smokers.

1.5.8 Functional Magnetic Resonance Imaging (fMRI) Study of Working Memory in Schizophrenia

In this study, 14 patients with schizophrenia and 12 healthy comparison participants were tested on a spatial working memory task with two difficulty levels (Driesen et al., 2008). Brain activation during three distinct phases (encoding, maintenance, and response) was recorded using fMRI. The study assessed phase-specific deficits in cortical function that contribute to cognitive impairments in schizophrenia. The relationship between task performance and brain activation was also assessed. Herein, we focus on averaged activation measures in pre-specified regions of interest (SMFG=superior medial frontal gyrus, MFG=middle frontal gyrus, IFG=inferior frontal gyrus, and VIFG=ventral inferior frontal gyrus) in the pre-frontal cortex as dependent measures.

This is an example of clustered data with the individual being the cluster. There are several sets of correlations within the cluster: correlations between the three different phases, the four different regions, and the two different task difficulty levels. Furthermore, variances in the different regions, phases, and difficulty levels are different. A proper statistical model for the analysis of these data needs to take all these features into consideration. We use this data set to illustrate how mixed models can be used to account for the complicated variance–covariance pattern of the data so that testing of the main hypotheses involving group differences can be accomplished.

Table 1.3 shows the means, variances, and covariances of a subset of the data. We provide descriptive statistics only for the encoding phase (eight repeated measures: one for each region by difficulty level combination), since it is difficult to visually inspect all 24 repeated measures simultaneously. In general, to obtain a preliminary impression of data with many repeated measures, one needs to separate the data into meaningful parts, examine the parts one at a time, and then assess the interrelationships between the different parts. More detailed exploration of these data is undertaken in subsequent chapters. From Table 1.3, we see that means in some regions (e.g., IFG) appear higher than means in other regions (e.g., VIFG) across task difficulty levels. Standard deviations are in general similar, although in regions with lower average they tend to be slightly lower. Also, all correlations within individuals are positive and sizeable, especially correlations within the same region and within the hard-working memory task.

TABLE 1.3

Means (M), Standard Deviations (SD) and Correlations (*r*) between Repeated Measures during Hard and Easy Working Memory Tasks in Four Different Brain Regions in the Schizophrenia Data Set

	Hard MFG	Hard IFG	Hard VIFG	Hard SMFG	Easy MFG	Easy IFG	Easy VIFG	Easy SMFG
Hard MFG	*M*=0.49 SD=0.23	*r*=0.57	*r*=0.59	r=0.17	r=0.63	r=0.44	r=0.35	r=0.24
Hard IFG		M=0.42 SD=0.25	r=0.71	r=0.62	r=0.56	r=0.80	r=0.52	r=c0.56
Hard VIFG			M=0.27 SD=0.16	r=0.38	r=0.55	r=0.63	r=0.79	r=0.52
Hard SMFG				M=0.44 SD=0.32	r=0.42	r=0.62	r=0.44	r=0.75
Easy MFG					M=0.35 SD=0.17	r=0.59	r=0.57	r=0.65
Easy IFG						M=0.32 SD=0.16	r=0.70	r=0.70
Easy VIFG							M=0.24 SD=0.16	r=0.70
Easy SMFG								M=0.35 SD=0.25

1.5.9 Association between Unemployment and Depression

These data are from a study of 254 recently unemployed individuals who were followed for up to 16 months after a job loss (Ginexi et al., 2000). At each of three interviews after the initial job loss, conducted at different times for different individuals, depression symptoms were measured using the Center for Epidemiologic Studies Depression (CES-D) questionnaire, which asks participants to rate the frequency with which they experience each of twenty symptoms of depression. The total CES-D score was calculated as the sum of the answers to the 20 individual questions with a possible range of 0–80. Unemployment status at each interview was also recorded.

Figure 1.13 shows the change in individual depression scores over time for subjects who were re-employed by the end of the study and for subjects who were unemployed at the last available interview. Visually, the range of CES-D scores for those who remained unemployed (or were employed and then laid off again) is wider than for those who were re-employed. Thus, the study hypothesis that depression is associated with higher levels of depressive symptoms appears plausible. Appropriate statistical models for these unbalanced data are presented in Chapter 3, whereas Chapter 8 uses the same data to illustrate the use of time-dependent covariates.

1.6 Historical Overview of Approaches for the Analysis of Repeated Measures

The first method for analysis of repeated measures data was the analysis of variance (ANOVA) model with a single random subject effect that dates back to the work of

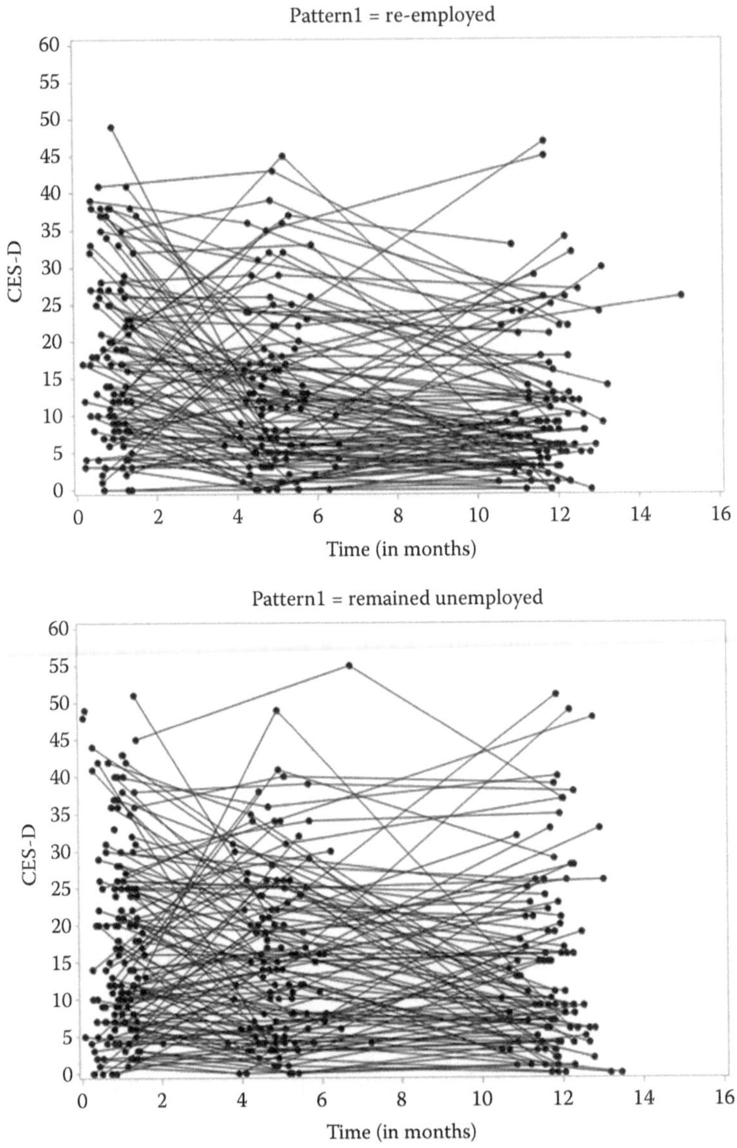

FIGURE 1.13
Profile plots of CES-D scores of all subjects by employment pattern in the study of the association between unemployment and depression.

R. A. Fisher (Fisher, 1925). This approach is also known as the *univariate repeated measures ANOVA* (rANOVA) and assumes equal variances of the repeated observations and equal correlations among all repeated observations within individuals or clusters. This assumption is likely to be satisfied in randomized block designs where the observational units within a block are deemed exchangeable, but is unlikely to be satisfied in more complicated clustered or longitudinal designs where variances and correlations can differ within individuals or clusters. Recognizing this problem, Greenhouse and Geisser (1959) and Huynh and Feldt (1976) developed corrections to the statistical tests in univariate repeated measures ANOVA so that this approach could be used for hypothesis testing when variances and correlations vary within individuals. Despite the correction, this approach is not very flexible for the analysis of longitudinal data and, as incorporated in most statistical packages, does not allow for missing data on an individual. It is also appropriate when the number of occasions per individual or cluster is the same while in many studies with longitudinal and clustered data, the number of observations may differ.

A modification of the ANOVA approach that requires more extensive computations, is *the multivariate repeated measures analysis of variance* (rMANOVA) model. MANOVA was developed for testing between-group differences on multiple distinct response measures simultaneously. The repeated measures situation is different from the situation with distinct response measures in that the same response variable is measured repeatedly over time or within clusters. Nevertheless, in both situations the response observations are correlated and both situations fall within the same framework. An advantage of the rMANOVA approach over the rANOVA approach, is that it allows the variance–covariance structure to be completely general. However, when there are missing data on an individual it excludes all data on this individual from analysis. It is also less powerful than the rANOVA approach when exchangeability is in fact satisfied. Like rANOVA it also requires that the number of repeated occasions per individual is constant.

A special case of rMANOVA analysis is *profile analysis* (Box, 1950) which constitutes a MANOVA analysis of multiple derived variables that are linear combinations of the repeated observations on an individual. This approach is most commonly used with longitudinal data and allows simultaneous testing of mean differences across occasions and trends over time between groups.

For the sake of simplicity of interpretation, often studies with repeated measures data are analyzed based on single summary measures of the observations within individuals. In clustered data studies, one can calculate the means for each cluster and then compare these means between groups using usual ANOVA models. In longitudinal data studies, one can calculate the change from baseline to endpoint and then perform ANOVA comparison on these derived measures. Alternatively, scores at the end of treatment can be compared using ANOVA or ANCOVA (analysis of covariance) with control for baseline scores. This approach has severe limitations, as it ignores a large portion of the data and often requires imputation of missing data. Missing data are very common in longitudinal studies and one of the earliest approaches for dealing with missing data was to impute missing values with baseline values carried forward, last observation carried forward, or mean values calculated based on all individuals. The observation carried forward approaches virtually always lead to biased estimates of effects and, although they were originally proposed as being conservative (i.e., having lower probability of false positive results) in clinical trials and observational studies, they can also be anti-conservative or too liberal (i.e., having higher probability of false positive results). Recently, more sophisticated methods, such as multiple imputation approaches, have been used, which provide valid conclusions under general assumptions about missing data.

The state-of-the-art approaches for analysis of repeatedly measured data nowadays are *mixed-effects models*. They are also known as *random effects models* (Laird and Ware, 1982; Ware, 1985), *random regression models* (Goldstein, 1987), *hierarchical linear models* (Bryk et al., 1987) and *empirical Bayes models* (Casella, 1985). Random effects models assume that individuals deviate randomly from the overall average response. The correlation between repeated observations on the same individual can arise from common random effects or the pattern of variance and correlations can be directly specified. A combination of both approaches is also possible. The specified structures can vary in complexity, from equal variances at all time points and equal correlations between any two measurements on the same individual (i.e., the structure assumed in rANOVA models), to no restrictions at all (i.e., the structure assumed in rMANOVA models). As an intermediate complexity, one can assume that correlation between observations decreases with increasing time lag. Mixed models are very flexible because they can consider many different variance–covariance structures and select the best-fitting one in the process of selecting the best model. They also use all available data on an individual and give unbiased estimates when data are missing at random. Chapters 3 and 4 present mixed-effects models in detail. Different missing data assumptions are discussed in Chapter 7. A more detailed historical overview at a non-technical level of methods for the analysis of repeated measures data can be found in Gueorguieva and Krystal (2004). Other fairly non-technical books on longitudinal data are Singer and Willett (2003) and Twisk (2013a).

1.7 Basic Statistical Terminology and Notation

For simplicity of explanation, we consider that the repeated observations occur within the individual. That is, the individual is the clustering factor. The relevance of the notation to other clustering situations (e.g., individuals nested within families or other larger units) is clear when in the rest of this section "individual" is replaced by "cluster." We also consider the *augmentation treatment for depression* study (Example 1.5.1) in order to illustrate the concepts.

The technical notation is kept to a minimum in this presentation. If, even at that level, it presents a challenge, the book of Altman (1991) can be consulted for a review of basic concepts. For more comprehensive notation and technical details, interested readers are referred to other books: Lindsey (1999), Weiss (2005), and Hedeker and Gibbons (2006). Fitzmaurice et al. (2009) provides a very comprehensive reference for longitudinal data analysis.

1.7.1 Response

The response (outcome, dependent) variable is denoted by Y. When there is a single observation per individual, the individual responses are denoted as Y_i where i corresponds to the ith individual and there are n individuals in the sample. The average of all observations in the sample is the sample mean and is calculated as

$$\bar{Y} = \frac{1}{n}\sum_{i=1}^{n} Y_i,$$

That is, all observations are summed and the sum is divided by the number of observations.

The sample variance reflects the entire variability in the sample and is calculated as follows:

$$s^2 = \frac{1}{n-1}\sum_{i=1}^{n} (Y_i - \bar{Y})^2.$$

That is, it represents an average of the squares of the deviations of the individual observations from the sample mean. In the denominator, we use $n - 1$ rather than n in order to take into account that we estimate the mean rather than use the true unknown value. The more spread out the observations are, the more variability there is and the larger the calculated variance will be. Since the variance is measured in squared units compared to the response, a more interpretable measure of variability is the standard deviation of the observations, which is measured in the same units as the mean and is obtained as the square root of the variance:

$$s = \sqrt{\frac{1}{n-1}\sum_{i=1}^{n}(Y_i - \bar{Y})^2}.$$

The formulae for variance and standard deviation are presented for completeness but are not crucial for understanding the material presented in this book.

In repeated measures data, we have multiple observations per individual and an additional subscript is needed to annotate the responses. The response is Y_{ij}, where i corresponds to the ith individual and j corresponds to the jth observation within the individual. The number of individuals in the sample is usually denoted by N and the number of observations within the ith individual is n_i. The subscript here is necessary to indicate that the number of observations within the individual does not need to be the same.

The simplest case that we consider in Chapters 2 and 3, is with a quantitative (continuous) response, that is, the response takes values over an interval of possible values. For example, weight and height measurements, rating scales over large intervals, are considered quantitative responses. Chapter 4 presents models for responses that are dichotomous (binary), ordinal, or represent counts. All responses are assumed to be random variables, that is, there is uncertainty in the values that are observed.

In the considered example of the augmentation study in depression, the response is a measure of depression severity (HDRS). We usually start the statistical analysis by calculating means and standard deviations for each group at each time point and visualize the data. In statistical notation, since we have as many means as there are repeated occasions, we denote the sample means and standard deviations as follows:

$$\bar{Y}_j = \frac{1}{N}\sum_{i=1}^{N} Y_{ij}$$

$$s_j = \sqrt{\frac{1}{N-1}\sum_{i=1}^{N}(Y_{ij} - \bar{Y}_j)^2}$$

Herein, we used N to denote the number of individuals on each of the repeated occasions but the number of individuals does not need to be the same. In longitudinal data especially, participants drop out so the number of individuals decreases over time. Figure 1.5 shows the means and standard deviations by treatment group in the depression example.

1.7.2 Predictors

In statistical notation, the predictors are usually denoted by X and can vary between or within individuals. This dependence is often reflected in the subscripts of the predictor. X_i usually denotes the value of a predictor for the ith individual and the subscript i means that the covariate has the same value on all repeated occasions within the individual, but in general, has different values for different individuals. In this case, the predictor is said to vary between individuals but not within individuals. In the considered example, the treatment group is a predictor that varies between individuals but not within individuals.

Similarly, X_{ij} denotes the value of a predictor for the jth observation on the ith individual. The additional subscript j is used in order to distinguish different values of this predictor on different observation occasions within individuals. In this case, the predictor is said to vary within individuals and it can also vary between individuals. In the depression example, time is a within-subject predictor as it varies within each individual (i.e., each individual has observations at several different time points). The time points may or may not be the same for different individuals. Other subject characteristics can vary over time, such as blood pressure or weight, or subjects can switch treatments over time and hence treatment can also vary within individuals. This is the case in cross-over studies.

When there are multiple predictors, a third subscript k can be used to denote the kth predictor. Time and group are almost always present as predictors in repeated measures studies with longitudinal data. Additional variables that may be affecting the response are usually referred to as covariates and they are also considered predictors. For example, history of depression and concurrent medication use may be additional covariates in the depression study.

Predictors are assumed to be exactly observed, that is, there is no uncertainty in the values of the predictors and they are considered fixed, not random. Time and group are usually exactly observed but other predictors may be measured with error and may need to be considered as random variables themselves. For example, self-reported medication compliance may be imprecisely ascertained. When predictors are also assumed to be random variables, estimation and inference are more complicated. Interested readers are referred to Fuller (1987) since this situation is not considered in this book.

1.7.3 Linear Model

The statistical relationship between the predictors and the response in the population and its change by occasion or time can be described using a statistical model. This represents our theoretical understanding and assumptions about the relationship between the predictors and the response and may or may not correspond to reality. The linear model assumes that the association is linear in the coefficients (betas in the formula below) and that the effects of the predictors are additive (i.e., they add onto one another rather than multiply or act together in another fashion). This can be expressed using the following formula:

$$Y_{ij} = \beta_0 + \beta_1 X_{ij1} + \beta_2 X_{ij2} + \ldots + \beta_p X_{ijp} + \varepsilon_{ij},$$

Where some of the predictors vary between individuals, and some vary within individuals, the beta coefficients are unknown parameters that can be estimated from the data and reflect the direction and magnitude of the association between the predictors and the response, and the epsilons denote the errors that describe the uncertainty or residual variability of the measurements, apart from what the predictors explain.

In the depression example, the equation describes how each observation varies depending on the predictors and can be written as

$$HDRS_{ij} = \beta_0 + \beta_1 Group_i + \beta_2 Time_j + \beta_3 Group_i \times Time_j + \varepsilon_{ij},$$

where:

> $Group_i$ takes the value of 1 if the ith individual belongs to the augmentation group and 0 if this individual belongs to the control group
> $Time_j$ is the week (coded 0 through 6) when the jth observation is taken
> $Group_i$*$Time_j$ denotes the interaction between $Group_i$ and $Time_j$ (i.e., is the product of $Group_i$ and $Time_j$)

The interaction reflects how the responses for the different groups differ from one another over time. Each individual's response can be described by substituting the appropriate values for $Group_i$ and $Time_j$ in the equation. For example, the baseline (i.e., Time=0) response for an arbitrary chosen patient i from the augmentation group is described as $HDRS_{i0}=\beta_0+\beta_1+\varepsilon_{i0}$ while the response at week 6 for another arbitrary chosen patient l from the control group is described as $HDRS_{l6}=\beta_0+\beta_2\,6+\varepsilon_{l6}$. The errors reflect the expected deviations for particular individuals and particular occasions from the average response of all patients in the corresponding hypothetical population measured on the corresponding occasion.

1.7.4 Average (Mean) Response

The average response for a particular combination of values of the predictors is described according to the linear function above and is

$$EY_{ij} = \beta_0 + \beta_1 X_{ij1} + \beta_2 X_{ij2} + \ldots + \beta_p X_{ijp}$$

Here, E stands for expectation and this formula describes how the expected (average) response in the population varies depending on the predictors. The predictors may appear by themselves in the formula or two (or even more) predictors can multiply each other (for example the *kth* predictor can be a product of some of the other predictors, e.g., $X_{ijk}=X_{ij1}X_{ij2}$). When predictors appear by themselves, they represent main effects. The beta coefficients are then interpreted as the differences in mean response that correspond to a unit change in the predictor (for continuous predictors) and the difference in mean response that corresponds to comparing a particular level of a categorical predictor to a reference level of this predictor (e.g., experimental to control group, or later time point to an earlier time point). When there are interactions between the predictors (i.e., when the predictors multiply each other, e.g., $X_{ijk}=X_{ij1}X_{ij2}$ in the formula above), the interactions need to be interpreted first. Interactions may involve two or more predictors and become increasingly complex to explain, especially in designs with multiple factors. We consider different interactions and their interpretations in subsequent chapters. Herein, a simple situation is considered in the context of the depression example.

In the depression example, the average response can be described as

$$E\{HDRS_{ij}\} = \beta_0 + \beta_1 Group_i + \beta_2 Time_j + \beta_3 Group_i \times Time_j.$$

Let us assume for a moment that β_3 is equal to 0, which means that there is no interaction between group and time, that is, the change over time in the two groups has the same form (i.e., average responses in the two groups can be described by parallel lines). The coefficient β_1 is interpreted as the difference in mean HDRS scores between the two groups averaged over the entire time period. Using the specified coding above for a group (1 for the augmentation group and 0 for the control group), positive values mean that the augmentation group has higher scores on average, while negative values mean that the control group has higher scores on average. The coefficient β_2 is interpreted as the change in average HDRS score per week (i.e., one unit change in time). To estimate how much the HDRS scores change on average over the entire study period, we need to multiply β_2 by the study duration in weeks (i.e., β_2 times 6). Note that this model assumes that the rate of change stays constant over the study period, that is, the change over time is described by a straight line. This is often an untenable assumption although, in some situations, it may be a convenient approximation.

If β_3 is not equal to 0, then there is an interaction between group and time. In this case, slopes of average change in the two groups over time are different and the average between-group differences change depending on which time points we consider. At time 0, the difference in average response between the two groups is described by β_1 but at time 6, for example, the difference in average response between the two groups is described by β_1+β_3.6. Depending on the signs of β_1 and β_3 the difference may be smaller or larger. The β_3 coefficient is interpreted as the difference in slopes (linear rates of change) between the two groups over time. When change over time is described by a more complicated function, rather than linear change, interpreting between-group differences becomes more challenging.

In the general linear model, a unique linear combination of the predictors corresponds to each observation time point and group. For the control group, the average response at baseline (time 0) is $HAMD_{i0}$=β_0, while for the experimental group, the average response at week 6 is

$$E\{HDRS_{i6}\} = \beta_0 + \beta_1 + \beta_2.6 + \beta_3.6.$$

In repeated measures data, estimation of the relationship between predictors and the mean response is usually of primary interest. In order to assess this relationship, all beta parameters need to be estimated. The deviations from the mean response need to be taken into account but are often of secondary interest.

1.7.5 Residual Variability

To perform statistical inference (i.e., construct confidence intervals or test hypotheses about the beta parameters), certain assumptions need to be imposed on the errors in the statistical model formulation above. Usually, when the response is continuous, the errors are assumed to be normally distributed with zero mean. Note that the distribution of the errors determines the distribution of the response in the sample when there are no other random effects. Thus, if the errors are normally distributed then the response is also normally distributed. A histogram of the responses on each occasion and within a group indicates whether the data are indeed approximately bell-shaped distributed and hence whether the normal distribution is appropriate.

The zero mean assumption is reasonable if we have included all important predictors of the response in the linear predictor and have specified the nature of the relationship correctly. That is, we have not omitted predictors that substantially affect the response and have used the appropriate form of each predictor. A classic example of miss-specified form is if the relationship between time and the response when plotted seems to be curvilinear but we include only the linear effect of time in the model. In this case, on some occasions the errors will have means that are larger than 0 and on some other occasions they will have means that are smaller than 0. Such a discrepancy will need to be corrected in order to reach justifiable conclusions for the relationship between predictors and response.

In classical regression and analysis of variance models, where each individual contributes a single observation, the errors are assumed to be independent of one another and to have equal variances. However, in repeated measures situations, error variances often vary by occasion and errors are correlated within individuals. In the depression example, and in similar longitudinal studies, it is likely that variances increase over time because individuals are usually selected to satisfy certain conditions for study entry, and then, some individuals show significant improvement in their response, some show no change, and some deteriorate. Thus, models that assume equal variances may not be appropriate.

Furthermore, the errors ε_{ij} corresponding to different individuals are assumed to be independent while different ε_{ij}'s corresponding to the same individual are assumed to be related. This is reasonable, as we expect repeated observations on the same individual on different occasions to deviate in a systematic way from the average for similar individuals. Thus, the errors for the same individual are more likely to be in the same direction (i.e., mostly positive or mostly negative) and their magnitudes are likely to be related. To assess whether the data support such assumptions, correlations of repeated observations on different occasions can be calculated and examined, either in table form or in figures. The *sample correlation* between repeated measures on occasion k and l within the individual is calculated as follows:

$$r_{kl} = \frac{\sum_{i=1}^{n}(Y_{ik} - \bar{Y}_k)(Y_{il} - \bar{Y}_l)}{\sqrt{\sum_{i=1}^{n}(Y_{ik} - \bar{Y}_k)^2}\sqrt{\sum_{i=1}^{n}(Y_{il} - \bar{Y}_l)^2}}$$

Correlations measure the degree of linear dependence between variables. Correlations vary between –1 and 1 with 0 corresponding to no linear relationship, –1 corresponding to a perfect negative relationship, and 1 corresponding to a perfect positive relationship. Figure 1.14 shows these three situations, as well as an example of a strong positive correlation, weak negative correlation, and curvilinear relationship, where the correlation is close to 0 but the two variables are related. When there are repeated measures within individuals some degree of linear dependence is expected and the dependence is usually positive.

The statistical notation for the error distributions in models with repeated observations is $\varepsilon_{ij} \sim N(0, \sigma_j^2)$, where σ_j^2 may be different for different occasions within individuals, N denotes normal distribution and errors are randomly spread out around 0. The errors for measurements on occasion k and l within a randomly chosen individual in the population are assumed to be correlated, that is $Corr(\varepsilon_{ij}, \varepsilon_{il}) = \rho_{jl}$ and this correlation is most often

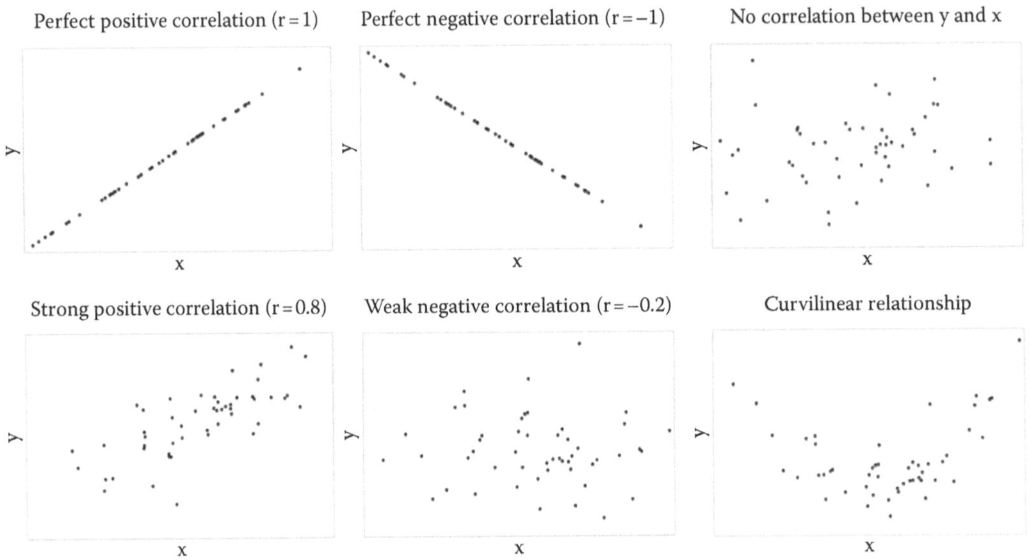

FIGURE 1.14
Examples of different corrections between two variables.

positive. With longitudinal data, the correlation is generally stronger for observations that are closer to each other in time and decreases with increasing time lag. Examining sample correlations between any two repeated measurements, either in table form or in a graph, provides information about appropriate correlation structures in the population. Plots to examine correlations in longitudinal data are described in Weiss (2005) and in Dawson et al. (1997).

In the depression example, if an individual starts with a HDRS score that is significantly higher than the average HDRS score in the sample, this individual's HDRS scores are more likely to stay above the average on the next few occasions, compared to the scores of an individual who starts with below average HDRS scores (see Figure 1.4). With increasing time lag, however, the probability of such systematic deviation becomes weaker and weaker.

1.7.6 Estimation

Estimates of the beta parameters are obtained using some statistical method so that the residual variability in the data is minimized. The method of *maximum likelihood* is the most commonly used approach and it finds the values of the beta parameters that maximize the likelihood that we observe the data in the sample, given our assumptions about how the data were generated, as reflected in the model formulation. Substituting the estimated beta values in the linear model, instead of the true unknown beta values, gives an estimate of the average response from the data. The obtained estimates are *unbiased* in large samples (i.e., they do not deviate in a systematic way from the true values of the parameters) and they are *efficient* (i.e., the uncertainty of these estimates is as small as possible). Uncertainty is measured by the standard errors of the estimates of the beta parameters and the standard errors are obtained in the estimation process. The parameter estimates are also approximately normally distributed which makes construction of confidence intervals and hypothesis tests straightforward.

1.7.7 Statistical Inference

Traditionally, the type of statistical inference of most interest in the subject-matter literature, has been testing whether one or more of the beta coefficients are zero, which corresponds to testing whether there is any effect of the corresponding predictor(s) on the response when keeping the values of the other predictors in the model constant (commonly referred to as controlling for the effects of the other predictors). In the simplest case of *testing a hypothesis* concerning a single beta coefficient, the null hypothesis is that the coefficient is zero. The alternative hypothesis is that this coefficient is different from zero if a two-sided test is performed, or that it is greater (or smaller) than zero in the corresponding one-sided tests. One-sided tests are rarely used because if the direction of the relationship between the predictor and the response is opposite to the hypothesized one, a one-sided test will fail to find a significant effect. For example, if an experimental treatment is compared to a standard treatment and the alternative hypothesis is that the experimental treatment is better than the standard treatment, there is no possibility to conclude based on a one-sided hypothesis test that the experimental treatment is worse than the standard treatment.

Test statistic, for testing whether a single beta coefficient is zero, is usually just the estimate of this coefficient over its estimated standard error. Large absolute values of this ratio indicate that it is unlikely that the beta parameter is zero. In such a case, the interpretation is that the predictor is significantly associated with the response.

Most statistical testing is based on the calculated *p-value,* which is the probability that the test statistic is at least as extreme as observed if there is no relationship between the predictor and the response. Note that if there is no true relationship, we would expect the parameter estimate to be close to zero and the test statistic to be small. If the p-value is smaller than a pre-specified cut off called significance level α (0.05% or 5% is most commonly used), then the conclusion is that it is unlikely that there is no relationship between the predictor and the response, and the relationship is declared to be statistically significant.

Two types of error can occur in this inference. When there is no relationship (of the form specified in the model) between the predictor and the response, but the hypothesis test concludes that the relationship is statistically significant, a *type I error* has occurred. This is a false positive result and by selecting a low significance level, we guard against this type of error. At 5% significance level, we would expect 5% of tests, when there is no significant relationship between the predictor and the response, to result in this type of error.

The other error occurs if there is a relationship between the predictor and the response but the hypothesis test results in failure to reject the null hypothesis of no relationship and the conclusion is that the relationship is not statistically significant. This type of error is called *type II error* and is a false negative result. How large the probability of this error is depends on the magnitude of the beta coefficient and the population variability. When the beta coefficient is small and/or the variability is large, there is a higher chance to commit this type of error. This type of error is also directly related to the power of the statistical test.

Power is the probability to reject the null hypothesis (i.e., declare that a statistically significant relationship exists) when the alternative is true (i.e., there is a relationship between the predictor and the response). Power changes with changing values of the beta coefficients and changing variability. It increases with increasing beta values and decreases with increasing variability. Issues of significance level and power of tests are considered in more detail in Chapter 11.

Hypothesis tests provide clear conclusions regarding the significance of the relationship between predictors and response. However, they are heavily dependent on sample size and do not provide estimates of the magnitude of the effects and the uncertainty in the estimates. *Confidence intervals* contain more information than hypothesis tests as they give a range for the magnitude of the effect of the predictor on the response with a certain level of confidence. Most commonly, 95% confidence intervals are constructed as the corresponding beta estimate plus/minus 1.96 times the standard error of this estimate. The confidence level 95% means that 95% of the time the true parameter falls within the limits of the confidence interval and is interpreted as the level of confidence that we have that we have captured the true underlying parameter in the confidence interval. Confidence intervals can also be used to evaluate whether the corresponding beta coefficient is statistically significantly different from zero (or any other value) or not, i.e., they can be used to perform the corresponding hypothesis test. If the confidence interval contains zero then the beta coefficient is declared not to be significantly different from zero and if the confidence interval does not contain zero then the beta coefficient is declared to be significantly different from zero.

In recent years, more emphasis is placed on reporting confidence intervals rather than p-values and for a very good reason. Rather than giving a yes/no answer to a sometimes contrived or overly simplified question as hypothesis tests do, they provide an estimate of the magnitude of an effect with an associated level of confidence. Thus, the reader or independent researcher can make their own judgment call on whether a particular result is clinically or practically meaningful or not. As a simple example, consider a hypothetical situation with two treatments (A and B) for depression. A very large clinical trial finds that treatment A improves a measure of depression severity on average by 0.1 standard deviations more than treatment B over a period of 8 weeks with a 95% confidence interval between 0.05 and 0.15. While this corresponds to a statistically significant result because the confidence interval does not contain 0, most doctors would probably not consider such a change as clinically meaningful and they would decide which treatment to use based on other considerations than differences in clinical efficacy.

Hypothesis tests are still useful in situations when some guidance is needed as to which effects to estimate, as in models with multiple possible interactions or in multiple comparison problems. But even in these cases, confidence intervals are still recommended as post-hoc analyses in order to obtain estimates of the magnitudes of effects. The discussion of the choice between hypothesis tests and confidence intervals and the joint use is continued in further chapters of the book.

1.7.8 Checking Model Assumptions

The errors in the linear model formulation are not directly observable. However, when estimates of the beta coefficients are obtained, these allow estimation of the errors by taking the difference between the individual responses and the predicted mean: $Y_{ij} - \hat{Y}_{ij}$. These quantities are called *residuals* and they give information about the fit of the model to the data. Since they are estimates of the unknown errors, assessing their distribution and variability can help assess whether the corresponding assumptions about the errors are approximately satisfied. Residual plots can be used to assess whether the assumptions of linearity, normality, and variance pattern are appropriate. If assumptions about the errors are not satisfied then remedial measures must be taken by either considering a more general model, adding covariates, transforming the data, or using statistical methods that make fewer assumptions about the data, such as non-parametric methods. A good reference for checking model assumptions and remedial measures for linear models is Kutner et al. (2005). Model diagnostics for models for repeated measures data are briefly considered in Chapters 3 and 4 where further references are also provided.

1.7.9 Model Fit and Model Selection

Many different models can be fit to any particular data set. Statistical criteria can be used in order to select the best-fitting model among a set of different possible models fitted to the same data set. Perhaps the most commonly used are different versions of information criteria such as the Akaike Information Criterion (AIC) and the Schwartz-Bayesian Information Criterion (BIC). We consider these in more detail in Chapters 3 and 4.

1.8 Summary

In this chapter, we described what repeated measures are, introduced different types of studies with repeated measures, discussed advantages of such studies, provided a brief historical overview of statistical methods for clustered and longitudinal data, reviewed some basic statistical terminology and notation, and introduced several data examples that are further considered in subsequent chapters. We focused on issues of describing mean response across repeated measures and accounting for variability and interdependence in the data. In Chapter 2, we consider the traditional methods for repeated measures analysis in more detail, while the rest of the book focuses on the state-of-the-art methods for such analysis and on different aspects of the analysis and design of studies with repeated measures.

2

Traditional Methods for Analysis of Longitudinal and Clustered Data

In this chapter, we describe methods for repeated measures analyses that have been traditionally used, but which are appropriate only in special situations (e.g., fixed measurement times, complete data, specific pattern of variances and covariances, normally distributed measures). Gold standard approaches for normal data, such as mixed-effects models, are introduced in Chapter 3, and extensions of these approaches for non-normal data are presented in Chapter 4. Readers who are only interested in the more flexible and general approaches, can skip the current chapter. Readers who would like a refresher on the more basic statistical models for analysis of variance, and a gentler transition from simple to more complicated methods for longitudinal and clustered data, should read this chapter where the techniques and limitations of traditional approaches are presented, and where situations in which it is acceptable that such methods are used, are described.

The simplest possible approach to analyzing data with repeated measures, is to calculate summary measures for each individual or cluster (e.g., mean response over repeated occasions or change from baseline to endpoint), and then use statistical methods for uncorrelated observations with the summary measure as the dependent variable, in order to make inferences regarding group differences or magnitudes of change from baseline to endpoint. Methods for uncorrelated data can also be directly applied to endpoint measures in longitudinal studies. The appeal of this approach (i.e., reducing the complexity of repeated measures data by focusing on a single measure) is its simplicity and straightforward interpretation. However, it is usually associated with loss of power to detect differences, decreased efficiency of statistical analysis, potential bias when there are missing data on key occasions (e.g., endpoint in longitudinal studies), and inability to characterize change or pattern of responses across different occasions. Especially problematic are situations when some repeated measures are ignored (e.g., when all intermediate data points in longitudinal studies are excluded from analysis).

In the first section of this chapter, we focus on methods for assessment of change, from baseline to endpoint, and for testing and estimation of group differences in longitudinal studies. This is done via methods for analysis of independent data such as t-test, ANOVA, or ANCOVA. In the second section, we focus on between-group comparisons of other summary measures using the same set of statistical approaches for independent data (t-test, ANOVA, ANCOVA). We focus on the assumptions of the methods and explain the disadvantages of these approaches, especially when some data are missing.

When observations are made at multiple intermediate time points, some studies still report results from a t-test or ANOVA performed separately at each time point. However, if a 5% significance level test is used for each test, then the probability of type I error becomes considerably greater than 5% and this may lead to falsely declaring groups to be different when differences do not exist. On the other hand, if a procedure for correcting for multiple testing is used (e.g., Bonferroni correction), then this leads to loss of power and increase in the probability of type II error (not detecting treatment differences when they do exist).

Performing separate tests at each time point also does not allow for direct comparison between treatment groups over time. This approach is not considered in this chapter as it rarely makes sense for longitudinal data.

More appropriate approaches for longitudinal and clustered data (when the assessment occasions are the same for all individuals/clusters and when the focus is on comparison of group means), are repeated measures analysis of variance (rANOVA, considered in Section 2.3), and repeated measures multivariate analysis of variance (rMANOVA, considered in Section 2.4). These methods use information from all repeated occasions and allow testing of hypotheses regarding change over time or pattern of responses within clusters or individuals. When assessment occasions are the same for all clusters or individuals (i.e., the design is *balanced*), when data are complete (i.e., there are no missing observations), there are no extreme outliers, and in the case of rANOVA, when the appropriate correction to the degrees of freedom is used, these methods provide valid hypothesis tests of main effects and interactions.

However, these methods can't be used when assessment occasions are different for different individuals (i.e., the design is *unbalanced*, e.g., one subject is assessed at weeks 1 and 4, another—at weeks 2 and 8, a third—at weeks 3 and 11). Furthermore, the multivariate approach (rMANOVA) can't be used when there are too many repeated occasions, compared to the sample size of the data set. Both methods can be severely affected by missing data. If there are missing data on one or more occasions within the individual or cluster, the entire individual or cluster is excluded from rMANOVA analyses and, although there are methods to handle such a situation in rANOVA, most software packages also exclude subjects with missing data. Thus, both rANOVA and rMANOVA analyses may produce biased results, since the resulting sample of individuals or clusters with complete data may not be representative of the entire population. Last but not least, these methods focus on hypothesis testing rather than effect size estimation, which is of primary interest in clinical studies. Thus, our descriptions of rANOVA and rMANOVA emphasize the assumptions and limitations of each method. In Chapter 3 we show that rANOVA and rMANOVA correspond to special cases of mixed-effects models and recommend that analyses of repeatedly measured data are performed within the framework of mixed models. Nevertheless, presenting these approaches first allows us to review the traditional methods for normal data with which readers may be more familiar, and provide a gentle lead-in to mixed models so that the reader can fully appreciate their advantages.

Data sets, SAS code, and output for all considered data examples in this chapter are available in the online materials.

2.1 Endpoint Analysis and Analysis of Summary Measures

2.1.1 Change from Baseline to Endpoint

Change-point analysis makes use of the change from the first (baseline) to the final observation on each subject ($Y_{iT} - Y_{i0}$). A very simple question that can be addressed with such data is to ascertain whether there is any change in response over time. This is accomplished by performing a *paired t-test*. The null hypothesis in this test is that there is no change over time while the alternative is that there is some change over time. In the case of a two-sided test, the change may be either positive or negative. When a one-sided test is used, we are specifically interested in whether there is significant increase (or decrease) over time. If the resulting p-value of the paired t-test is smaller than the selected significance threshold (usually 0.05) then we declare that there is a statistically significant change over time. Depending on the sign of the test statistic (which corresponds to the sign of the difference between baseline and endpoint means), we can claim that there is either significant increase from baseline (when the sign is positive) or significant decrease (when the sign is negative).

As an example, in the augmentation study in depression from Section 1.5.1, a paired t-test results in the test statistic $t(37) = 13.94$ with a p-value < 0.0001. The mean HDRS score at baseline is 30.14 with a standard deviation of 6.16. This is commonly denoted as M (SD) = 30.14 (6.16). At week 6, the mean HDRS score is 10.29 with a standard deviation of 6.62 (M (SD) = 10.29 (6.63)). Based on the paired t-test, we conclude that there is a significant decrease in average depression severity from baseline to endpoint as measured by the HDRS, which is not surprising since both treatment groups receive an active treatment. Note that the paired t-test is based on the ratio of the mean change over the standard deviation of the change. Whereas the mean change is simply the change of the means, the standard deviation of the change is not only determined by the standard deviations at the individual time points, but depends on the correlation of repeated observations within the individual as well.

The paired t-test, by itself, provides only evidence of whether there is statistically significant effect of time. In general, it is more important to estimate the magnitude of the observed effect. We can do this by constructing a confidence interval for the difference in means between baseline and endpoint. In the augmentation depression example, the mean change in HDRS score is estimated to be 20.39 points with a 95% confidence interval with bounds of 17.43 and 23.36 (i.e., 95% CI: (17.43, 23.36)). This is loosely interpreted as having 95% confidence that we have captured the true decrease in the population of subjects with major depression in our confidence interval. Thus, we estimate that the improvement in depression severity is between 17.43 and 23.36 points with 95% confidence. There is still 5% probability that the true mean change is outside of the constructed interval, but given how much larger even the lower bound of the confidence interval is than zero, we can confidently infer that the mean change is substantially greater than zero. The latter illustrates how we can use the confidence interval for the mean change to directly test the corresponding two-sided hypothesis whether the mean change is zero. Since the confidence interval not only allows us to test the corresponding hypothesis test but provides an estimate of effect size, it is the preferred approach.

A few cautionary notes are in order for this analysis:

First, it is appropriate when the outcome is quantitative and takes on a range of values. We can't use a paired t-test or construct the corresponding confidence interval to test for change in binary or categorical outcomes. Methods for categorical data need to be used in this situation and are described in Agresti (2002, 2007).

Second, the paired t-test and the confidence interval for mean change is valid when the sample size is large and/or the distribution of the change scores is approximately normally distributed (i.e., bell-shaped). If the sample is small and the distribution is not bell-shaped, then a non-parametric equivalent such as the Wilcoxon signed-rank test (Hollander and Wolfe, 1999) should be used for hypothesis testing. The Wilcoxon signed-rank test does not make assumptions of the shape of the distribution and hence can be used even with skewed data. Confidence intervals can be constructed for medians rather than means or medians are often reported with interquartile ranges (i.e., the 25th and the 75th percentile of the observations).

Third, sometimes percent change, rather than absolute change, may be of interest. In this case a one-sample t-test on percent change can be used to assess whether there is change over time or confidence interval can be constructed for percent change from baseline. Whether to focus on absolute change or percent change depends on the application. Percent change outcomes are usually used when the measurements are positive and when relative rather than absolute change is of interest. Note also that when the distribution of the original observations is not bell-shaped, sometimes a transformation such as log or square root can be applied to normalize the data. When log transformation is used, the difference in log-transformed observations is actually the log of the percent change of the original observations. Thus, interpretation of analysis of change scores can be made in terms of log-transformed percent change rather than absolute change.

Fourth, the paired t-test requires that each subject has baseline and endpoint observations. If one of the two observations is missing, then the corresponding subject is dropped from the analysis, which may lead to bias and/or loss of efficiency in the confidence interval estimate and the hypothesis test. A common "solution" to this problem is to impute the last available observation of each individual for the endpoint observation which can improve efficiency but almost surely results in bias of the estimate since this imputation assumes that there is no change in the subject's response after dropout. Other forms of imputation, such as imputing the mean value for the entire sample for the missing individual's value, are also possible but also lead to problems (e.g., increase in type I error rate). More sophisticated imputation approaches, such as multiple imputation, can be used and are more appropriate. Such methods are considered in the context of statistical modeling in Chapter 7.

Note that the number of degrees of freedom for the test statistic of the t-test is one less than the number of subjects used in the analysis, and thus, can indicate whether the analysis was performed on the entire sample or on a subsample of individuals. This is useful to know, in order to be able to interpret results from published papers in cases when sample sizes for individual tests are not directly presented. For example, in the t-test for the depression data, the degrees of freedom are 37 which means that the number of subjects this test is based on is 38. Thus, of the entire sample size of 50, 12 subjects are excluded from analysis because they have missing endpoint data.

2.1.2 Group Comparison in Endpoint Analysis

While, in some situations, hypothesis testing or estimation of mean change for the entire group of individuals may be of interest, more often there are multiple groups that need to be compared in terms of average change over time or response at the end of the study. This is especially pertinent when an experimental treatment needs to be evaluated in comparison to a control treatment. If there is no control group, there is no way of knowing whether the change over time is due to treatment or to other factors, such as spontaneous improvement or some other change in the environment.

When two groups need to be compared, the simplest approach is to use a two-sample t-test or construct a confidence interval for difference of two independent means. These approaches can be used either for comparisons of mean change between groups or comparison of mean response at the end of the study. When there are more than two groups, *one-way ANOVA* allows us to assess whether there are any differences among the groups. Post hoc tests can then be used to ascertain which groups may be different and confidence intervals allow us to estimate the magnitudes of the effects. We first consider the two-group scenario and illustrate how to perform a hypothesis test and construct a confidence interval for the difference in mean change between groups on the augmentation study in depression.

In hypothesis testing, most often the null hypothesis is that the mean (either mean change or mean response at the end of study) in the two groups is the same, while the alternative is that the two groups are different or that one is better than the other. However, it is also possible to test whether the mean in one of the groups is higher/lower than the mean in the other group by a certain amount. This scenario is rarely of interest and is not considered here.

In the depression example, we are interested in testing for significant differences between the control and augmentation group on change in depression severity. Usually, the more conservative approach for this test is to use a two-sided alternative hypothesis (i.e., that the two groups are different from one another). Using a one-sided alternative (in this case, that the change in the augmentation group is greater than the change in the control group) is slightly more powerful in finding a statistically significant difference but does not allow for the possibility that the response in the augmentation group may be worse than in the control group (i.e., the mean change in the augmentation group may be smaller than in the control group). The generally preferred approach is to use a two-sided alternative.

Similarly to the assessment of overall change in response over time, in the group comparison, a confidence interval of the difference in mean change from baseline to endpoint between groups provides more information than the corresponding hypothesis test. In the depression example, the t-test for the between-group comparison of change over time results in a small test statistic and a non-significant p-value ($t(36)=0.23$, $p=0.82$), thus leading to the conclusion that there are no significant differences in improvement in depression severity between the two groups. The confidence interval for the difference in mean change between the augmentation and control groups (mean change = 0.68, 95% CI: (−5.33, 6.70)) also contains 0, leading to the same conclusion. It also indicates that the change in the augmentation group is estimated to be slightly more than in the control group (by 0.68 points) but could be by up to 6.70 points more and by up to 5.33 points less than in the control group.

While there is significant overall improvement as evidenced by the analyses in the previous section, the magnitude of this improvement does not vary significantly by group, as evidenced by the confidence interval and the independent samples t-test. Note that these analyses of change are also based only on data from individuals with both baseline and endpoint observations ($N=38$), rather than the entire sample size ($N=50$). If imputation is used, then all individuals will be included in the analysis. However, we do not advocate this approach and defer discussion about missing data till Chapter 3, where mixed models are introduced, and Chapter 7, where missing data are discussed in detail.

When comparing two independent groups, there are two versions of the t-test. One assumes that the variances of the two groups are equal (pooled method) and the other estimates each group variance separately (Satterthwaite's approximation method). An additional test to compare the variances between groups could be performed in order to decide which version of the t-test to use. This is the F-test for equality of variances and is widely available in software packages. There is some disagreement in the statistical literature as to whether a two-stage approach with testing the equality of the variances prior to comparison of the means, or a direct use of the t-test based on an *a priori* decision about the version of t-test, is better. Often, both versions of the t-test lead to the same conclusion, but in case when there is discrepancy, the F-test could be used to decide between the two versions.

In the augmentation depression data set, the equality of variance test does not indicate that the variances are significantly different ($F(18,18)=1.37$, $p=0.51$) and hence the pooled variance version of the t-test is used. In contrast, in the serotonin transport study in maternal-child pairs from Section 1.5.5, the variances of the observations in mothers and in children after treatment are significantly different ($F(13,13)=94.69$, $p<.0001$) and hence the Satterthwaite's version is used to compare serotonin levels in mothers to serotonin levels in children after maternal treatment for depression. This test results in a highly significant p-value ($t(13.28)=7.74$, $p<.0001$) and leads us to declare that there are significant differences in serotonin levels in the mothers, compared to their children, after maternal treatment for depression. Thus, medication is significantly changing serotonin transport in the mothers but not in their children.

Note that Satterthwaite's version of the t-test has, in general, fractional degrees of freedom. This is due to the use of an approximation and this situation must be distinguished from situations when test statistics have two sets of degrees of freedom such as the F-test for equality of variances. In both the augmentation treatment for depression study and in the serotonin transport study, regardless of which version of the test is used, the substantive conclusions are the same.

When the two groups are comparable at baseline, it is likely that the comparison of the scores at endpoint will lead to the same result as the comparison of the change scores from baseline to endpoint. This is the case in both considered data sets. But quite often, especially in observational studies, the results can be quite different. Even small differences at baseline may increase to become larger and statistically significant differences at endpoint, especially if subjects selectively drop out of the study. Focusing on change scores, rather than on endpoint scores, is, in general, more appropriate for assessment of treatment effects although control for baseline covariates may be necessary as discussed further in this chapter.

Similar to the paired t-test and corresponding confidence interval, the two independent sample comparisons on change from baseline or endpoint depend on a number of assumptions:

- The data to which they are applied needs to be quantitative, with bell-shaped distribution in small samples, possibly after a transformation. If the data are not bell-shaped and can't be transformed to normality, a non-parametric method, such as Wilcoxon rank sum test (Hollander and Wolfe, 1999), should be used.
- The appropriate version for equal or unequal variances should be selected based on an *a priori* decision or examination of the variances.
- Measurements on different subjects are assumed to be independent.
- These methods use only individuals who have both baseline and endpoint data unless imputation is applied.

The depression data are approximately normally distributed and the sample size is modest, hence we are justified to apply the independent samples t-test and to construct the corresponding confidence interval for the mean change. However, as we saw above, the results were based on the subsample of individuals with both baseline and endpoint data.

Note that change-point analysis may be entirely adequate in simple situations with only pre- and post-measurements, no missing data, and comparable groups at baseline. However, such simple designs are rare in most subject-matter areas and dropout is almost inevitable in longitudinal studies, and thus, more complex methods are necessary to analyze longitudinal data sets.

2.1.3 Multiple Group Comparisons in Endpoint Analysis

When there are more than two groups of subjects whose responses need to be compared, ANOVA is the natural extension of the two-sample t-test. We first consider the simplest ANOVA situations with only one factor with multiple levels, each level corresponding to a different group of subjects (one-way ANOVA). ANOVA with multiple factors (multiway ANOVA) is considered further along in this section. We focus on statistical testing of the overall effects in the models, followed up by group comparisons, in order to explain the nature of the discovered differences. Many details regarding ANOVA models are available in Montgomery (2013).

The main hypothesis that is tested in one-way ANOVA, in this context, is that the mean endpoint (or change from baseline to endpoint) scores are the same for all groups. If this hypothesis of an *overall group effect* is rejected, then follow-up comparisons are necessary in order to explain which groups are different. Usually, the follow-up analyses are *pairwise comparisons* of means among the different groups. Note that it is possible that the overall test of group differences is significant but none of the pairwise comparisons between groups are significant. Conversely, the overall test of group differences may not be statistically significant, but some pairwise differences between groups may be significant. Thus, if there are *a priori* hypotheses regarding certain pairwise differences that are pre-specified, these can be performed at a pre-specified significance level even if the overall group test is not significant.

We use part of the COMBINE data introduced in Section 1.5.3 to illustrate the one-way ANOVA approach. This study assessed the effects of treatments for alcohol dependence over approximately four months. For the sake of simplicity, in this first analysis we ignore whether subjects received active or placebo acamprosate (which was not shown to be an effective treatment in this trial) and initially assess whether there are any differences in the average number of drinks per day at month 4 for those who drink. Four groups of individuals are considered, depending on whether they received naltrexone or CBI: naltrexone and CBI, naltrexone only, CBI only, or neither. We apply log transformation to the dependent variable (drinks per day) in order to make the data more closely adherent to the normal distribution. The null hypothesis is that the four treatment combinations have the same means, while the alternative is that some of the means are different. We perform this test by calculating the F-statistic which compares the between-group and the within-group variances in the data. Large F-values correspond to small p-values and lead to rejection of the null hypothesis of no difference in means. In this data set, the overall test of the group effect results in a small p-value ($F(3,717)=3.34$, $p=0.02$) and thus we conclude that there are significant differences among the treatment groups. However, this overall test does not show which mean(s) are different and how much they differ. To understand the nature of the treatment effect, one needs to perform post hoc comparisons of *least square means* and/or to visualize the data.

The least square means are estimated means for each group in the ANOVA model that are adjusted for other effects in the model. Post hoc pairwise comparisons of these means (Table 2.1) reveal that all active groups are associated with lower intensity of drinking than not receiving either treatment. The other pairwise comparisons are not statistically significant. The p-values from the tests of the pairwise differences succinctly summarize whether the differences are statistically significant, but do not indicate the

TABLE 2.1

Least Square Means, Associated Standard Errors and Adjusted p-Values for Pairwise Comparisons of Log Transformed Drinks Per Day During Month 4 for Those Who Drink in the COMBINE Study

Group Least Square Mean (standard error)	Naltrexone+CBI 1.04 (0.06)	Naltrexone Only 1.04 (0.06)	CBI Only 1.01 (0.06)	Neither 1.23 (0.05)
naltrexone+CBI		p=0.99	p=0.69	p=0.02
naltrexone only	p=0.99		p=0.70	p=0.02
CBI only	p=0.69	p=0.70		p=0.005
neither	p=0.02	p=0.02	p=0.005	

direction and the magnitude of the differences. One needs to look at the mean estimates and their standard errors in order to judge in what direction the differences are and how much uncertainty there is in the mean estimates. Better yet, 95% confidence intervals for the mean differences can be constructed in order to show in what range we are confident the mean difference lies. The intervals are provided in Table 2.2 and from them we can easily reach the same substantive conclusions, but we also have a possible range for the difference in means.

Note that correction for multiple comparisons should be used for the post hoc analyses (whether p-values or confidence intervals), especially when the comparisons are not pre-planned. Correction needs to be applied because otherwise the probability of making a type I error (i.e., declaring a statistically significant difference for one or more post hoc comparisons when no differences exist) is increased. In Chapter 6 we consider different correction methods and illustrate them on the COMBINE data.

We ignored acamprosate in order to simplify our illustration of the one-way ANOVA procedure. If we considered all eight treatment combinations as levels of the group factor with the one-way ANOVA approach and had a significant overall group effect, there are 28 post hoc pairwise comparisons that one can do and many of those are not of specific interest. A more appropriate approach, and one that reflects the design of the COMBINE study, is multiway (factorial) ANOVA, which allows assessment of main effects and interactions of the different treatments. The interaction tests evaluate the hypotheses that the effect of one factor varies at the levels of the other factors, while the tests of the main effects

TABLE 2.2

Confidence Intervals for Pairwise Comparisons of Log Drinks per Day During the Last Month of the Study Period for Subjects Who Drink in the COMBINE Study

Treatment Group	versus Treatment Group	Least Square Mean Difference (95% CI)
naltrexone+CBI	naltrexone only	0.001 (−0.16, 0.17)
naltrexone+CBI	CBI only	0.03 (−0.13, 0.19)
naltrexone+CBI	neither	−0.19 (−0.35, −0.03)
naltrexone only	CBI only	0.03 (−0.13, 0.19)
naltrexone only	neither	−0.19 (−0.35, −0.03)
CBI only	neither	−0.22 (−0.38, −0.07)

TABLE 2.3

Test Statistics and Corresponding p-Values of the Tests of Main Effects and Interactions in the Factorial ANOVA Analysis of Log Drinks per Drinking Day at Month 4 for Subjects Who Drink in the COMBINE Study

Effect	Test Statistic	p-value
acamprosate	F(1,713) = 0.00	0.96
naltrexone	F(1,713) = 1.86	0.17
CBI	F(1,713) = 3.64	0.06
acamprosate × naltrexone	F(1,713) = 0.41	0.52
acamprosate × CBI	F(1,713) = 0.11	0.75
naltrexone × CBI	F(1,713) = 3.77	0.05
acamprosate × naltrexone × CBI	F(1,713) = 0.01	0.93

evaluate whether there are differences in the mean response between the levels of one of the factors when response is averaged across the levels of the other factors.

In COMBINE, we assess the effects of the three factors (naltrexone, acamprosate, and CBI) by testing all possible interactions (one three-way interaction and three two-way interactions) and the three main effects. In this case the multiway ANOVA is a 3-factor model, each factor with two levels (i.e., 2 × 2 × 2 factorial). Table 2.3 presents the results from the three-factor ANOVA analysis of the log-transformed number of drinks per day at month 4 among subjects who drink in COMBINE. All tests of main effects and interactions are based on type III test statistics and are performed at 0.05 significance level.

When interpreting results from factorial experiments, first the significant interactions are interpreted and then the main effects could also be interpreted, especially if the interactions appear to be quantitative (i.e., the direction of the effect of one factor does not vary by the levels of the other factors), rather than qualitative (i.e., the direction of the effect of one factor varies by the levels of the other factors). Thus, if there is a significant three-way interaction, post hoc tests to explain such an interaction are necessary. If the three-way interaction is not significant, but some two-way interactions are significant, the significant two-way interactions are interpreted first.

Table 2.3 includes the test statistics and corresponding p-values for all effects in the three-factor ANOVA. The results show that only the interaction between naltrexone and CBI ($F(1,713) = 3.77$, $p = 0.05$) is statistically significant at 0.05 significance level. The interaction test indicates that the effect of CBI varies depending on whether naltrexone was given or not, and the effect of naltrexone varies depending on whether active CBI was provided or not. To understand this interaction, the least square means are examined, either in table or graph form, and *simple effects* of one factor at all the levels of the other factor are assessed. The simple effects of naltrexone to explain the naltrexone by CBI interaction are simply comparisons between the least square means on active naltrexone and on placebo naltrexone at each level of therapy (CBI and no CBI). Similarly, the simple effects of CBI are comparisons between the least square means on CBI and without CBI at each level of naltrexone (active and placebo).

Figure 2.1 visualizes these simple effects in a convenient way by plotting the effect of each factor at the levels of the other factor. The top panel of the figure shows that among subjects who did not receive CBI, those on active naltrexone when compared to those on placebo naltrexone drank less on average, while the difference when CBI was given was slight and in the

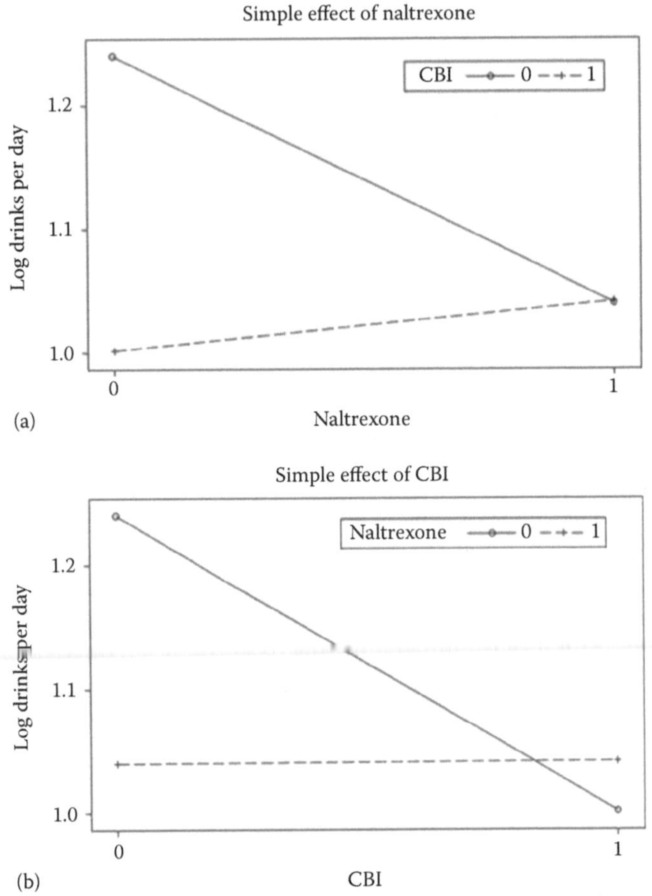

FIGURE 2.1
Least square means for the simple effect of naltrexone on average drinks per day at month 4 at each level of CBI (on the top) and for the simple effect of CBI at each level of naltrexone in the COMBINE study.

opposite direction. Table 2.4 shows the confidence intervals for these simple effects and since the intervals both overlap zero, the simple effects are not statistically significant at 0.05 level. Similarly, the bottom panel of Figure 2.1 shows that among subjects on placebo naltrexone, those on CBI compared to those not on CBI drank significantly less, while there was no difference between CBI and no CBI when naltrexone was given. The corresponding confidence

TABLE 2.4
Estimates and 95% Confidence Intervals for the Simple Effects Explaining the Significant Naltrexone by CBI Interaction on Number of Drinks per Day in the COMBINE Study

Simple Effect	At level	Least Square Mean Difference (95% CI)
naltrexone versus placebo	CBI	0.04 (−0.13, 0.20)
naltrexone versus placebo	no CBI	−0.19 (−0.35, −0.03)
CBI versus no CBI	naltrexone	0.00 (−0.16, 0.17)
CBI versus no CBI	placebo	−0.22 (−0.38, −0.07)

interval estimates of the simple effects of CBI in Table 2.4 indicate that CBI was effective in reducing drinking when placebo but not when naltrexone was given. Note that these estimates and associated 95% CI from Table 2.4 are a subset of all pairwise comparisons that are shown in the second-to-last column in Table 2.2. By focusing only on the simple effects, we reduce the need to correct for all possible comparisons although some correction may be necessary (see Chapter 6 for more discussion and guidance on multiple comparisons).

The interaction between naltrexone and CBI is an example of a *qualitative interaction*. That is, the effect of one factor is categorically different depending on the level of the other factor. In this case, CBI is effective if naltrexone is not given but not if naltrexone is given. When there are qualitative interactions, it is of limited use to interpret main effects. In contrast, when there are *quantitative interactions* (i.e., the effect of one factor is in the same direction at each level of the other factor but the magnitude is different), main effects should also be interpreted.

The general rule of interpreting interactions and main effects is to interpret the significant interaction of the highest order first by testing and/or estimating simple effects of each factor at the levels or combination of levels of the other factor(s). Depending on the nature of the interaction, lower order interactions and main effects could also be interpreted. In particular, if the higher order interactions are quantitative rather than qualitative, then testing lower order effects of this factor makes sense. However, one needs to be careful to use type III tests of effects for hypothesis tests and appropriate linear contrasts for estimation of effects that take into account all the interactions in the model, rather than parameter estimates taken directly from the output. Such estimates for lower order effects when there are higher order effects can be easily misinterpreted. More details about interpretation and testing of interactions in ANOVA models are available in Montgomery (2013). Further discussion is included in Chapter 6.

The assumptions underlying ANOVA analyses of change from baseline data are similar to the assumptions underlying two-sample t-test and confidence interval analyses:

- The data need to be quantitative with approximately normal distribution in small samples, possibly after a transformation. If the data are not normally distributed then non-parametric tests should be used. The Kruskal–Wallis test (Hollander and Wolfe, 1999) is the non-parametric equivalent of ANOVA analysis for quantitative data with non-normal distributions.
- Measurements on different subjects should be independent of one another.
- In ANOVA variances of observations in different groups are assumed to be the same. While ANOVA is fairly robust to deviations from the equal variance assumption, there are a number of options if variances are vastly different. Details can be found in Kutner et al. (2005).

Like the two-group comparisons, ANOVA on change-point values may be entirely adequate in simple situations with only pre- and post-measurements, no missing data, and comparable groups at baseline. Small imbalances on baseline covariates can be handled by analysis of covariance methods, as shown in the next section, and discussed in more detail in the context of mixed models for repeated measures data in Chapter 8.

2.1.4 Controlling for Baseline or Other Covariates

When there are potentially confounding variables at baseline that might affect the outcome, ANCOVA can be used to compare the final measures or the change from baseline to endpoint measures between groups. Traditional ANCOVA involves adding the baseline response measure or other covariate(s) to the ANOVA model as main effects. This approach can reduce variance in the analysis when there is imbalance on potentially confounding measures, due to chance. In such situations, ANCOVA may increase power to detect treatment differences without introducing bias. However, it is a common misconception that ANCOVA can be applied in any scenario to control for systematic differences between groups at baseline. When treatment or exposure is completely or substantially confounded with a predictor at baseline, ANCOVA can result in even more bias in analyses than ANOVA since variance due to treatment\exposure and variance due to the predictor are overlapping and can't be distinguished. Thus, it is very important at the design stage to consider potential confounders carefully and limit their effects, either by using randomization in experimental studies or matching in observational studies.

The same assumptions regarding the distribution of the response and the independence of the errors apply to ANCOVA as to ANOVA. Additionally, in traditional ANCOVA it is assumed that there are no interactions between the predictors of interest (treatment/exposure) and the baseline measures, and the model for the average is correctly specified (i.e., there are additive effects between treatment/exposure and the relationship between the covariate and the response variable is known and the same for each treatment). The covariates must not be affected by the treatments, which means that there is substantial overlap of the covariate distributions for the different treatment/exposure groups. If there is no overlap then treatment/exposure estimates from ANCOVA will be biased because of complete confounding. Also, if the distributions of the continuous covariates are skewed, extreme observations may have undue effect on the inferences, so transformations of the covariates prior to analysis may need to be performed. Finally, if the relationship of covariates and outcome varies by treatment\exposure, interactions between the covariate and treatment\exposure should be assessed, in addition to main effects. The covariates in ANCOVA should be pre-specified and not based on multiple assessments of baseline differences. Controlling for covariates is considered in more detail in Chapter 8 and design issues are considered in more detail in Chapter 11. Milliken and Johnson (1984) provide detailed information about covariate control.

We illustrate the traditional ANCOVA approach on the augmentation depression study and on the COMBINE data. Analysis of endpoint depression severity when controlling for baseline depression severity results in non-significant effect of treatment ($F(1,35)=1.56$, $p=0.22$) and the effect of baseline severity is also not statistically significant ($F(1,35)=0.03$, $p=0.87$). Thus, we conclude that there are no differences between the two treatment groups when controlling for baseline depression severity (i.e., when considering the outcome at the same level of baseline depression severity) and that endpoint depression scores are not significantly associated with depression severity at study entry.

In COMBINE, there is increased evidence for the interaction between naltrexone and CBI ($F(1,712)=4.83$, $p=0.03$) and for the main effect of CBI ($F(1,712)=6.70$, $p=0.01$) after controlling for baseline drinks per drinking day. Also, baseline drinks per day (log-transformed) is statistically significantly associated with the outcome during treatment ($F(1,712)=56.49$, $p<.0001$). Thus, in COMBINE there is a gain in power when controlling for baseline, which allows us to more confidently claim that there is an interaction between naltrexone and CBI. Also, we have evidence that individuals who drink more at baseline also drink more during treatment. The online materials show all results before and after controlling for the covariate. The increased power and precision of estimates of least square means is evident in this outcome. Note that in ANCOVA, if least square means are estimated and confidence intervals constructed, this needs to be done at a pre-specified value of the covariate. By default the mean covariate value is used.

2.1.5 Summary

In summary, all methods for endpoint or change-point analysis are simple and results are easy to interpret. However, all such methods are vulnerable to large effects from missing values or imputation. If subjects with missing data are dropped from analysis, bias may be introduced as the reduced sample may no longer be representative of the population of interest. If missing data are imputed, as is most commonly used with last observation carried forward, then bias is introduced because it is rarely the case that the last observation and the missing endpoint observation are the same. Regardless of whether there are missing data or not, efficiency and power are decreased in endpoint analysis because all intermediate data points are ignored. Finally, patterns of change over time can't be estimated with this simple form of analysis. Endpoint analysis is acceptable only in simple designs with baseline and endpoint observations when data are complete. Also, confidence intervals, rather than hypothesis tests, should be used to explain significant overall tests, since they provide estimates of the magnitudes of effects.

2.2 Analysis of Summary Measures

The most commonly used summary measure in data sets with repeated measures is the mean over all repeated observations. For example, in COMBINE one of the primary outcome measures was percent days abstinent, which is actually the mean of the binary measures of any drinking on each day over the entire study period. In imaging studies, often responses are averaged over regions of interest and the means in these regions are considered as the dependent measures in analyses.

In longitudinal data, summaries like the individual regression slopes over time can be directly analyzed with methods for independent data. For example, in the augmentation depression study individual slopes of change over time can be estimated and then compared between groups using t-test or ANOVA. This approach ignores the uncertainty in the estimation of slopes and may lead to incorrect conclusions.

In laboratory studies, summary measures, such as peak response or area under the curve, may be of interest in order to characterize maximum achieved response and combined intensity/duration of response. For example, in the study of menthol effects on nicotine reinforcement (Section 1.5.7) subjective effects can be characterized in terms of peak response or area under the curve during the infusion session. Depending on the goals of the study and the available data, univariate analyses of some of these summary measures may be appropriate.

2.2.1 Mean Response

One of the simplest summary measures for clustered or longitudinal data is the mean response over all repeated occasions. This is denoted as $\bar{Y}_i = (Y_{i1} + Y_{i2} + \ldots + Y_{im}) / m$ where m is the number of repeated occasions within the individual/cluster. Note that the summation is over the repeated observations of the same individual, not across individuals. Also, the number of observations for each individual/cluster need not be the same. If the response does not change in a systematic way from occasion to occasion, then the mean, compared to individual measures, has the advantage of having smaller variance. It can also be calculated even if there are some missing data on individuals as long as each individual has at least one recorded value. Once individual means are calculated, methods for independent data such as t-test, ANOVA, or ANCOVA can be used to analyze the means.

However, when the response changes systematically, which is the case in almost all longitudinal data sets, then the individual mean is not a useful measure. For example, in the augmentation study of depression, HDRS scores change significantly from baseline to endpoint. Taking their average does not provide information about change over time, which is of primary interest. Even in clustered data sets, taking the average over different occasions may not be very meaningful. For example, in the schizophrenia data set, we can calculate average percent signal change measures across several different regions, but each of these regions has its own mean and variance, and hence further averaging of the data across regions does not necessarily decrease variability of the data. Although specific region effects may not be of primary interest in the analysis, analyzing all repeated measures, rather than the mean, helps separate the different sources of variability and provides greater power to detect group differences. This is illustrated in subsequent chapters.

2.2.2 Slope over Time

One of the earliest approaches for analyzing change over time was estimating a slope for each individual and then using standard statistical techniques, such as t-tests or ANOVAs, to compare the slopes between groups. Slopes describe the constant rate of increase or decrease over time.

To illustrate, we consider the augmentation depression study. In the context of this study, each subject's slope is estimated by fitting a separate simple linear regression model with HDRS score as the dependent variable, and week as a continuous predictor. Each of the 50 individual models (one for each subject) has the following form:

$$Y_{ij} = \beta_{i0} + \beta_{i1}week_{ij} + \varepsilon_{ij} \quad (2.1)$$

with the usual assumptions about independence and identical normal distributions of the errors. Separate intercept (β_{i0}) and slope (β_{i1}) is estimated from each model. The averages of the slope estimates of β_{i1} in the two treatment groups are then compared using t-tests. Figure 2.2 presents box plots of the slopes in the augmentation and control groups. On average, the slope estimates in the augmentation group are more negative than in the control group, suggesting faster rate of improvement over time on the augmentation treatment. The difference is statistically significant as indicated by a two-sample t-test comparison ($t(48) = -2.20$, $p = 0.03$). However, four of the subjects have HDRS measured at only two time points and these values entirely determine the individual slopes for these subjects. In these four cases, estimates of the uncertainty of the slopes are missing and the slopes may provide very poor prediction of future observations.

Furthermore, the uncertainties of the slope estimates of the other subjects are not taken into account in the t-test and thus the variance used in the t-test is often underestimated, thus potentially leading to an increase in type I error rate. It is possible to put different weights on the slope estimates based on these uncertainties in order to correct the

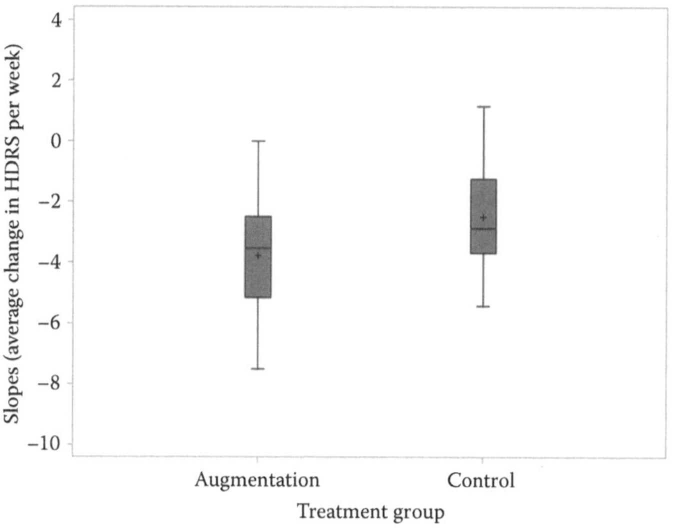

FIGURE 2.2
Box plots of individual slopes of change in HDRS scores over time in the augmentation depression study.

two-group comparison. However, this is rarely done. The most appropriate approach for comparison of slopes is to fit mixed-effects models to the data that seamlessly take into account the uncertainty of the slope estimates. Details of this approach follow in Chapter 3.

2.2.3 Peak Response and Area under the Curve

In some studies, the maximum achieved response or a combined measure of intensity and duration of response may be of particular interest. In such cases, the corresponding summary measure can be calculated for each individual and then statistical inference can be applied to this measure, as shown previously for mean and slope estimates. As an example, consider the human laboratory study presented in Section 1.5.7. In this study, nicotine is infused intravenously and a number of physiological and psychological measures are collected repeatedly over time on each participant. The *peak response* $\left(Y_i^p = \max(Y_{i1}, Y_{i2}, Y_{im}) - Y_0\right)$ and *the area under the curve* formed by connecting all repeated responses over the observation interval for an individual are two important summaries, which might be of primary interest for statistical analysis. If primary hypotheses are formulated for these measures, then performing univariate analysis on these measures may be appropriate.

For example, if one is interested in the maximum reduction in craving achieved after nicotine infusion in smokers, then peak change can be calculated and methods for uncorrelated data applied to make inferences. Or if one wants to estimate the overall effects of nicotine on drug liking measures, then the area under the curve can be calculated for each individual and confidence intervals or hypothesis tests for uncorrelated data can be performed.

However, peak response and AUC assess particular aspects of the response and do not provide information about other aspects (e.g., shape of response over time). They are also easily affected by missing data. Thus, if the goals of the study are broader and missing data are a concern, a more complete analysis of all repeated measures is preferred.

2.2.4 Summary

Similar to endpoint analysis, all methods for analysis of summary measures are simple, results are easy to interpret, but the methods may be vulnerable to large effects from missing values or imputation. Patterns of change also can't be estimated with this simple form of analysis. Analyses of summary measures are appropriate only when a particular aspect of the data is of primary interest and when the uncertainty in the calculation of the measures is properly accounted for.

2.3 Univariate rANOVA Models

The simplest approach to analyzing all repeated measures on an individual, or within a cluster, is the univariate rANOVA model. This approach provides more complete description of the average pattern of change over time or within cluster than endpoint analysis and analysis of summary measures. In longitudinal data, the response over time may take a variety of shapes: for example, little or no improvement, steady improvement, larger improvement in the beginning followed by leveling off of the response, or a U-shaped curve. There may be the same total improvement between baseline and endpoint in different treatment groups but faster response in one of the groups. In the latter case, endpoint analysis, even with complete data, will not find a difference while rANOVA may detect a statistically significant time by treatment effect.

However, rANOVA requires that correlations among measurements on the same individual on any two occasions or correlations among measurements on different units within a cluster satisfy a restrictive condition called *sphericity* or *circularity*. Usually (but not always), this amounts to having equal variability of the measurements and equal correlations between every two measurements within the same individual or cluster. While this assumption may be reasonable for clustered data, where units within a cluster may be considered interchangeable, it is rarely satisfied for longitudinal data where observations on the same individual that are closer in time are expected to be more highly correlated than observations that are further apart. Other assumptions of this approach are that all repeated measures are approximately normally (bell-shaped) distributed, observations on different individuals/clusters are independent of one another, and that individuals/clusters are randomly sampled from the population. To apply rANOVA to a data set, we also need to have data on the same occasions for all individuals in the sample (i.e., balanced design). When there are missing data on an individual, usually all the data on this individual are dropped from the analysis.

We focus on the rANOVA approach with one between-subject factor (referred to as group) and one within-subject factor (referred to as time). We also use the augmentation depression study as a simple example with longitudinal data. In this study, group is a between-subject factor because its levels vary between subjects. That is, each subject is assigned to a particular group and stays in that group for the purposes of analysis throughout the study. Time, on the other hand is a within-subject factor, which means that its levels vary within individual. That is, repeated observations on an individual are taken at multiple time points. This distinction is important because in rANOVA models different error terms are used to test hypotheses relating to between-subject factors and within-subject factors. This distinction carries into all further methods for repeated measures that are considered (rMANOVA, mixed models, and non-parametric methods).

In this situation with one between-subject and one within-subject factor, the rANOVA model can be formulated as shown below for observation *j* on subject *i* in group *t*:

$$Y_{ij} = \mu + \alpha_t + \beta_j + (\alpha\beta)_{tj} + b_i + \varepsilon_{ij},$$

where μ is the overall mean, α_t is the effect of group *t*, β_j is the effect of time *j* and $(\alpha\beta)_{tj}$ is the interaction between group *t* and time *j*. The random subject effect $b_i \sim i.i.d.N(0,\sigma_b^2)$ introduces correlations between the repeated observations on the same individual and is independent of the errors $\varepsilon_{ij} \sim i.i.d.N(0,\sigma^2)$. The variance σ_b^2 captures the variability in responses between subjects while the variance σ^2 corresponds to the variability unaccounted for by differences between subjects. Here *i.i.d.* is an abbreviation for independent and identically distributed and it means that the random effects for different subjects are independent of one another and have the same statistical distribution, and that the errors of all observations that capture residual variability are independent and have the same statistical distribution. The means of both normal distributions are zero and each has a distinct variance to be estimated from the data.

With one between-subject factor and one within-subject factor, there are three hypotheses of primary interest: testing the interaction between the two factors (i.e., whether all $(\alpha\beta)_{tj}$ are zero) and testing the main effect of each factor (group and time). In the context of the depression study, the test of the interaction between group and time shows whether the patterns of average response over time in the two groups are significantly different. The test of the main effect of time shows whether there is significant change over time when observations at each time point are averaged across groups, and the test of the main effect of group shows whether there are significant differences between groups when all repeated observations over time are averaged within group. If there are additional between-subject or within-subject factors, all additional main effects and all possible interactions among factors are tested too.

Unlike the usual ANOVA model, where all observations are assumed to be independent of one another, the rANOVA model usually assumes that the variances on all occasions are the same $\left(Var\left(Y_{ij}\right) = \sigma_b^2 + \sigma^2\right)$ and that the correlations between all repeated observations within individual are the same $\left(Corr\left(Y_{ij}, Y_{ik}\right) = \sigma_b^2 / \left(\sigma_b^2 + \sigma^2\right)\right)$. Note that the correlation between repeated observations on the same individual is due to the shared random effect for subject. This is the *compound symmetry assumption* and it follows from the model definition above. This compound symmetry assumption is a special case of the sphericity/circularity assumption, which states more generally that the variances of the differences between any two observations within individual are the same. The sphericity assumption is tested by Mauchly's test, but the test is not considered very useful since in small samples it tends to miss sphericity violations while in large samples it is often significant even for trivial violations of sphericity. Thus, a more practical approach to dealing with deviations from sphericity is to apply one of the two widely available corrections to the degrees of freedom of the tests of the within-subject factors in rANOVA: the corrections of Greenhouse and Geisser (1959) or Huynh and Feldt (1976). They adjust the tests by reducing the numerator degrees of freedom so that the p-values are usually adjusted upward and type I error is closer to the target level when sphericity is violated. Both tests correct the type I error rate when there is serial correlation in the data (observations closer in time are more highly correlated than observations further apart) but the Greenhouse-Geisser

TABLE 2.5

Univariate Structure of a Repeated Measures Data Set

Subject id	Occasion	Group (or other between-subject predictor)	Response
S001	1	1	Y_{11}
S001	2	1	Y_{12}
S001	3	1	Y_{13}
.....	....	....	....
S002	1	2	Y_{21}
S002	2	2	Y_{22}
.....	....	.....	.....
S003	1	1	Y_{31}
.....	....	.....	....

also corrects when the variability of the measurements increases over time but the correction tends to be very conservative.

The data structure in rANOVA can be in the *long format* or in the *wide format*, depending on which statistical program and module is used for data analysis. The *long format* means that each repeated observation is in a separate row of the data set and implies that there are as many rows per individual as there are repeated occasions. Table 2.5 represents this structure. In the augmentation depression example, the last column contains the corresponding HDRS measures for each subject and occasion. This representation is also known as the *univariate repeated measures structure.*

The *wide format,* where all repeated observations on an individual are included in the same row but in different columns, also known as *the multivariate repeated measures structure,* is presented in the next subsection as it is a requirement for the use of the repeated measures MANOVA considered therein. More details on data format for rANOVA (and also for rMANOVA considered in the next subsection) can be found in Hedeker and Gibbons (2006). In the online materials we illustrate how data sets can be restructured from the long to the wide format and vice versa and how either format can be used for rANOVA analysis in SAS.

We fit the rANOVA model to the depression severity ratings in the augmentation study in depression data and obtain the results shown in Table 2.6. The results show that the interaction between group and time is not statistically significant according to the F-test for this effect ($F(6,198)=0.37$, $p=0.90$, G-G adjusted p-value = 0.78, H-F adjusted p-value = 0.80). Thus there are no significant differences in the patterns of mean change over time in the two groups. The main effect of group is also not statistically significant ($F(1,33)=1.45$, $p=0.24$). However, there is a statistically significant effect of time ($F(6,198)=75.49$, $p<.0001$, G-G adjusted p-value < .0001, H-F adjusted p-value < .0001). We already know that HDRS scores in both groups decrease significantly over time from the graphical representation of the data in Chapter 1. Figure 1.5 shows raw means and standard errors but a similar plot of least square means (the estimated means on each occasion for each group, which may differ from the raw means because of missing values) and their standard errors shows the same trend. Since the interaction between group and time is not significant, post hoc comparisons by time point are not performed. If the interaction was significant, separate comparisons between the groups at each time point would have allowed us to identify

TABLE 2.6

Repeated Measures ANOVA Analysis of Augmentation Depression Study

	Test Statistic	p-Value	Greenhouse-Geisser Adjusted p-Value	Huynh-Feldt Adjusted p-Value
Group	F(1,33) = 1.45	0.24	—	—
Time	F(6,198) = 75.49	<.0001	<.0001	<.0001
Group by time	F(6,198) = 0.37	0.90	0.78	0.80

when the two groups had significantly different response. The significant main effect of time could be further investigated by testing hypotheses of linear and quadratic trend over time, or comparing each subsequent time point to baseline. We discuss such post hoc tests in more detail in the following chapters of the book, in the context of the more general mixed models.

Note that only 35 of the 50 subjects are used in the rANOVA analysis of the depression example. This is because the remaining 15 subjects have at least one missing value over time. This leads to a decrease in power and potential bias in the analysis. While it is possible to perform data imputation and then fit rANOVA models on the imputed data set, a more straightforward and fully efficient approach is to use mixed models, which use all available data on an individual.

This illustrates that similar to endpoint analysis, rANOVA may be severely affected by missing values or imputation. Most statistical packages automatically drop subjects with even one missing observation from the analysis and researchers may use imputation of missing data without acknowledging it. As explained previously, omission of subjects can introduce sample bias, as the group of people with complete data may not be representative of the entire population. Imputation by using the last available observation on each subject in place of all subsequent missing observations leads to biased treatment estimates usually (but not always) in the direction of making them more conservative. Another disadvantage of rANOVA is that repeated observations need to be made on the same occasions. For example, individuals need to be assessed at the same points in time.

However, rANOVA may be entirely appropriate for clustered data where the sphericity assumption is approximately satisfied and there is no missing data.

2.4 Multivariate rMANOVA Models

Unlike rANOVA, the multivariate approach to repeated measures (rMANOVA) does not impose any restrictions on the patterns of means, variances, and covariances of the repeated observations within individual or cluster. This approach is also known as *multivariate growth curve analysis*. Like rANOVA, it assumes that all repeated measures are approximately normally (bell-shaped) distributed, observations on different individuals/clusters are independent of one another, individuals/clusters are randomly sampled from the population, and the repeated observations are taken on the same occasions for all individuals. When there are missing data on an individual, this individual is dropped from the analysis.

In the rMANOVA approach, the entire set of repeated observations on the same individual is considered as a multivariate response. The mean values of this response can be expressed in the same way as in rANOVA (as effects of group, time, group by time in the case of one between and one within-subject factor). However the errors within individual (and hence the repeated observations for an individual) have multivariate normal distribution. This is denoted as $(\varepsilon_{i1},\varepsilon_{i2,...}\varepsilon_{iJ}) \sim i.i.d.MVN(0,\Sigma)$, where the errors are randomly distributed around 0 on each occasion and the variance–covariance matrix Σ is expressed as

$$\Sigma = \begin{pmatrix} \sigma_{11} & \cdots & \sigma_{1J} \\ \vdots & \ddots & \vdots \\ \sigma_{J1} & \cdots & \sigma_{JJ} \end{pmatrix}.$$

The variances of the response on the different occasions are on the main diagonal of this matrix $(\sigma_{11,}\sigma_{22,...,}\sigma_{jj})$ and the covariances σ_{kl} between any two repeated observations are in the off-diagonal elements. The element in row k and column l of Σ is the covariance between the observations on occasions k and l within the individual/cluster: $\sigma_{kl}=Cov(\varepsilon_{ik,}\varepsilon_{il})$. Note that $cov(\varepsilon_{ik},\varepsilon_{il}) = corr(\varepsilon_{ik},\varepsilon_{il})\sqrt{\sigma_{kk}\sigma_{ll}}$ so there is direct correspondence between the covariance between two observations and the correlation. Correlations are bounded by 1 and −1, while the magnitudes of the covariances depend on the magnitudes of the variances. The variance–covariance matric is symmetrical so the elements in the lower left of the matrix are mirror images of the elements in the upper right with the diagonal from upper left to lower right as the "mirror" (that is $\sigma_{kl}=\sigma_{lk}$).

The rMANOVA approach requires that the data are structured in the *wide format* rather than the long format. This is the *multivariate representation of repeated measures data* and it requires that all data on an individual are in the same row of the data set. Table 2.7 shows how this is done. SAS code to transfer from one format to another is included in the online materials and more details can be found in Hedeker and Gibbons (2006). In the multivariate format the response on each occasion is coded in a different variable and is in a different column of the data set. In the context of the augmentation depression study this means that there are seven different columns with HDRS scores of the subjects at baseline and the six post-baseline assessment points.

The rMANOVA model is actually equivalent to the most general mixed-effects model for complete data (to be introduced in Chapter 3), since no restrictions are imposed on the variances and correlations of the repeated observations. This approach is often preferable to the rANOVA approach because of the lack of restrictions. However, it requires complete data on all subjects and, like rANOVA, can show significant loss of power and sample bias if individuals with missing data are dropped from the analysis. Imputation of missing observations also usually leads to conservative estimates and rMANOVA is less powerful

TABLE 2.7

Multivariate Structure of a Repeated Measures Data Set

Subject id	Group (or other between-subject predictor)	Response_1	Response_2	....	Response_m
S001	1	Y_{11}	Y_{12}	....	Y_{1m}
S002	2	Y_{21}	Y_{22}	....	Y_{2m}
S003	1	Y_{31}	Y_{32}	....	Y_{3m}
.....	....	....			

than rANOVA when the sphericity assumption is approximately satisfied. rMANOVA may not work in small samples when the number of repeated observations is large as there are too many parameters to be estimated (all parameters describing the means, and also all variances and correlations).

In rMANOVA, the same set of hypotheses can be tested as in rANOVA. In the context of the augmentation study in depression, these are the interaction between group and time, and the main effects of group and time. There are several different multivariate test statistics for testing the effects of the within-subject factors and the interactions of between-subject and within-subject factors (Wilks' Lambda, Pillai's Trace, Hotelling-Lawley Trace, Roy's Greatest Root) but they all are converted to an F-statistic. In simple designs they all lead to the same F-value and p-value.

In the augmentation depression study, all four tests of the interaction between treatment group and time result in a non-significant p-value ($F(6,28)=0.51$, $p=0.79$). All four tests of the main effect of time show a significant effect of time ($F(6,28)=26.99$, $p<.0001$). There is also no significant effect of group ($F(1,33)=1.45$, $p=0.24$). Note that the test of the group effect in rMANOVA is exactly the same as the test of the group effect in rANOVA. That is, the procedure for testing the effects of between-subject factors does not vary whether the univariate or the multivariate approach to repeated measures analysis is taken.

In general, the rMANOVA approach is preferable to the rANOVA approach when there are sizeable differences in the variances and correlations between repeated observations and when the number of observations within the individual/cluster is relatively small compared to the number of individuals in the sample.

2.5 Summary

Traditional methods for analysis of longitudinal and clustered data include analysis of summary measures, endpoint and change-point analysis, rANOVA, and rMANOVA models. Summary measures, such as means, AUCs, peak change, or slope, may be appropriate if one is interested only in the particular aspect of data. However, missing data may introduce sample bias if subjects with missing data on key occasions are dropped from analysis and may lead to loss of efficiency in statistical estimation and inference.

Endpoint analysis for longitudinal data has been traditionally used because of its ease of interpretation and implementation. However, it ignores all intermediate data and hence can't be used to estimate trends over time. Furthermore, it suffers even more from the effects of missing data than analyses of summary measures and is not as efficient. If analysis is done only on these subjects who have been measured at the last time point, then the sample may not be representative of the population and serious sample bias may occur. If the analysis is performed with some simple imputation method, such as last observation carried forward, there is a serious risk of estimation bias. Thus, endpoint analysis can yield misleading results, especially regarding comparisons between treatment groups, when dropout rates differ between the groups. Univariate and multivariate methods for repeated measures analyses based on rANOVA and rMANOVA, respectively, use information from all occasions and allow testing of hypotheses regarding change over time or pattern of responses within the cluster or individual. With complete data and balanced designs, these methods provide valid tests of main effects and interactions. However, these methods are not appropriate when assessment occasions are different for different individuals, lose power, and may produce biased results in the presence of missing data. rMANOVA also can't be used when there are too many repeated occasions. In general, rANOVA is preferable to rMANOVA when the sphericity/circularity assumption is approximately satisfied. However, both methods are focused on hypothesis testing of group effects. Both rANOVA and rMANOVA are special cases of mixed-effects models, which provide much greater flexibility in modeling longitudinal and clustered data.

3

Linear Mixed Models for Longitudinal and Clustered Data

The ANOVA-based approaches for analysis of data from Chapter 2, focus on average response, require balanced designs and complete data, and either make an overly simplifying assumption about the correlations between repeated measurements or estimate a full set of variances and covariances. These features severely limit the situations when traditional ANOVA-based approaches provide valid results. In this chapter, we explain how linear mixed models overcome these limitations and provide a very flexible framework for the analysis of longitudinal and clustered data.

The assumption that all individuals follow the same average response is overly stringent, especially in the context of longitudinal data where individual responses may be higher or lower than the average response at baseline and the individual rates of change over time may also be higher or lower than the average rate of change. When the response over time can be approximated by a straight line, this situation can be described by one of the simplest *random effects models*: a model with a random intercept (response at baseline) and a random slope (rate of change over time). Figure 3.1 shows hypothetical data on five individuals generated from a *random intercept and random slope model*. Dashed lines denote individual responses over time while the solid line denotes the average response over time. Three of the individuals start higher than the average response, and all but one of the individuals shows decrease over time. The rates of change vary considerably around the mean rate of change.

The random intercept and slope model is a fairly simple model, but based on the same principle, one can describe more complicated patterns of change over time. For example, adding a quadratic random effect allows to model J- or U-shaped change over time. Note that, unlike the ANOVA approaches we considered in the previous chapter, random effects models do not require repeated observations to be made at the same time points for all individuals. With random effects it is possible to model individual response data measured at unique or partially overlapping sets of time points.

In the random effects approach, the individual random effects imply a certain correlation pattern between repeated observations within subject. However, it is also possible to model different variance–covariance structures of the repeated observations within individuals directly and to use the data to estimate the parameters describing the variances and covariances. Such models are known as *covariance-pattern models*. The rANOVA model is the simplest covariance-pattern model with equal variances across time points and equal correlations between repeated observations on the same individual at any two time points. The rMANOVA model is the most unrestricted covariance-pattern model as it assumes different response variance at each observation occasion and different covariances between responses at any two occasions. Other structures are possible, for example, decreasing correlations with increasing time lag.

While the name "mixed effects" comes from the combination of random and fixed effects in the model specification, for normally distributed data covariance-pattern models are

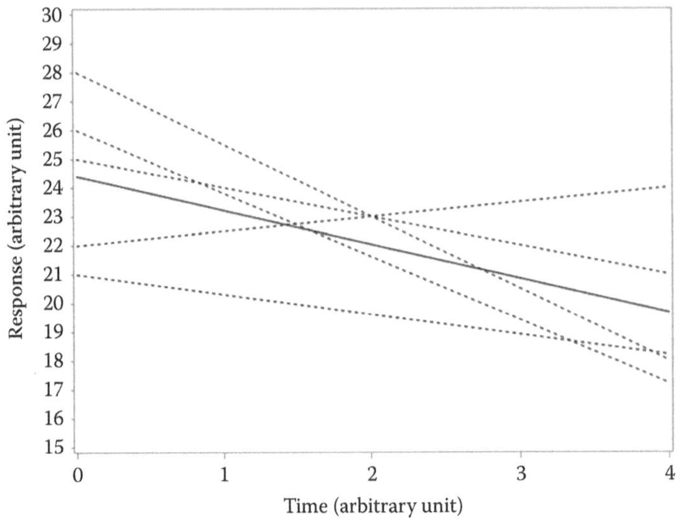

FIGURE 3.1
Profile plot of hypothetical data generated according to a random intercept and random slope model. The five dashed lines correspond to responses over time of five hypothetical subjects. The solid lone shows the average response over time

usually fit using the same software as random effects models, even if random effects are not specified. In this chapter, we consider random effects, covariance-pattern models and combinations thereof as different subclasses of mixed-effects models. Combining random effects and different covariance patterns leads to an incredible variety of mixed models that can describe a wide range of scenarios. This flexibility of modeling the correlation structure of the data is one of the main advantages of mixed models.

All models considered in this chapter are linear mixed models (LMM) (Harville, 1977; Laird and Ware, 1982) because the expression that describes the response is a linear function of the regression coefficients (whether fixed and/or random). In these models, the response is assumed to be normally distributed. Extensions of this approach to binary data, count data, and other outcomes in the exponential family (McCullagh and Nelder, 1989; Agresti, 2015). are considered in Chapter 4. Non-linear mixed- effects models are not considered in this book and interested readers are referred to Davidian and Giltinan (1995) and Vonesh and Chinchilli (1997).

In addition to flexibility in modeling the correlation structure of the data and ability to account for both balanced (i.e., with the same set of observations points for each individual) and unbalanced (i.e., with different observations points for different individuals) designs, another major advantage of LMM is how they handle missing data. Specifically, the mixed-effects approach does not require a complete set of observations on each individual, rather, it uses all available data on each individual. If a participant drops out of the study, all the data collected up to the time of dropout are used in the model fitting. If a subject has intermittent missing data, or subjects/clusters have different numbers of repeated observations, again all available data are used. Furthermore, in scenarios with missing data when the model is approximately correctly specified and missingness is random (i.e., whether an observation is missing depends only on the observed data and not on the actual unobserved values, to be discussed in more detail in Chapter 7), the obtained parameter estimates and the corresponding statistical inferences are unbiased and maximally efficient. These properties, together with the flexibility of modeling the correlation structure and the wide availability of software for fitting LMM, is the basis of the current popularity of mixed-effects models as the preferred approach for the analysis of longitudinal and clustered data.

In this chapter, we explain how to specify the different aspects of LMM. First, we focus on describing the average response with emphasis on modeling of the time trend in longitudinal studies. Situations when time is treated as a categorical and as a continuous predictor are considered. Second, we introduce random effects as a way of accommodating individual variations around the average trend and describe the implied correlations between repeated measures on the same individual due to the random effects. Third, we show how the variance–covariance structure of repeated observations can be specified directly by assuming different patterns and estimating the parameters of these patterns, based on the data. Several data examples are considered with focus on interpretation of results. We also briefly consider estimation, assessment of model fit, and selection of the best-fitting model. Throughout this chapter, we focus on quantitative response that is either approximately normally distributed or can be transformed to normality. Data sets, SAS code, and output for the considered data examples are available online. We keep the exposition at a non-technical level. Other non-technical descriptions with focus on psychiatry and mental health applications can be found in Gibbons et al. (1993) and Gueorguieva and Krystal (2004). Technical details can be found in Laird and Ware (1982), Ware (1985), Longford (1993), Lindsey (1999), Diggle et al. (2002), and Fitzmaurice et al. (2009), among others.

3.1 Modeling the Time Trend in Longitudinal Studies

This section shows different ways to model the average pattern of change over time. The primary focus is on situations with planned data collection at particular time points for all individuals, since in such balanced designs time can be treated either as a categorical or a continuous predictor. When individuals are observed at unique time points, time needs to be treated as a continuous predictor in order to be able to describe change over time. Such situations are considered in more detail in other books (Hedeker and Gibbons, 2006; Weiss, 2005). Note that when the design is unbalanced, the time points at which individuals are observed are assumed to be independent of the responses and random effects. If, on the other hand, observations are taken "as needed," i.e., driven by previous observations, bias can occur if the data are analyzed as is.

For simplicity of presentation, we again consider a simple situation with one between-subject factor (treatment group) and one within-subject factor (time) and use the *augmentation depression study* from Chapter 1 for illustration on modeling of time trends. As a reminder, in this study two groups of patients were randomized either to a standard or to an augmentation treatment and depression severity was assessed once per week for six weeks after baseline. In the previous two chapters, we already presented two specifications of the average response for this example. In Section 1.7, we specified that the average response over time depended on the main effects of group, time, and the interaction between group and time where time was treated as a continuous predictor. The expression for the average Hamilton Depression Rating Scale (HDRS) response (denoted as Y in order to show how the model generalizes to other data sets, averaged over individuals in the same group) is as follows:

$$E\{Y_{ij}\} = \beta_0 + \beta_1 Group_i + \beta_2 Time_j + \beta_3 Group_i \times Time_j \tag{3.1}$$

Here, all predictors are fixed and the beta coefficients are fixed (unknown) parameters that describe the effect of group and time on average response. Interpretation of these coefficients was considered in more detail in Section 1.7. Implicit in this specification is that the average response changes linearly over time (i.e., the rate of change from week to week is the same). However, closer examination of Figure 1.5 shows some curvature of change in HDRS scores over time with greater initial improvement followed by decreased rate of change. Thus, it is possible that an addition of a quadratic term may more closely approximate the average response over time. This would lead to the following expression for the average trend where the group is coded as 1 for the active group and 0 for the control group and time takes values of 0 through 6, corresponding to baseline and post-randomization week, respectively:

$$E\{Y_{ij}\} = \beta_0 + \beta_1 Group_i + \beta_2 Time_j + \beta_3 Group_i \times Time_j + \beta_4 Time_j^2 + \beta_5 Group_i \times Time_j^2 \tag{3.2}$$

Two terms are added to the model: a quadratic effect of time and an interaction between group and the quadratic effect of time. As a result, two additional parameters need to be estimated, compared to the linear model (β_4 and β_5), that allow for different amounts of curvature in the two treatment groups. The expression for the quadratic model implies that the average HDRS score over time in each group can be described as part of a parabola. Figure 3.2 shows the resulting curves from the linear model and the quadratic model fit to the data, and their correspondence to the raw means by time point in the augmentation depression data set. From the top panel of Figure 3.2, we see that the linear model overestimates the average HDRS score in both groups during weeks two and three and slightly underestimates the average HDRS score in the augmentation group at week six. The quadratic model from the bottom panel of Figure 3.2 shows a very good fit to the raw means in the augmentation group but somewhat overestimates the average HDRS score in the control group at the end of the study. Since some patients in the study possibly drop out because of lack of efficacy, especially in the control group, it is feasible that the true underlying response at the end of treatment is more in line with the quadratic model than with the linear trend or even the raw mean trend. The raw means are calculated only based on the available measurements of subjects who have data at each particular time point and thus may be biased toward better response if subjects with worse outcome selectively drop out. However, the prediction of the quadratic model at endpoint is the least precise and it is quite possible that the parabola is forced to curve in a certain way by a model that may not fit very well. We delay discussion of model fit and assessment of goodness of fit until subsequent sections. For now, we just illustrate the complexity of interpretation of time effects even in relatively simple models. The quadratic model appears to fit the average trend over time in HDRS scores a little bit better than the linear model, since there is an initial sizeable response and then gradual slowing down of improvement.

While in the linear model the beta coefficients β_2 and β_3 are interpreted as the average rate of change in HDRS scores in the control group per week, and the difference in the average rate of change per week in the active group, compared to the control group, respectively, in the quadratic model the same coefficients no longer have the same meaning since the rate of change is not constant. Rather, the three coefficients (intercept β_0, linear β_2 and quadratic β_4) describe the parabola over time for the control group (because Group = 0 for subjects in the control group). The linear β_2 and quadratic β_4 determine where the parabola

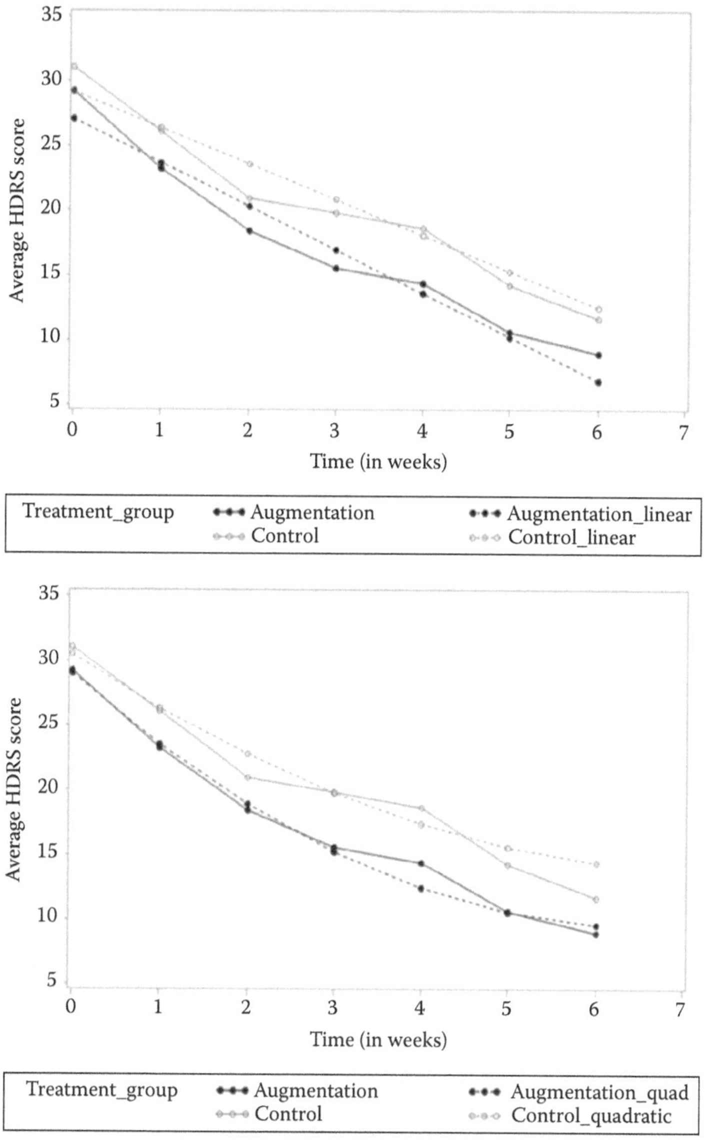

FIGURE 3.2
Raw (solid line) and estimated (dashed lines) mean HDRS scores over time based on liner (on the left) and quadratic (on the right) model in the augmentation depression study.

for the control group achieves its minimum or maximum and the intercept β_0 shows the average HDRS score at week 0 for the control group. To get the corresponding numbers for the active group (coded as Group = 1), one needs to add the regression coefficients in front of the corresponding terms involving the group factor. Thus, $\beta_0+\beta_1$ is the intercept, $\beta_2+\beta_3$ is the slope, and $\beta_4+\beta_5$ is the quadratic term for the active group. Note that in this particular example, the intercepts for each group can be interpreted since they correspond to the average HDRS score at baseline. But depending on how time is coded (e.g., the first time point may be time 1), the intercept may not be interpretable since it is outside of the range of the data. Sometimes, the time variable is centered by subtracting the average time point (week three, in this particular example) and then the intercept is interpreted as the average response at this mid time point. More information on the benefits of centering with examples can be found in Hedeker and Gibbons (2006).

Both the linear and the quadratic models are special cases of *polynomial models*. The linear model is a polynomial model of the first degree and the quadratic model is a polynomial model of the second degree. The degree refers to the highest power of time in the expression for the average response (first degree in the linear, and second degree in the quadratic model). If we add terms with higher powers of time to the models above (time cubed, time to the fourth power, and so on), we allow the trend over time to go up and down and to have inflection points. Note that in order for the model to be well-defined, we must include all sequential degrees in the model. For example, if the highest degree in the model is third then we should have terms of second and first degree and an intercept in the model.

It is a well-known mathematical fact that a polynomial of nth degree can go through $(n+1)$ pre-specified points and thus we can perfectly describe the means over time in any situation with a fixed set of observation times with a polynomial of a sufficiently high degree. However, the predictions of the average response, with such a high degree polynomial in between points, are highly inaccurate as the polynomial is forced to wiggle extensively in order to perfectly match the means at the pre-specified time points. In practice, usually the highest degree that is considered is quadratic, although a polynomial of third degree can occasionally be encountered. Information about polynomial models and the use of orthogonal polynomials (centered and rescaled polynomials) can be found in Hedeker and Gibbons (2006). More sophisticated models for describing change over time are based on piecewise approximations to different time windows called splines. Consult Weiss (2005) for a fairly non-technical description and Fitzmaurice et al. (2009) for more technical details.

Curvilinear trends over time can also be accommodated by transforming the time variable and then fitting a straight line model. For example, one can take natural log of time and fit a linear model with log-transformed time, rather than time as a predictor. Note that logarithmic transformation can be applied only to positive values. Thus, if zeros are used to code time on some occasions (which is usually the case when baseline is included), a small constant may need to be added to all the time points before applying a logarithmic transformation. In the augmentation depression study, the linear predictor with time transformed using natural log is as follows:

$$E\{Y_{ij}\} = \beta_0 + \beta_1 Group_i + \beta_2 \log(Time_j) + \beta_3 Group_i \times \log(Time_j) \tag{3.3}$$

Since baseline is coded as time 0, we add 1 to all time points before taking natural log. We choose 1 because this constant keeps baseline coded as 0. The rest of the time points are small positive numbers. Log-transforming time and then fitting a linear model may appear unnatural but it does in fact describe reality reasonably well in many longitudinal studies (especially clinical trials) where there might be an initial fast change in outcome and then slowing down as response/remission status is reached or further improvement is not likely/possible.

Figure 3.3 shows the estimated average response from Equation 3.3 applied to the augmentation depression study. The top panel of the figure has log-transformed time on the horizontal axis and on this time scale the average response in both groups appears as a straight line. However, the lags between successive time points vary so that later time points appear to be closer together. This panel represents exactly how the average response

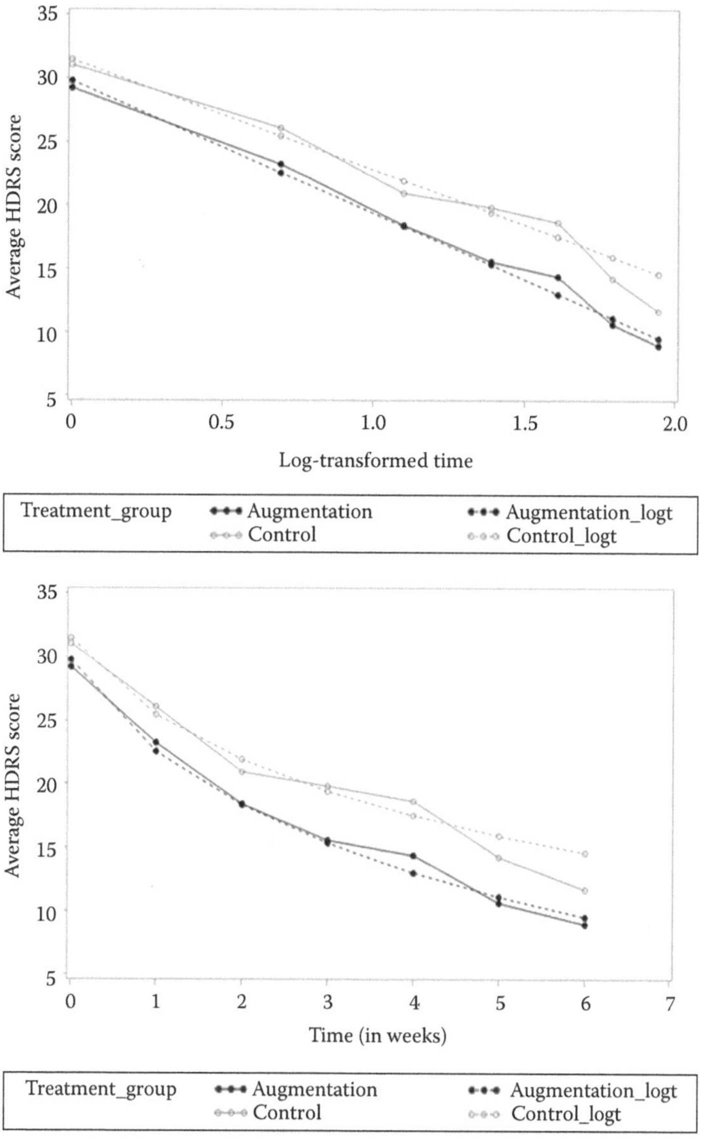

FIGURE 3.3
Raw (solid line) and estimated (dashed lines) mean HDRS scores over time based on liner model with long-transformed time in the augmentation depression study. On the top the horizontal axis in nature log transformed time, on the bottom the horizontal axis is time (in week).

was modeled. However, it is not as easily interpretable as the panel on the bottom, which shows the exact same fit but has the original time scale on the horizontal axis. Although only an intercept and a slope are included in the expression for the mean, the graph shows curvature on the original scale, which is due to the transformation of time prior to entering it in the model. At least, by visual inspection the model with log-transformed time provides a very similar fit to the data as the quadratic model considered previously. This illustrates how different models can provide almost the same fit to the raw data. Selection of the best model is usually based not only on statistical considerations but on practical considerations related to interpretability.

We now turn our attention to incorporating individual variability around the time trend in the models.

3.2 Random Effects for Individual Variability in Response

The primary focus in many longitudinal studies is estimating the average trend and testing the effects of predictors on this trend. However, it is also important to properly account for individual variation in participant response and sometimes estimation and prediction of individual response is of interest in itself. An intuitively appealing approach to dealing with this issue, is to introduce random effects in the model formulation that describe the inter-individual variability. To illustrate the concept, we continue working with the augmentation depression study as a simple example and initially assume a linear trend over time. That is, we consider Equation 3.1 for the average trend.

3.2.1 Random Intercept Model

The simplest random effects model is the random intercept model. It is specified as follows:

$$Y_{ij} = \beta_0 + \beta_1 Group_i + \beta_2 Time_j + \beta_3 Group_i \times Time_j + b_i + \varepsilon_{ij}, \qquad (3.4)$$

where b_i denotes the random intercept for subject i and is assumed to be normally distributed with mean 0 and unknown variance σ_b^2 (i.e., $b_i \sim i.i.d.N(0, \sigma_b^2)$) to be estimated from the data. The parameter σ_b^2 describes the between-subject variability in the data. The random effects b_i are assumed to be independent of the random errors ε_{ij}, which describe the residual variability in the responses at the jth occasion for the ith subject (in addition to what is accounted for by the average trend and the systematic individual deviation from the average trend represented by the random intercept). In the simplest case, the errors are also assumed to be independent and normally distributed with equal variance (i.e., $\varepsilon_{ij} \sim i.i.d.N(0,\sigma^2)$). We consider different structures of the errors in the next subsection of this chapter.

The random intercept model has an intuitive interpretation. It assumes that individuals vary around the average trend in a systematic way. If b_i is positive, then the responses of the ith individual are likely to be above the average for the group to which the subject belongs. If b_i is negative, then the responses of the ith individual are likely to be below the average of the group. The larger b_i is, the further above the average the observations for this subject are. Since there are also random errors, the individual responses over time do not all fall on parallel lines to the average trend, but fluctuate up and down around subject-specific parallel lines away from the average. When the errors are independent of one another, the deviations from the straight subject-specific line are random and do not depend on one another. Figure 3.4 shows a schematic with hypothetical data for two individuals (one with a positive random intercept and one with a negative random intercept). The circles represent the observed response values at each of four time points. The dashed lines correspond to the individual trends for each of the two subjects. The trends

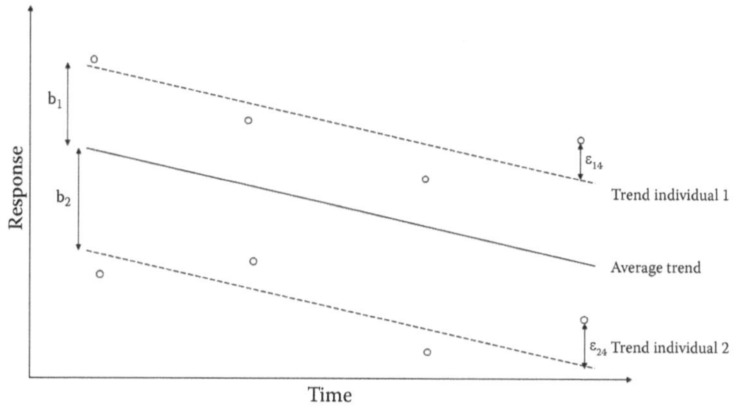

FIGURE 3.4
Hypothetical trends and observations of two individuals with response changing according to a random intercept model.

are parallel to the average trend but the trend for the first individual (with a positive random intercept) is above the average trend, while the trend for the second individual (with a negative random intercept) is below the average trend.

The normal distribution assumption of the random intercepts, with zero mean and constant variance, implies that the individual intercepts are equally spread and centered around 0, forming a bell-shaped distribution when plotted with a histogram. Note that since the random intercept is an additional random variable that is added to the model and it is assumed uncorrelated with the errors, the variance of an individual response is the sum of the variance of the random intercept and the variance of the random errors: $Var\left(Y_{ij}\right) = \sigma_b^2 + \sigma^2$. The random intercept model with *i.i.d.* errors also implies that the correlation (and the covariance) between any two observations Y_{ij} and Y_{ik} on the same individual is the same. In fact,

$$Cov\left(Y_{ij}, Y_{ik}\right) = \sigma_b^2,$$

$$Corr\left(Y_{ij}, Y_{ik}\right) = \frac{\sigma_b^2}{\sigma_b^2 + \sigma^2}.$$

This is the compound symmetry assumption that we discussed in Chapter 2, in the context of rANOVA, with the added restriction that the covariance and correlation can't be negative since the variance of the random intercept σ_b^2 can't be negative (although it can be 0 if individual responses do not vary systematically from the average trend). We previously discussed that the compound symmetry assumption may hold for clustered data where the observations within the cluster are considered inter-chargeable, but is rarely satisfied for longitudinal data. While rANOVA provides a way of correcting the tests of the effects of the within-subject factors for deviations from this assumption, there is no such correction in the mixed model. Hence, the random intercept model should be chosen only if data conform reasonably well to the assumption of compound symmetry. If this is the case, the random intercept mixed-model approach is preferable to the rANOVA approach, since all available data on an individual are included in model fitting and thus the sample needs not be restricted only to individuals with complete data. More flexible mixed models are necessary when the compound symmetry assumption is not satisfied.

The correlation between any two repeated observations, within individuals or clusters $Corr(Y_{ij,}Y_{ik})$, is one of the simplest measures of intra-class correlation (ICC). It is the ratio of the variance of the random intercept to the total variance of the response and is referred to as the proportion of variance (unexplained by fixed predictors) due to between-subject variability. The ICC is a commonly used measure of test-retest reliability for quantitative variables when the same instrument is administered repeatedly to the same individuals. High values of ICC (i.e., values close to 1) mean that the subject's repeated responses are consistent with one another and hence the instrument that is evaluated is reliable. Low values of ICC mean that there is considerable variability in repeated responses of the same subject and hence the instrument is not reliable. More information on ICC can be found in Snijders and Bosker (2012) and Muller and Buttner (1994).

3.2.2 Random Intercept and Slope Model

In longitudinal data, subjects often not only start higher or lower than the average trend, but the rate of change is faster or slower than the average rate of change. To accommodate such a scenario, a random slope can be added to the model specified above. Thus, we consider the random intercept and slope model:

$$Y_{ij} = \beta_0 + \beta_1 Group_i + \beta_2 Time_j + \beta_3 Group_i \times Time_j + b_{i0} + b_{i1} Time_j + \varepsilon_{ij}. \tag{3.5}$$

The only difference between this model and the random intercept model in Equation 3.4, is the addition of the random slope term $b_{i1}Time_j$. Here, b_{i1} is the random slope and like the random intercept b_{i0}, it is assumed to be normally distributed with mean 0 and constant but unknown variance (to be estimated from the data). Since the random slope and the random intercept can be correlated, it is assumed that the two have a multivariate normal distribution $(b_{i0,}b_{i1})$~MVN$(0,\Sigma_b)$ where

$$\Sigma_b = \begin{pmatrix} \sigma_{b0}^2 & \sigma_{01} \\ \sigma_{01} & \sigma_{b1}^2 \end{pmatrix}.$$

The diagonal elements of Σ_b (namely σ_{b0}^2 and σ_{b1}^2) are the variances of the random intercept and the random slope, respectively, while σ_{01} is the covariance between the random intercept and the random slope. The covariance is related to the correlation ρ between the random intercept and the random slope as follows: $\sigma_{01} = \rho\sigma_{b0}\sigma_{b1}$. In some programs, the random intercept and the random slope are assumed to be uncorrelated by default. This may be a restrictive assumption for some data and, in general, needs to be checked by comparing the fit of a model in which the random intercept and slope are correlated to the fit of a model in which they are not correlated. Assessment of model fit is considered further in this chapter.

Figure 3.5 shows a schematic with hypothetical data for two random individuals (one with a positive random intercept and steeper slope, and one with a negative random intercept and flatter slope). The circles represent the observed response values at each of four time points. The dashed lines correspond to the individual trends for each of the two subjects. Unlike the situation described in Figure 3.4, here both the intercepts and the rates of change of the two individuals differ from the corresponding means, and the individual trends are no longer parallel to the average trend. The assumption about normal distribution of the random intercepts and slopes, means that the individual intercepts form a

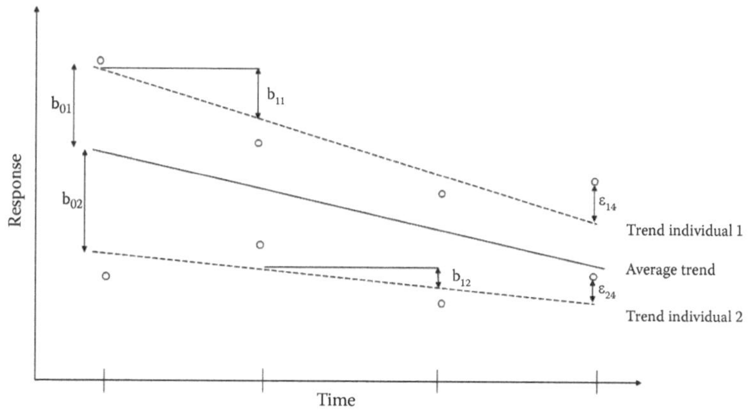

FIGURE 3.5
Hypothetical trends and observations of two individuals with response changing according to a random intercept and random slope model.

bell-shaped distribution around the average intercept, so that about half of the individual intercepts are above the average and half are below, and most of the individual intercepts are within two standard deviations of the average intercept. Similarly, individual slopes form a bell-shaped distribution around the average slope.

If the correlation between the random intercept and slope is negative, then subjects with larger intercepts (i.e., subjects who are initially above the average) have smaller slopes and subjects with smaller intercepts have larger slopes. The two left panels of Figure 3.6 illustrate negative correlations between the random intercept and slope when the slopes are, in general, negative (on the top), and when the slopes are, in general, positive (on the bottom). Note that in most longitudinal studies, one would expect to see negative association between the intercepts and slopes because of the phenomenon known as regression to the mean. Individuals who are further away from the mean at one point in time, are expected to move closer to the mean. In this case, the variance is unlikely to increase dramatically over time.

The two panels on the right in Figure 3.6 illustrate the situation when there is positive correlation between the random intercept and slope. Although not as frequently encountered, it is quite possible that subjects with larger intercepts have larger slopes and subjects with smaller intercepts have smaller slopes. This leads to a noticeable increase in variance over time as seen in both panels.

While the random intercept model implies that the variances of the observations on all occasions are the same, and that the correlations between any two repeated measures within individuals are the same, the random intercept and slope model implies that the variances change (usually increase) over time, and that the correlation between repeated measures within individuals changes, depending on the lag between the two time points. Exactly how much the variances increase depends on the time scale and on the relative magnitudes of the different variances (the variance of the random intercept, the variance of the random slope, and the variance of the random error). The pattern of the correlations between repeated measurements on the same individual also depends on the time scale, the magnitudes and ratios of the variances, and additionally, on the correlation between the random intercept and the random slope. It may be difficult to judge from the raw data whether the pattern of the correlations in the data set is consistent with the random intercept and slope model. Once the model is fit, the observed variances and covariances

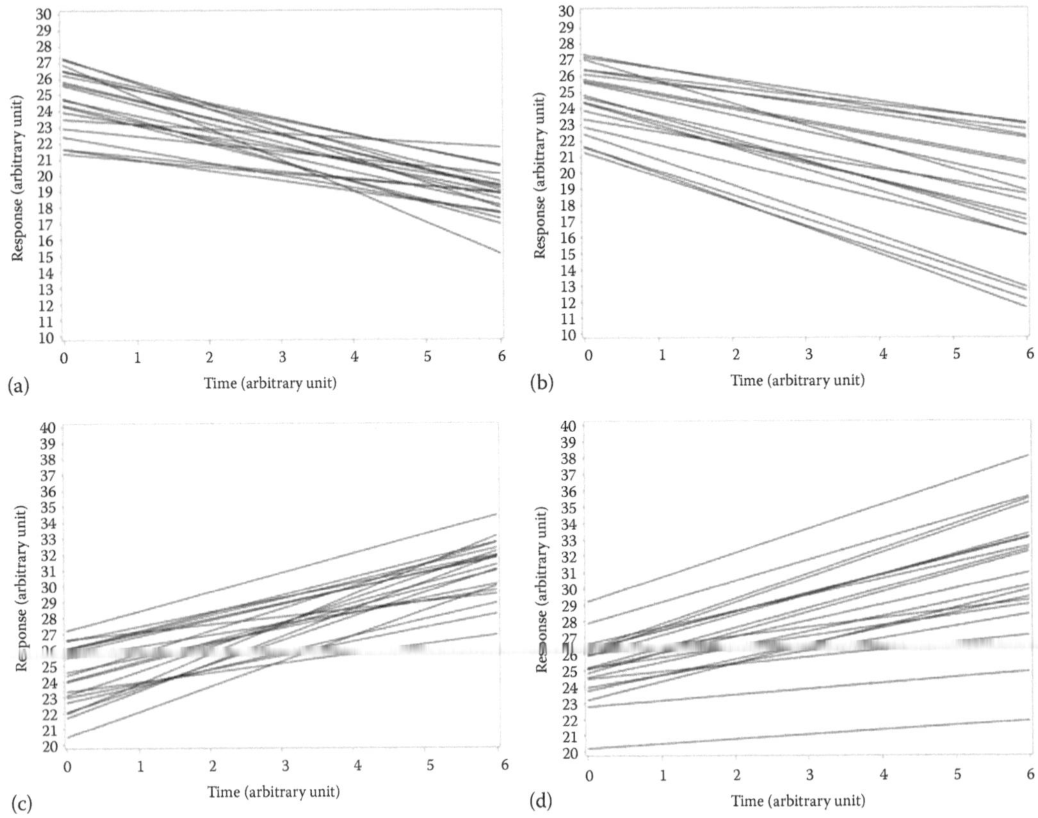

FIGURE 3.6
Four hypothetical situations with data for 20 individuals generated according to random intercept and slope model.

between responses at different time points can be compared to the estimated variances and covariances based on the model, to see whether there is good correspondence. Model selection should be used to choose the best-fitting model.

3.2.3 More Complex Random Effects Models

As we saw in the analysis of the augmentation depression study, a linear trend over time may not be describing the change over time sufficiently well and it may be necessary to account for curvature in response over time. This can be accomplished by adding quadratic terms to the model. The *random intercept, slope and quadratic model* is defined as follows:

$$Y_{ij} = \beta_0 + \beta_1 Group_i + \beta_2 Time_j + \beta_3 Group_i \times Time_j + \beta_4 Time_j^2 + \beta_5 Group_i \times Time_j^2 + b_{i0} + b_{i1} Time_j + b_{i2} Time_j^2 + \varepsilon_{ij} \quad (3.6)$$

Note that we added both fixed and random quadratic effects. We also have an interaction term between group and time squared in order to allow for different curvature in the two groups. The assumptions of the random intercept and slope model naturally extend to this more complicated scenario. We assume that the random intercept b_{i0}, the random slope b_{i1}, and the random quadratic term b_{i2}, are jointly normally distributed and are independent of

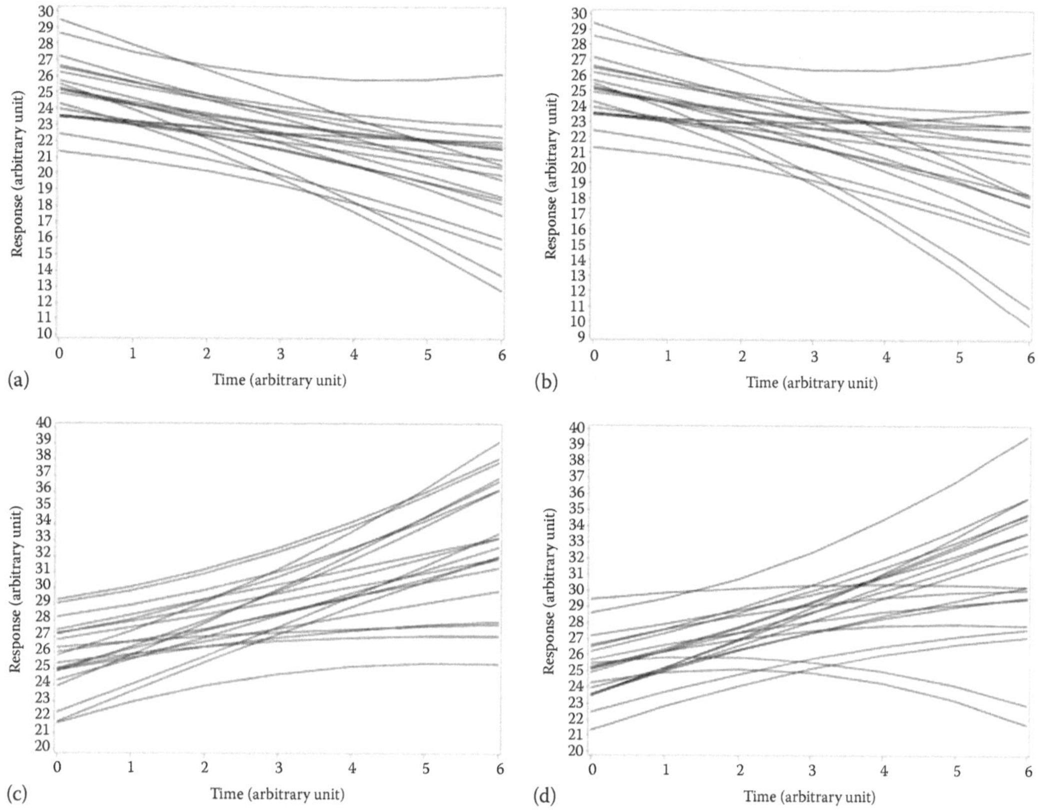

FIGURE 3.7
Four hypothetical situations with data for 20 individuals generated according to random intercept, slope and quadratic models.

the errors. Since there are three random effects, three separate variances and three different covariances (one for each pair of random effects) need to be estimated for the random effects. Figure 3.7 shows hypothetical examples of individual trajectories generated based on the random intercept, slope and quadratic models. There are many possible combinations of positive or negative slopes, positive or negative quadratic coefficients, and correlations among the three random effects (intercept, slope, and quadratic). Figure 3.7 shows only some of them, in order to illustrate that in all cases there is curvature in individual trajectories and increasing variability over time.

Although it is theoretically possible to add higher order fixed and random effects, the models become increasingly more complicated as the total number of variance and covariance parameters rapidly increases. Furthermore, the model-fitting algorithm may not converge for higher order models and interpretation becomes very difficult. Thus, from a practical perspective the quadratic random effects model is the highest order polynomial random effect that is useful in most applications.

Random slopes (and higher order terms) can be added on the log-transformed scale, rather than on the original scale. For example, the following random intercept and slope model can be constructed:

$$Y_{ij} = \beta_0 + \beta_1 Group_i + \beta_2 \log(Time_j) + \beta_3 Group_i \times \log(Time_j) + b_{i0} + b_{i1} \log(Time_j) + \varepsilon_{ij}$$

As shown for the mean portion of this model (Figure 3.3), each individual trajectory will be a straight line on the log-transformed time scale but will display curvature on the original scale.

3.3 Multilevel Models

So far, we considered models with repeated observations where there was only one level of clustering. In many situations, however, there are multiple levels of clustering. Models that consider different levels of clustering are usually known as *multilevel* or *hierarchical* models. Often individuals in longitudinal studies may be clustered in families or may receive treatment in a group setting. For example, in the Health and Retirement Study, introduced in Section 1.5.4, survey participants and their spouses are repeatedly interviewed over time. Thus, two levels of clustering may be considered: individual (these are repeated measures within individuals over time) and family (individuals are clustered within family units). Usually, the individual is referred to as the level 1 cluster, and it is nested within the level 2 cluster (in this case, the family). Correlations are expected to be strongest within individuals, but positive correlations are also expected on some measures within families.

Another scenario with multiple levels of clustering is when responses on individuals participating in a longitudinal study are repeatedly measured on the same day and the process is repeated on different days. In this case, observations within the same day are expected to be more highly correlated than observations on different days within the same individual. Because there are repeated measures within each day on an individual, here the level 1 cluster is the day within the individual, and the level 2 cluster is the individual. Level 1 clusters are nested within level 2 clusters. An example of such a situation is the *human laboratory study in smokers*, introduced in Section 1.5.7. This study is a two-level cross-over experiment in which different doses of menthol are given in random order on three different test days (level 1 clusters) to all participants (level 2 clusters) and responses are repeatedly measured on each test day (repeated observations within level 1 clusters).

In imaging studies, there can be even more levels of clustering. For example, in the *fMRI study of working memory in schizophrenia*, introduced in Section 1.5.8, where individuals complete different tasks at different difficulty levels, brain activation during three distinct working memory phases is recorded for each task and there are multiple brain regions from which a signal is extracted for all working memory phases for each task.

In all these situations, fitting a random effects model with a single random intercept (or random intercept and slope) is not adequate to describe the correlations in the data. Additional random effects should be considered to account for the correlations within each level of clustering. Herein, we consider some simple multilevel models. More information on multilevel and hierarchical linear models is available in Goldstein (1987), Snijders and Bosker (2012), and Twisk (2013b).

The two-level random intercept model is specified as follows:

$$Y_{ijk} = Mean_{ijk} + b_i + b_{ij} + \varepsilon_{ijk}$$

Here, we do not specify exactly how the fixed effects affect the average response. This can be done by specifying a linear combination of predictors that is deemed adequate to describe the average response, as shown previously for the depression example. We introduce an additional subscript k so that the different levels of clustering can be clearly identified. To illustrate, we consider specific examples. In the context of the *Health and Retirement Study*, i denotes the family pair, j denotes the individual within the family pair and k denotes the wave at which the measurement is taken on each individual. In the context of the *human laboratory study in smokers*, i denotes individual, j denotes test day within individual, and k denotes repeated observation within test day within individual. Thus, in addition to the random intercept for the first level of clustering b_i, we have an additional intercept for the second level of clustering b_{ij}. Each of these intercepts is assumed to be *independently* normally distributed: $b_i \sim i.i.d.N\left(0,\sigma_{b1}^2\right)$, $b_{ij} \sim i.i.d.N\left(0,\sigma_{b2}^2\right)$, and, to be independent of the errors, $\varepsilon_{ijk} \sim i.i.d.N(0, \sigma^2)$. This implies that the variability of each individual observation can be parceled out as the variability due to the first level clustering, variability due to the second level clustering, and residual variability, i.e., $Var\left(Y_{ijk}\right) = \sigma_{b1}^2 + \sigma_{b2}^2 + \sigma^2$. Since each measure of variability is non-negative, this also implies that the correlation between repeated observations within the level 1 cluster $\left(\text{i.e., } Corr\left(Y_{ijk}, Y_{ijl}\right) = \dfrac{\sigma_{b1}^2 + \sigma_{b2}^2}{\sigma_{b1}^2 + \sigma_{b2}^2 + \sigma^2}\right)$ is higher than the correlation between repeated observations on different level 1 clusters within a level 2 cluster $\left(\text{i.e., } Corr\left(Y_{ijk}, Y_{igl}\right) = \dfrac{\sigma_{b1}^2}{\sigma_{b1}^2 + \sigma_{b2}^2 + \sigma^2}\right)$, and that observations from different level 2 clusters are uncorrelated (i.e., $Corr(Y_{ijk}, Y_{hgl}) = 0$).

In the context of the *Health and Retirement Survey*, this means that the variability of each individual response is parceled into variability due to family, variability due to the individual, and residual variability. Also, the correlations between repeated observations on the same individual are implied to be higher than the correlations between repeated observations on different individuals in the same family, and observations on different individuals are uncorrelated.

In the context of the *human laboratory study in smokers*, variability of individual observations is the sum of variability due to the individual, variability due to the day within the individual, and residual variability. The correlations between repeated observations taken on an individual on the same day are higher than correlations between repeated observations taken on the same individual but on different days, and there is no correlation between observations on different individuals.

Note that since there are only random intercepts, the repeated observations within the level 1 cluster are equally correlated. This may not be reasonable if the repeated measures at this level are taken over time, as it is in the *human laboratory study in smokers*, for example. Also, any two observations from different level 1 clusters, but the same level 2 cluster, are equally correlated. This may also not represent reality, in some cases. More flexibility in accounting for such complicated structures can be achieved by adding additional random effects (e.g., adding a random slope term $b_{ij1}Time_{ij}$ for longitudinal observations on the same day) or by combining random effects and covariance-pattern models, as discussed further in this chapter.

Mixed-effects models with more than two nested levels of clustering can be constructed by adding random effects at additional levels of clustering. This is necessary in situations like the *fMRI study of working memory in schizophrenia*, where there are more factors introducing correlation between repeated observations on the same individual.

A random intercept model with three levels of clustering is defined as follows:

$$Y_{ijkl} = Mean_{ijkl} + b_i + b_{ij} + b_{ijk} + \varepsilon_{ijk},$$

where the additional random effect b_{ijk} is also assumed to be normally distributed with zero mean, some unknown variance, and is uncorrelated with the other random effects and the random errors. In the context of the *fMRI study of working memory in schizophrenia*, the clustering level indexed with i is the individual, the clustering level indexed by j is the task, and it is nested within the individual, clustering level indexed by k is the phase (encoding, retention, response), and l indexes individual observations in different regions. If we fit such a model to these data, we assume that observations within the same phase, during the same task, on the same individual, are more highly correlated than observations from different phases, during the same task, on the same individual, which in turn are more highly correlated than observations from different tasks on the same individual. We are also assuming equal variances and exchangeability between observations within each level of clustering. This may not be reasonable as observations within different regions may have different variances and correlations across phases, and regions may also differ. More sophisticated models based on both random effects and structured variances and covariances should be considered. This is presented in more detail further in this chapter. We now focus on a different approach to accounting for the correlations between repeated observations on the same individual—namely, directly assuming a certain pattern of the error variances and covariances.

3.4 Covariance-Pattern Models

So far in this chapter, we assumed that the random errors have equal variances on all occasions and are uncorrelated with one another. This is usually inconsistent with the pattern of data variability in clinical trials where subjects are selected according to a strict set of inclusion/exclusion criteria and then show divergent trajectories over time. However, it is possible that variability does not follow this pattern and then the models may not provide a good fit to the data. Making alternative assumptions about the errors (e.g., assuming unequal variances across time and/or additional correlations between observations on different occasions) may help in such situations. Instead of using random effects to model individual variability around the average trend, and to account for correlations within individuals or clusters, we can directly consider different patterns of variances and correlations for the random errors.

This is similar to the approach taken in rMANOVA where we assume that the errors across repeated occasions on the same individual follow a multivariate normal distribution $(\varepsilon_{i1}, \varepsilon_{i2}, \ldots \varepsilon_{ij}) \sim MVN(0,\Sigma)$ where the mean consists only of zeros and the variance–covariance matrix Σ is expressed as follows:

$$\Sigma = \begin{pmatrix} \sigma_{11} & \cdots & \sigma_{1J} \\ \vdots & \ddots & \vdots \\ \sigma_{J1} & \cdots & \sigma_{JJ} \end{pmatrix}.$$

There are a number of patterns for the variance–covariance matrix that we can consider. They vary in complexity by the number of parameters that are used to describe all the variances and covariances between repeated observations on the same individual. The simplest structure that we can specify is *compound symmetry*. That is, we assume that all variances are equal and all covariances (correlations) are also equal:

$$\Sigma = \begin{pmatrix} \sigma^2 & \cdots & \rho\sigma^2 \\ \vdots & \ddots & \vdots \\ \rho\sigma^2 & \cdots & \sigma^2 \end{pmatrix}$$

There are only two unknown parameters in this formulation (the variance σ^2 and the correlation ρ). This structure is almost identical to the structure imposed by the single level random intercept model but here the correlation ρ is not restricted to be positive (or 0) and can be negative. Although this structure is slightly more general than the structure of the random intercept model, it is likely that it is not well suited in most longitudinal situations where correlations between observations measured closer together within individuals are expected to be higher.

At the other extreme of complexity of the variance–covariance structure, we have the most general scenario with the *unstructured* (aka *unrestricted*) variance–covariance matrix, as assumed in rMANOVA. This structure can be considered only when the observation occasions are the same within individuals or clusters. In this case, we freely estimate the variances on all repeated occasions and the correlations between any two occasions. With t repeated occasions, there are $t(t+1)/2$ parameters that correspond to all the variances and correlations between repeated occasions. As the number of observation occasions increases, the number of parameters that need to be estimated drastically increases and the sample size in some data sets may be insufficient to estimate all the parameters. Unlike rMANOVA, where only subjects with complete data are used in the analysis, in the corresponding mixed model all available data on an individual are used, and hence, even subjects with missing values contribute to the estimation process.

Some variance–covariance structures of intermediate complexity include *the autoregressive structure, the Toeplitz structure, compound symmetry with heterogeneous variances, autoregressive structure with heterogeneous variances*, and *spatial power*. A tutorial on modeling the covariance structure of repeated measures data is available in Littell et al. (2000). Structures of varying complexity are available in software programs, which provide modules or procedures for fitting mixed-effects models. Herein, we consider the most commonly used structures.

The *autoregressive structure of first order* AR(1) is a parsimonious structure that assumes equal variances on all repeated occasions and exponentially decreasing correlations between repeated observations with increasing time lag. The correlation between observations at time points k and l is calculated, based on the following formula:

$$Corr\left(Y_{ik}, Y_{il}\right) = \rho^{|k-l|}.$$

Like the compound symmetry structure, the autoregressive structure uses only two parameters to describe all variances and correlations (namely the variance σ^2 and the correlation ρ). The further apart occasions k and l are from each other, the smaller the correlation between the repeated observations on these occasions is. For example, if $\rho = 0.5$, then the correlation between observations that are one unit of time apart is equal to 0.5. The correlation between observations that are two units of time apart is equal to $0.5 \times 0.5 = 0.25$. The correlation between observations that are three units of time apart is equal to $0.5 \times 0.5 \times 0.5 = 0.125$. The decrease in correlation, according to the AR(1) structure, is quite rapid, which may not reflect reality. In the next section we show how a combination of a random intercept model and AR(1) error structure can be used for longitudinal data. But first we focus on a few additional structures of intermediate complexity.

The *Toeplitz structure* assumes that variances are equal on all occasions and that correlations between observations m occasions apart are also equal. With three time points the structure is as follows:

$$\Sigma = \begin{pmatrix} \sigma^2 & \rho_1\sigma^2 & \rho_2\sigma^2 \\ \rho_1\sigma^2 & \sigma^2 & \rho_1\sigma^2 \\ \rho_2\sigma^2 & \rho_1\sigma^2 & \sigma^2 \end{pmatrix}$$

Here, ρ_1 denotes the correlation between neighboring repeated observations on the same individual, while ρ_2 denotes the correlation between repeated observations on the same individual that are two occasions apart. Subsequently, $\rho_1\sigma^2$ denotes the covariance between two neighboring observations and $\rho_2\sigma^2$ denotes the covariance between repeated observations that are two occasions apart. In the general case with t occasions, the variance–covariance structure is

$$\Sigma = \begin{pmatrix} \sigma^2 & \rho_1\sigma^2 & \rho_2\sigma^2 & & \rho_{t-3}\sigma^2 & \rho_{t-2}\sigma^2 & \rho_{t-1}\sigma^2 \\ \rho_1\sigma^2 & \sigma^2 & \rho_1\sigma^2 & \cdots & \rho_{t-4}\sigma^2 & \rho_{t-3}\sigma^2 & \rho_{t-2}\sigma^2 \\ \rho_2\sigma^2 & \rho_1\sigma^2 & \sigma^2 & & \rho_{t-5}\sigma^2 & \rho_{t-4}\sigma^2 & \rho_{t-3}\sigma^2 \\ & \vdots & & \ddots & & \vdots & \\ \rho_{t-3}\sigma^2 & \rho_{t-4}\sigma^2 & \rho_{t-5}\sigma^2 & & \sigma^2 & \rho_1\sigma^2 & \rho_2\sigma^2 \\ \rho_{t-2}\sigma^2 & \rho_{t-3}\sigma^2 & \rho_{t-4}\sigma^2 & \cdots & \rho_1\sigma^2 & \sigma^2 & \rho_1\sigma^2 \\ \rho_{t-1}\sigma^2 & \rho_{t-2}\sigma^2 & \rho_{t-3}\sigma^2 & & \rho_2\sigma^2 & \rho_1\sigma^2 & \sigma^2 \end{pmatrix}$$

and uses t parameters to describe all variances and covariances (namely the variance σ^2 and the correlations ρ_1, ρ_2, …, and ρ_{t-1}). If the observations are not equally spaced over time, this structure may not fit well as it imposes the same correlation for observations that are a different number of units of time apart. The autoregressive structure AR(1) is actually a special case of the Toeplitz structure for equally spaced repeated occasions when the correlations decrease exponentially. In the special case when the repeated occasions are one unit in time apart, the Toeplitz structure reduces to AR(1) when $\rho_2 = \rho_1^2$, $\rho_3 = \rho_1^3$, and so on.

Another possible generalization of the AR(1) structure is the *spatial power* structure. For 3 repeated occasions, it is represented as follows:

$$\Sigma = \begin{pmatrix} \sigma^2 & \rho^{d_{12}}\sigma^2 & \rho^{d_{13}}\sigma^2 \\ \rho^{d_{12}}\sigma^2 & \sigma^2 & \rho^{d_{23}}\sigma^2 \\ \rho^{d_{13}}\sigma^2 & \rho^{d_{23}}\sigma^2 & \sigma^2 \end{pmatrix},$$

where:

d_{12} is a measure of the distance between occasion 1 and 2
d_{13} is a measure of the distance between occasion 1 and 3
d_{23} is a measure of the distance between occasion 2 and 3

When the repeated measures are taken over time, this distance is simply represented by the number of units (hours, days, weeks, years) that separate the corresponding time points. If the repeated measures are taken over a spatial map (as may be the case with some imaging data, measurements taken on a subject's body, or measurements taken over a specific area), then distance is measured as actual physical distance. Such a structure may also be used in order to model correlations among measurements on people who are related (e.g., a distance of 1 may denote a first degree relative, a distance of 2 may denote second degree relatives, etc.). As can be easily seen, the AR(1), structure is a special case of the spatial power structure when distances are measured in time units.

So far, all structures that we considered, except the unstructured, assume that the variances on repeated occasions are the same. However, this may not reflect the variability in the data well and it may be judicious to assess whether this assumption is satisfied. One way to do this is to consider more general structures and compare the fit of models with the same mean specification and the same correlation structure, but allowing the variances to be different. The following structures with unequal variances correspond to structures we already considered: *compound symmetry heterogeneous* (CSH), *autoregressive heterogeneous* (ARH(1)), *Toeplitz heterogeneous*, and *spatial power heterogeneous* (SPH). The only difference between these and their homogeneous variance counterparts, is that the variances on all occasions are allowed to vary freely. For the simple case of an autoregressive heterogeneous pattern, the structure for three time points is as follows:

$$\begin{pmatrix} \sigma_1^2 & \rho\sigma_1\sigma_2 & \rho^2\sigma_1\sigma_3 \\ \rho\sigma_1\sigma_2 & \sigma_2^2 & \rho\sigma_2\sigma_3 \\ \rho^2\sigma_1\sigma_3 & \rho\sigma_2\sigma_3 & \sigma_3^2 \end{pmatrix}$$

In general, the number of parameters that characterize the variance–covariance matrices increases substantially as the number of repeated occasions t increases and is equal to:

For CSH: $t+1$ (t variances and 1 correlation)
For ARH(1): $t+1$ (t variances and 1 correlation)
For Toeplitz heterogeneous: $2t-1$ (t variances and $t-1$ correlations)
For SPH: $t+1$ (t variances and 1 correlation)

3.5 Combinations of Random Effects and Covariance-Pattern Models

Different variance–covariance structures can be used either alone or in combination with random effects. The most commonly used combination that often provides a good fit for longitudinal data is *random intercept plus autoregressive structure* ($r.i.+AR(1)$). The model is formulated as follows:

$$Y_{ij} = \beta_0 + \beta_1 Group_i + \beta_2 Time_j + \beta_3 Group_i \times Time_j + b_i + \varepsilon_{ij},$$

where the usual assumptions for the random intercept and the errors hold and where $Var(b_i) = \sigma_b^2$, $Var(\varepsilon_{ij}) = \sigma^2$ and $Corr(\varepsilon_{ik}, \varepsilon_{il}) = \rho^{|k-l|}$. The resulting variance–covariance structure for t repeated occasions is then

$$\Sigma = \begin{pmatrix} \sigma^2+\sigma_b^2 & \rho\sigma^2+\sigma_b^2 & \cdots & \rho^{t-2}\sigma^2+\sigma_b^2 & \rho^{t-1}\sigma^2+\sigma_b^2 \\ \rho\sigma^2+\sigma_b^2 & \sigma^2+\sigma_b^2 & & \rho^{t-3}\sigma^2+\sigma_b^2 & \rho^{t-2}\sigma^2+\sigma_b^2 \\ \vdots & & \ddots & & \vdots \\ \rho^{t-2}\sigma^2+\sigma_b^2 & \rho^{t-3}\sigma^2+\sigma_b^2 & & \sigma^2+\sigma_b^2 & \rho\sigma^2+\sigma_b^2 \\ \rho^{t-1}\sigma^2+\sigma_b^2 & \rho^{t-2}\sigma^2+\sigma_b^2 & \cdots & \rho\sigma^2+\sigma_b^2 & \sigma^2+\sigma_b^2 \end{pmatrix}$$

While the AR(1) structure assumes a fast decrease of correlations with increasing time lag, and the random intercept model assumes equal correlation between any two repeated measures on the same individual, the structure of the combined model shows decreasing correlation with time lag, but at a slower rate than in the AR(1) structure because of the addition of σ_b^2 to each covariance. Littell et al. (2000) demonstrate that this structure is often best-fitting in medical studies with longitudinal data.

The *r.i. + AR(1)* structure assumes that the variances at all occasions are the same. If this is not a reasonable assumption, then one can consider *r.i. + ARH(1)* structure or add a random slope in addition to the random intercept in the model. Many more combinations of random effects and structured variances and covariances can be considered, especially when there are different levels of clustering. We consider some such combinations in Section 3.8 and refer interested readers to Brown and Prescott (2006) for more systematic exploration of such combinations. Note, though, that certain combinations may over-specify the variances and covariances (i.e., introduce more parameters than can be estimated from the data) and should not be considered. For example, in longitudinal scenarios without additional clustering and with fixed occasions, it is not possible to fit a random intercept model plus an unrestricted variance–covariance structure. The variance of the random intercept, in this situation, is completely absorbed in the individual variances on the different occasions. Thus, one needs to be careful when considering different variance–covariance structures since not all possible combinations of random effects and structures of the errors are reasonable.

With many different ways to specify the variances and covariances between repeated observations, it may be challenging to select the best-fitting one and it is often not a clear-cut decision. In the next section we consider statistical criteria that can be used to compare different models.

3.6 Estimation, Model Fit, and Model Selection

Estimation of fixed-effects coefficients in mixed models is accomplished using the method of *maximum likelihood* (ML), which finds the values of the parameters that maximize the likelihood of obtaining the observed data from the hypothesized model. This method turns out to be equivalent to the *generalized least squares* (GLS) method, which minimizes the sum of squares of the residuals (i.e., the differences between observed and predicted values) weighted by the inverse of the variances.

The variance parameters can also be estimated using maximum likelihood. However, in order to take into account that the fixed-effects coefficients are also estimated, a modification of the maximum likelihood approach, namely *restricted maximum likelihood* (REML) is preferred because it provides unbiased estimates of the variance parameters.

Empirical Bayes estimation of the random effects (e.g., intercept, slope) allows estimation and prediction of individual responses. The individual-specific estimates and predictions are weighted averages of the responses of the particular individual and the estimated mean responses for the group of individuals that are similar to that individual. Detailed information about the estimation process and properties of the estimates is beyond the scope of this book. We refer interested readers to Brown and Prescott (2006) and Hedeker and Gibbons (2006) for a relatively non-technical description.

The estimation procedures provide estimates not only of the coefficients and variance parameters, but also of the variability (uncertainty) of these estimates. General statistical theory then allows confidence intervals to be constructed and hypothesis tests evaluated for individual parameters or combinations of parameters. Thus, both the overall tests of the between-subject and within-subject effects in the model and post hoc tests are performed, and confidence intervals constructed for the effects of interest within the general model framework. In the subsequent sections with data examples, we focus on interpretation of the overall tests of main effects and interactions in the statistical models and on estimation of mean comparisons with confidence intervals, in order to provide effect size estimates.

The estimation procedure also provides the maximum value of the likelihood function achieved by each model when the parameters are equal to their estimated values. This function is at the basis of the statistical criteria for model comparison. In the special case of nested models, when the fixed effects of one model are a subset of the fixed effects of another model, the *likelihood ratio test* that compares the likelihood of the two nested models can be used to decide which model to select for a particular data set. However, the likelihood ratio test can't be used for models that are not nested. Thus, we focus on two statistical criteria that are most commonly used to compare different models fitted to the same data set: *the Akaike Information Criterion* (AIC) and the *Schwartz' Bayesian Information Criterion* (BIC).

Both the AIC and the BIC are based on the maximum likelihood value and include a penalty for the number of parameters estimated in the model. The AIC tends to favor models with more parameters while the BIC tends to favor more parsimonious models. Thus the BIC is considered to be more conservative and penalizes more for the number of parameters in the model. Among a set of alternative models, the model with the lowest AIC or the lowest BIC is selected. For selection of the best-fitting variance–covariance structure, the AIC is generally preferred as the BIC is considered too conservative (Fitzmaurice et al. 2011).

The idea behind the AIC and BIC measures is that we want to find the model that best describes the data and that provides results that generalize to the population of interest. By adding more and more parameters, we make the models fit the observed data better and better. But some parameters add little to the explanatory ability of the model. If too many parameters are added, the model may reflect random noise in the sample data set and may become less and less useful in terms of predicting response in the actual population. The information criteria include penalties for the number of parameters in order to favor selection of models with balance between explanatory power and parsimony. Because the information criteria can be applied to any set of models fit to the same data set (not just nested models) we focus on the AIC and BIC in deciding on the best-fitting model among those considered.

Other information criteria are also available, for example the *finite sample size adjusted AIC*. Detailed information about a variety of model selection criteria is available in Claeskens and Hjort (2008).

3.7 Residuals and Remedial Measures

As in other model classes, in mixed-effects models we can examine the residuals in order to assess whether the assumptions of the model (e.g., normality) are reasonably satisfied. *Raw (unstandardized) residuals* are just the differences between the observed values and the predicted values on each occasion for each individual. Residuals can be standardized in order to take into account that they do not have equal variances in most mixed models. *Studentized residuals* are standardized residuals so that extreme values (values larger than 3 or smaller than −3) are easily identifiable and indicative of deviations from the assumptions of normal distribution of the errors. In models with random effects, there are two types of studentized residuals: *marginal* and *conditional*. The two sets of residuals differ in the following way. To obtain the marginal residual, the predicted value for each individual observation, based only on the fixed-effects portion of the model, is subtracted from the observed value. To obtain the conditional residual, the predicted value based on the fixed effects and the random effects portion of the model is subtracted from the observed value. When there are several random effects, the predicted values are obtained by adding the mean prediction and the individual-specific estimates for the random effects obtained, using the empirical Bayes method. Thus, the conditional residual adjusts for systematic individual-level variation from the mean, due to random effects, while the marginal residual does not. In covariance-pattern models only marginal studentized residuals are calculated. The raw and studentized residuals should have approximately bell-shaped distributions, since they approximate the errors which are assumed to be normally distributed.

A *normal probability plot* of the residuals (i.e., plotting the ordered residuals against the expected values from the standard normal distribution given their ranks, see for example Kutner et al. (2005)), or a plot of the *residuals against their predicted values*, can be used to assess whether the normality assumption is approximately satisfied. In the normal probability plot we expect to see a straight line. Deviations from the straight line indicate skewness and lack of fit. In the residuals versus predicted plot, we expect randomly distributed residuals around zero with no obvious patterns. Both plots can also be used to check whether there are outlying observations. The residual versus predicted plot also shows whether the residual variance is constant across observations. These plots are illustrated on the data examples in the next section.

If there is an indication of non-normality (i.e., deviation from straight line in the normal probability plot), a transformation of the response can be considered. For example, taking a log of the response values often helps correct positive skewness. If there are outliers, the corresponding observations need to be double-checked. If no obvious reason for the outlying observations can be identified, results may need to be presented with and without the outliers, especially if there are significant differences in the results.

If variances are not approximately equal across occasions, an alternative variance–covariance structure can be considered, or sometimes, a transformation may help standardize the variance. If deviations from the assumptions are sizeable, non-parametric statistical methods may need to be used, as described in Chapter 5.

More detailed discussion of residuals and remedial measures in the context of mixed models can be found in Fitzmaurice et al. (2011) and Nobre and da Motta Singer (2007).

3.8 Examples

We now present several different examples that illustrate how to construct mixed models for longitudinal and clustered data, how to select the best model, assess whether model assumptions are satisfied, and perform statistical inferences based on the model. The SAS code for fitting all models is provided on the associated website.

3.8.1 Augmentation Treatment for Depression

This study was introduced in Section 1.5.1 and already repeatedly considered in order to illustrate simple methods for the analysis of longitudinal data, such as endpoint analysis, rANOVA, and rMANOVA, in the previous chapter, and mixed models with random effects, earlier in this chapter. Herein, we start by fitting a number of reasonable mixed models to these data and using the AIC and BIC to select the best-fitting model. For the best-fitting model, we present residual plots to assess if model assumptions are reasonably satisfied and show how to interpret overall tests, post hoc comparisons, and how to estimate and interpret the effects of interest.

We consider both models with random effects and with structured variance–covariance matrices appropriate for longitudinal data. Also, in some models time is treated as a continuous predictor and in some models it is treated as a categorical predictor. All models include main effects of time, treatment group, and the interaction between time and treatment group.

Table 3.1 shows the AIC and BIC for all considered models. The first five models are models with random effects and with time treated as a continuous predictor. The AIC and the BIC decrease steadily as we add higher order random effects to the model (i.e., include a random intercept, add a slope, then add a quadratic term), indicating that the random slope and quadratic term are necessary to describe the data well, if we consider time as a continuous predictor. Note that when comparing models with uncorrelated random effects (i.e., models 2 and 4) to the corresponding model with correlated random effects (models 3 and 5, respectively) the change in AIC and BIC is small and the AIC decreases while the BIC increases. Thus, it does not appear essential to include correlations between the random effects as the addition of extra parameters partially outweighs the gain in improvement of the fit of the model to the data.

The rest of the models in Table 3.1 treat time as a categorical predictor (i.e., six dummy variables are used to describe the time effect) and consider different structures for the variance–covariance matrix. In general, these models (models 6 through 12) fit better than the random effects models when time is treated as a continuous predictor (models 1 through 5) as most of them have lower AIC and BIC. The model with compound symmetry structure, which assumes equal variances and equal correlations of any two repeated observations on an individual, fits poorly compared to the other models. Also, the models with unequal variances at the different time points fit worse than the corresponding models with equal variances for the different time points. Thus, there is no indication in this data set that there is a substantial increase in variability with time.

According to both information criteria, the model with autoregressive structure of first order fits the data the best (model 7) as the AIC and BIC are the smallest. We also considered a model with a random intercept and autoregressive variance–covariance structure of the errors (r.i. + AR(1)) but since the estimated variance of the random intercept was zero, indicating that the random intercept was not needed, we do not include these results in the table and do not consider this model further. Additional models can be fit to these data,

TABLE 3.1

Model Fit Criteria for Mixed-Effects Models Fitted to the HDRS Scores in the Augmentation Depression Study

Model	Fixed Effects	Random Effects	Variance–covariance Structure of the Errors	AIC	BIC
Model 1: Random intercept	Group Time (continuous) Group × time	Intercept	Uncorrelated errors with equal variances	1980.7	1984.5
Model 2: Random intercept and slope	Group Time (continuous) Group × time	Intercept and slope (uncorrelated)	Uncorrelated errors with equal variances	1941.5	1947.2
Model 3: Random intercept and slope	Group Time (continuous) Group × time	Intercept and slope (correlated)	Uncorrelated errors with equal variances	1940.5	1948.2
Model 4: Random intercept, slope, and quadratic	Group Time (continuous) Time^2 Group × time Group × time^2	Intercept, slope and quadratic (uncorrelated)	Uncorrelated errors with equal variances	1917.5	1925.1
Model 5: Random intercept, slope, and quadratic	Group × Time (continuous) Time^2 Group × time Group × time^2	Intercept, slope and quadratic (correlated)	Uncorrelated errors with equal variances	1878.1	1891.5
Model 6: Compound symmetry with categorical time	Group Time (categorical) Group × time	None	Compound symmetry: CS	1927.1	1930.9
Model 7: Autoregressive with categorical time	**Group Time (categorical) Group × time**	**None**	**Autoregressive: AR(1)**	**1827.3**	**1831.1**
Model 8: Toeplitz with categorical time	Group Time (categorical) Group × time	None	Toeplitz: TOEP	1832.7	1846.1
Model 9: Compound symmetry heterogeneous with categorical time	Group Time (categorical) Group × time	None	Compound symmetry heterogeneous: CSH	1933.4	1948.7
Model 10: Autoregressive heterogeneous with categorical time	Group Time (categorical) Group × time	None	Autoregressive heterogeneous: ARH(1)	1829.7	1845.0
Model 11: Toeplitz heterogeneous with categorical time	Group Time (categorical) Group × time	None	Toeplitz heterogeneous: TOEPH	1834.5	1859.3
Model 12: Unstructured with categorical time	Group Time (categorical) Group × time	None	Unstructured: UN	1831.8	1885.3

Note: The best-fitting model (i.e., the model with the lowest AIC and BIC) is indicated in bold.

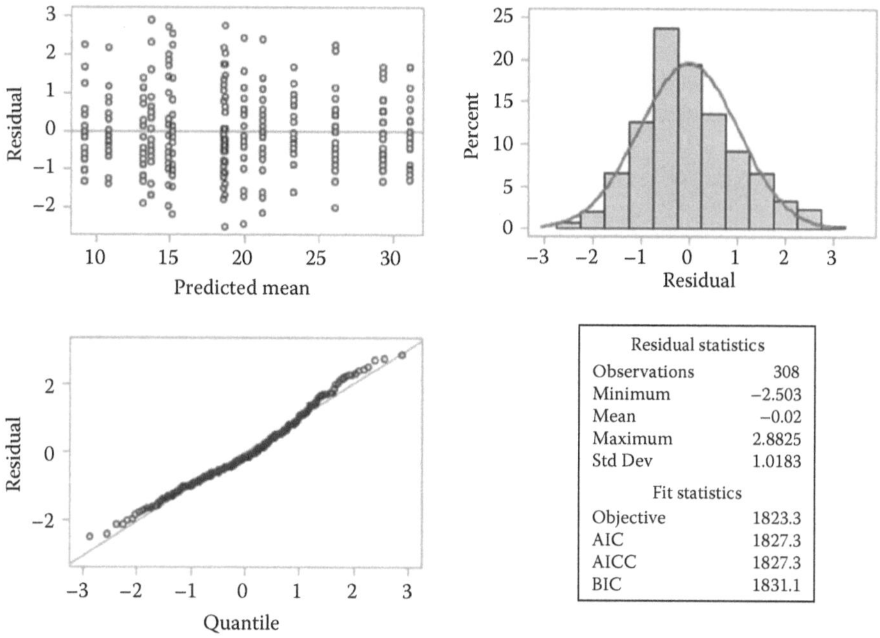

FIGURE 3.8
Plots of studentized residuals for the Hamilton Depression Rating Scale from the autoregressive model with categorical time fit to the data set from the augmentation study in depression.

especially when one considers combinations of random effects and structured variances and covariances. However, since a fairly simple structure, with decreasing correlations with increasing time lag, fits the data better than more complicated models, we consider this as our final model. We now focus on exploration of residuals in order to assess how well the model assumptions are satisfied and then proceed with interpretation of significant effects in the model with appropriate post hoc comparisons and estimates.

Figure 3.8 shows several residual plots with studentized residuals from the best-fitting model (Model 7). The plot in the upper left of Figure 3.8 is a scatter plot of residuals versus predicted values. We do not see studentized residuals larger than three in absolute value and the plot is fairly symmetrical around the zero horizontal line. Therefore, we conclude that the model provides a good fit to the data. Note that on the horizontal axis we have the predicted means, which are also equal to the predicted values for individual subjects because the model does not have random effects. There are, in fact, only 14 distinct predicted values corresponding to the seven time points for the two treatment groups. This is not an issue but it explains why the points are vertically aligned.

The plot in the upper right of Figure 3.8 is a histogram of the studentized residuals with the corresponding theoretical distribution of the residuals superimposed over the histogram. There is a slight discrepancy between the histogram and the theoretical distribution but no gross deviations, which would have indicated substantial lack of fit. The normal distribution plot in the lower left of Figure 3.8 confirms that there are no substantial deviations from normality of the errors as the circles indicating individual observations fall approximately on a straight line.

The bottom right of Figure 3.8 shows the number of studentized residuals (which corresponds to the number of non-missing response values in the sample) and some descriptive statistics (minimum, maximum, mean, and standard deviation). The mean of the studentized residuals should be close to zero if normality of the errors is approximately satisfied and it comes close at −0.02. The standard deviation should be close to 1 and it is 1.02. The minimum and maximum should be no larger than 3. All these conditions are satisfied in this example and hence we conclude that the model assumptions are fairly well satisfied.

Note that nothing can be determined from the plots of Figure 3.8 about residual patterns within an individual subject. We need to plot the residuals by week and by individual in order to see whether any patterns emerge within individuals over time. Figure 3.9 shows studentized residuals by treatment group, week, and individual. Although the residuals are again approximately symmetrical around the zero horizontal line, we see that residuals for the same individual tend to stay either above or below the zero horizontal line. Such systematic deviation can easily be accounted for by adding a random intercept to the model. However, our model selection procedure led to the conclusion that this is not needed.

After we have determined that model assumptions are reasonably well satisfied, and the best-fitting model among a set of plausible models is identified, we proceed with hypothesis testing, effect estimation, and interpretation of significant effects. Usually, the first step of statistical inference is to assess the significance of the main and interaction effects of the predictors in the model, followed by post hoc comparisons and effect estimation.

Table 3.2 contains the results from the tests of the three effects of interest in this example and post hoc comparisons to explain the significant effects. The interaction between treatment and time is not statistically significant ($F(6,231)=0.60$, $p=0.73$), but the main effects of treatment and time are statistically significant at 0.05 significance level ($F(1,57.4)=5.15$, $p=0.03$ and $F(6,231)=37.04$, $p<0.0001$). Thus, this model suggests that the differences in pattern of change over time in the two groups are not significant, but that average response changes significantly over time and there are significant differences between the groups when all time points are averaged together.

In order to understand what this means, we consider the estimated *least square means* (model-based estimates of the mean response at each combination of levels of the predictors) shown in Figure 3.10. They follow the same pattern as the raw means from Figure 1.5

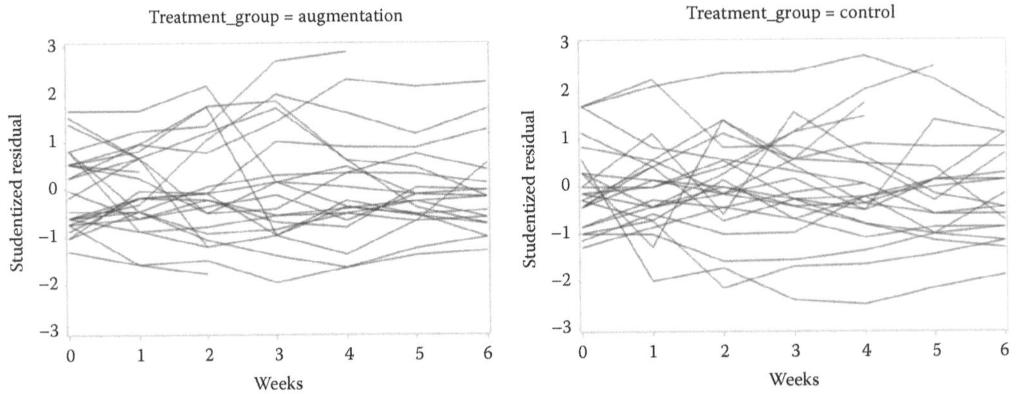

FIGURE 3.9
Plots of studentized residuals for the individual subjects by treatment group and week from the autoregressive model with categorical time fit to the Hamilton Depression Rating Scale scores in the data set from the augmentation study in depression.

TABLE 3.2

Test Results from the Autoregressive Model with Categorical Time Effect in the Augmentation Study in Depression

Effect	Test Statistic	p-Value
Treatment	**F(1,57.4) = 5.15**	**0.03**
Time	**F(6,231) = 37.04**	**<0.0001**
Treatment × time	F(6,231) = 0.60	0.73
Linear time trend	F(1,237) = 159.06	<0.0001
Quadratic time trend	F(1,276) = 13.90	0.0002
Cubic time trend	F(1,233) = 5.37	0.02
Week 1 vs. baseline	t(240) = 7.85	<0.0001
Week 2 vs. baseline	t(276) = 10.82	<0.0001
Week 3 vs. baseline	t(293) = 11.45	<0.0001
Week 4 vs. baseline	t(288) = 11.51	<0.0001
Week 5 vs. baseline	t(269) = 13.15	<0.0001
Week 6 vs. baseline	t(245) = 13.81	<0.0001

Note: Significant main effects are highlighted in bold.

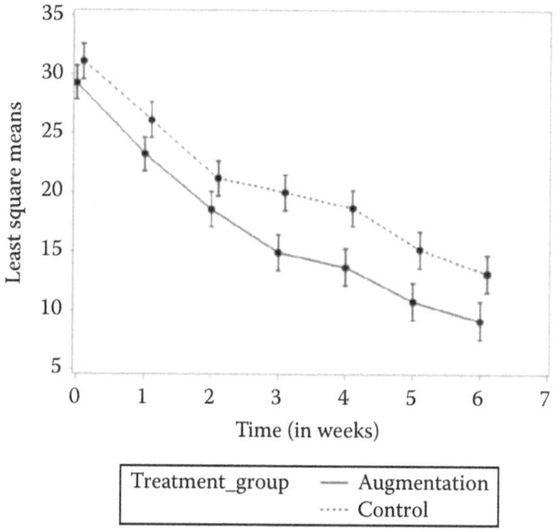

FIGURE 3.10
Estimated least square means and standard error for the Hamilton Depression Rating Scale by treatment group and week from the autoregressive model with categorical time fit to the data set from the augmentation study in depression.

and indicate that depression severity decreases steadily in both treatment groups and that the control group has higher depression severity scores on average than the augmentation group, with the between-group difference increasingly slightly (but not significantly) with time (i.e., there is no significant interaction between group and time). Since there are seven different time points, we attempt to interpret the time trend in a more parsimonious way by testing for linear, quadratic, and cubic trends in the least square means over time.

This is done by specifying individual contrasts within the mixed model using PROC MIXED in SAS, as shown in the online code for this example. As seen from Table 3.2, the linear, quadratic, and cubic trends over time are all significant, suggesting that the shape of response over time is fairly complex with a significant steady decrease, but with some leveling off of the response in the middle of the period. Since there are only seven time points and interpretation of cubic trends is somewhat complicated, for this particular example it seems judicious to continue treating time as a categorical factor rather than as a continuous predictor.

When time is a categorical variable, we can perform all pairwise comparisons among time points. In Table 3.2 we show the comparisons of all post-baseline time points to baseline. All these comparisons are statistically significant even at overall alpha level of 0.05 corrected for multiple comparisons using Bonferroni's adjustment (to be presented in detail in Chapter 6). Among all possible pairwise comparisons of different time points (not shown), only the comparisons between least square means at weeks 3 and 4, and between weeks 5 and 6, are not statistically significant, suggesting leveling off of response in these time periods.

Note that because the overall treatment by time interaction is not statistically significant, we are not performing post hoc tests to assess differences between groups at each time point. If there are *a priori* hypotheses about such differences at particular time points, they can be performed, but with appropriate adjustment for multiple testing. Although the overall treatment by time interaction is not significant, it is possible that a more focused interaction test (such as linear trend by treatment interaction or quadratic trend by group interaction) may be significant. We did perform three such tests (linear trend by treatment, quadratic trend by treatment, and cubic trend by treatment) but none of them were statistically significant (not shown here, but included in online code for this example).

The main effect of the group is statistically significant, but baseline is one of the repeated occasions in this model and, since the control group starts with slightly (not significantly) higher scores, on average, than the augmentation group at baseline, we can't interpret this as indicating that the augmentation treatment is more efficacious than the control treatment. One way to assess whether there are significant differences in post-treatment initiation between groups is to modify the model so that we covary for depression severity at baseline and drop baseline from the response set. This approach allows us to answer the question of whether controlling for baseline severity yields statistically significant differences between groups during treatment. Controlling for covariates is considered in detail in Chapter 8.

Since hypothesis tests only tell us whether there are statistically significant results, and the conclusions are heavily dependent on sample size, it is very important to estimate the magnitude of the effects and judge whether they are clinically meaningful. Because time is considered a categorical factor in the best-fitting model, we present estimates and 95% confidence intervals for mean change from baseline for each time point (Table 3.3). These estimates are shown for the entire sample, and not by group, because the overall group by

TABLE 3.3

Estimated Effects and 95% Confidence Intervals for Change from Baseline Based on the Best-Fitting Model in the Augmentation Study in Depression

Effect	Estimate (Difference of Least Square Means) with Standard Error	95% Confidence Interval
Decrease from baseline to week 1	5.48 (0.70)	(4.10, 6.85)
Decrease from baseline to week 2	10.30 (0.95)	(8.42, 12.17)
Decrease from baseline to week 3	12.73 (1.11)	(10.54, 14.91)
Decrease from baseline to week 4	14.00 (1.22)	(11.61, 16.40)
Decrease from baseline to week 5	17.20 (1.31)	(14.62, 19.77)
Decrease from baseline to week 6	19.02 (1.38)	(16.30, 21.73)

time interaction is not significant. Estimates can also be calculated by group in order to provide information that might be used in the planning of future studies.

The estimated average change from baseline to the end of the treatment period (week 6) is 19.02 with a standard error of 1.38. The corresponding 95% confidence interval is (16.30, 21.73). Thus, with 95% confidence, the change from baseline to week 6 is estimated to be between 16.30 and 21.73 points. This is a clinically meaningful change. All estimates in Table 3.3 show that there is a steady decrease in scores over time, but most of the change occurs in the first 2 weeks of the study. This is not surprising since there is more room for improvement in the beginning of the study and, as depression severity decreases, overall room for improvement is less.

The estimated variance of the random errors is 52.05 with a standard error of 6.86 (shown in the online materials). Because the estimate is several times larger than its corresponding standard error, there is substantial residual variability. The estimated variance corresponds to a standard deviation of 7.21, that is, the common standard deviation of individual observations is estimated to be 7.21. The correlation between neighboring observations is 0.77 with a standard error of 0.03. The variance and correlation estimates are in line with those from the raw data (the variances in the two groups at the different time points range between 34.36 and 78.26), with most estimates around 50. The correlation value is also in the range of raw correlations between consecutive observations (0.64–0.90). The strength of correlations in the raw data also steadily decreases with time (e.g., raw correlations between baseline and subsequent time points goes down from 0.64 for the first time point, to 0.06 for the last time point). Therefore, it is not surprising that the AR(1) structure fits the data well.

Since there are no random effects in the best-fitting model, the individual predicted values are the same as the average predicted values. If there were random effects, then we could obtain empirical Bayes estimates for the individual random effects and estimate individual-specific response trajectories over time.

Just for illustration, we consider the model with random intercept, slope, and quadratic time (Model 5 in Table 3.1) and show the estimated individual trajectories in Figure 3.11. We see that all predicted trajectories show some curvature, which is due to the inclusion of the quadratic term (both fixed and random). Also individuals differ considerably in change over time. While the majority of subjects are estimated to have initial faster decrease in severity with subsequent leveling of response, there are a few for whom there is no substantial change over time and some exhibit worsening of symptoms. It does appear that more subjects in the augmentation

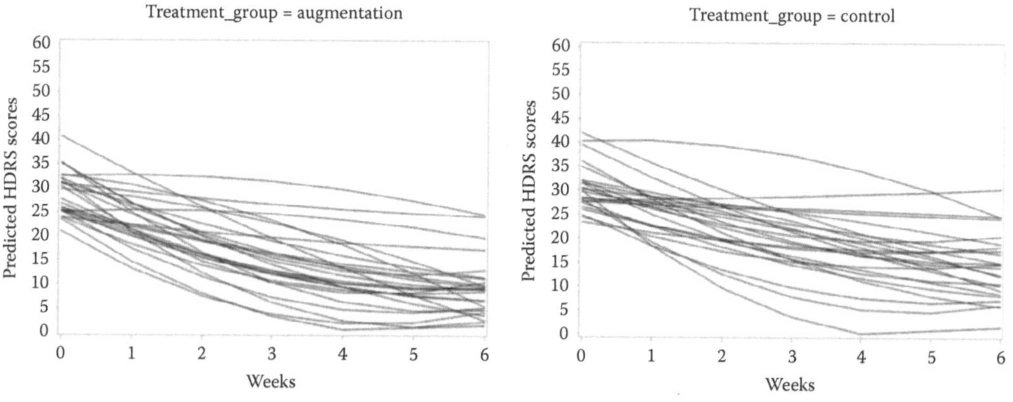

FIGURE 3.11
Predicted individuals trajectories for the Hamilton Depression Rating Scale by treatment group and week from the random intercept, slope and quadratic model fit to the data set from the augmentation study in depression.

group show improvement than in the control group but the statistical tests of the group effects in the model are not significant. Individual trajectories could be used to predict response for individuals with missing data and to classify individuals of groups, according to change over time. Individual-level inference is considered in more detail in subsequent chapters.

3.8.2 Serotonin Levels in Mother–Infant Pairs

In this study serotonin blockade was measured in breastfeeding mothers and their infants before and after maternal treatment with antidepressant medication. As shown in Section 1.5.5 where this study was introduced, there were sizeable correlations within mother–child pairs. The main hypothesis here is that there is significant change in serotonin levels in mothers from pre- to post-treatment, but not in their infants. To assess this hypothesis, we set up a mixed-effects model with the mother–infant pair as the clustering factor and with the individual (mother versus infant), time (pre- versus post-treatment), and the interaction, as fixed effects. The test of the interaction tells us whether the change in levels from pre- to post-treatment is the same in mothers and in their infants.

We assess several different variance–covariance structures within mother–infant pairs: unstructured, compound symmetry, and compound symmetry heterogeneous. The unstructured assumes different variances for all repeated observations within the mother–child pair and different correlations between any two observations within the pair. Thus, it has 4 freely estimable variances and 6 freely estimable correlations. The compound symmetry assumes equal variances of all four repeated observations within the cluster, equal correlations between any two, and thus has only two estimable parameters. The compound symmetry heterogeneous allows the variances to be different but keeps the correlations the same, and thus has 5 parameters that are estimated. Of the three mixed models, the one with the unstructured variance–covariance is the best-fitting (BIC = 548.7 compared to 597.4 for the compound symmetry model, and 553.7 for the compound symmetry heterogeneous model, AIC = 542.3 compared to 596.1 for the compound symmetry model, and 550.5 for the compound symmetry heterogeneous model). This is not surprising, since the variance of levels in mothers at post-treatment is much smaller than all other variances and the correlations between measurements on the same individual in the pair are larger than the correlations between measurements on different individuals in the pair, as shown previously in Chapter 1 (Table 1.1).

Table 3.4 presents the results from testing the model effects and the results from the corresponding post hoc tests. Both the main effects and the interaction are statistically significant (all p-values <0.0001). In such a situation the interaction needs to be interpreted.

TABLE 3.4

Test Results from the Unstructured Variance–covariance Mixed Model Fitted to Serotonin Levels in Mother–Infant Pairs

Effect	Test Statistic	p-Value
Individual (mother vs. infant)	**F(1,13) = 44.41**	**<0.0001**
Time	**F(1,13) = 43.02**	**<0.0001**
Individual × time	**F(1,13) = 73.54**	**<0.0001**
Mothers: pre vs. post	F(1,13) = 84.18	<0.0001
Infants: pre vs. post	F(1,13) = 0.09	0.77
Pre-treatment: Mother vs. infant	F(1,13) = 13.78	0.003
Post-treatment: Mother vs. infant	F(1,13) = 64.37	<0.0001

Note: The bold indicates significant main effects and interactions in the model.

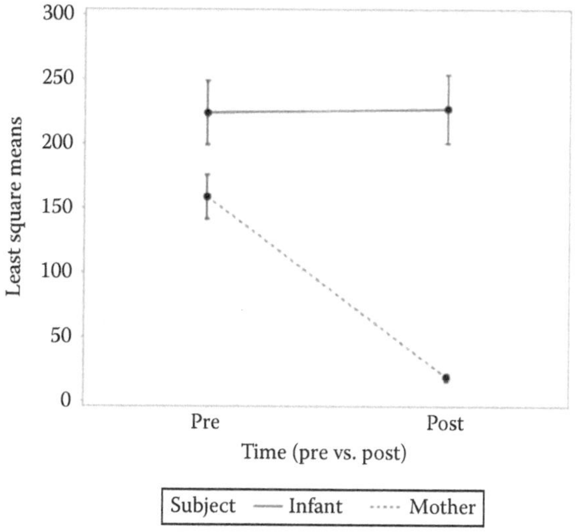

FIGURE 3.12
Estimated least square means and standard errors for the serotonin levels of mothers and infants before and after antidepressant treatment of the mother.

We perform four post hoc comparisons to assess changes in levels as a result of treatment in mothers and in infants separately, and differences between mothers' and infants' levels before treatment and after treatment. These are the *simple effects* where we evaluate the effect of each factor at all possible levels of the other factor. As expected, serotonin levels change significantly in mothers but not in their infants, with treatment. The mean change in mothers is estimated to be −140.00 (95% CI: (−172.96, −107.04)) while the mean change in infants is estimated to be 3.29 (95% CI: (−20.77, 27.34)). Both pre-treatment and post-treatment infants' levels are higher than the corresponding levels in their mothers.

Figure 3.12 shows the estimated least square means and their standard errors by type of individual and time. It is evident that infants' serotonin levels stay constant over time while mothers' levels decrease substantially. The variability of the mean of the maternal post-treatment measures is very small compared to the variability of the rest of the means.

Note that in this example we have two levels of clustering: mother–infant pairs, and individuals (mothers or infants) within a pair. Hence an alternative mixed model that we could consider is a three-level random intercept model with random intercepts for the pair and for the individual within the pair. The errors in this model are considered independent. This approach implies stronger correlations between measurements within individuals than between different individuals (mother and infant) in a pair. However, it implies that the variances of the repeated observations are the same on each occasion for both types of individuals, and this does not seem to correspond to reality. The structure that is implied is as shown below. The order of the rows/columns is as follows: mother pre-treatment, mother post-treatment, infant pre-treatment, and infant post-treatment.

$$\begin{pmatrix} \sigma^2_{pair}+\sigma^2_{ind.}+\sigma^2_{error} & \sigma^2_{pair}+\sigma^2_{ind.} & \sigma^2_{pair} & \sigma^2_{pair} \\ \sigma^2_{pair}+\sigma^2_{ind.} & \sigma^2_{pair}+\sigma^2_{ind.}+\sigma^2_{error} & \sigma^2_{pair} & \sigma^2_{pair} \\ \sigma^2_{pair} & \sigma^2_{pair} & \sigma^2_{pair}+\sigma^2_{ind.}+\sigma^2_{error} & \sigma^2_{pair}+\sigma^2_{ind.} \\ \sigma^2_{pair} & \sigma^2_{pair} & \sigma^2_{pair}+\sigma^2_{ind.} & \sigma^2_{pair}+\sigma^2_{ind.}+\sigma^2_{error} \end{pmatrix}$$

Thus, the variance of an individual observation is the sum of the variance due to the pair, the variance due to the individual within the pair, and the error variance. The covariance within the individual is just the sum of the variance due to the pair and the variance due to the individual within the pair. The covariance between observations on different individuals (mother and infant) within a pair is just equal to the variance due to the pair. This type of structure does not correspond well to the patterns seen with the sample variances and covariances, because the variance of observations on mothers, post-treatment, is markedly smaller than at pre-treatment and also compared to the variances of the observations on infants. Indeed the AIC and BIC for this model are 586.9 and 588.8, respectively—much larger than the AIC and BIC for the best-fitting unstructured covariance model (542.3 and 548.7).

A third type of mixed model that can be fit to these data is with a random intercept for mother–infant pairs and an unstructured variance–covariance matrix for the repeated observations within individuals in a pair. Such a structure allows for different variances by time point and stronger correlations within an individual. However, it still does not allow for different variances between corresponding measures for infants and mothers. It is possible to specify unstructured variance–covariance matrices with different parameters for mothers and for infants by using a special option in the model formulation. However, the current data set is fairly small, which limits the complexity of the structures that we can fit. The implied structure of this more general model is as follows:

$$\begin{pmatrix} \sigma_{pair}^2 + \sigma_{m1}^2 & \sigma_{pair}^2 + \sigma_{m12} & \sigma_{pair}^2 & \sigma_{pair}^2 \\ \sigma_{pair}^2 + \sigma_{m12} & \sigma_{pair}^2 + \sigma_{m2}^2 & \sigma_{pair}^2 & \sigma_{pair}^2 \\ \sigma_{pair}^2 & \sigma_{pair}^2 & \sigma_{pair}^2 + \sigma_{i1}^2 & \sigma_{pair}^2 + \sigma_{i12} \\ \sigma_{pair}^2 & \sigma_{pair}^2 & \sigma_{pair}^2 + \sigma_{i12} & \sigma_{pair}^2 + \sigma_{i2}^2 \end{pmatrix}$$

Here, m and i index the different structures for the mothers and the infants, respectively. Such a structure is reasonable for the data but the estimation procedure in PROC MIXED in SAS failed to converge. This is an issue that can be encountered with mixed models, especially as the models become more complicated. When this occurs one is forced to use a simpler model for which estimates can be obtained.

In summary, of all fitted models, the one with an unstructured variance–covariance matrix for the four repeated observations within mother–infant pairs was the best-fitting model and showed a statistically significant decrease of serotonin levels in mothers, but not in their infants. This suggests that antidepressant treatment with sertraline is safe for infants of breastfeeding mothers but, because of the limited sample size (only 14 mother–infant pairs), the conclusions are tentative.

3.8.3 fMRI Study of Working Memory in Schizophrenia

The already pre-processed data from this study introduced in Section 1.5.8 represent a complex repeated measures situation with multiple repeated measures factors. There is one between-subject factor, namely the group (schizophrenics versus normal controls), and three within-subject factors (task difficulty level, region of interest, and phase). The response variable is the activation levels measured during the three distinct phases of the working memory task (encoding, maintenance, and response) within each region of interest (SMFG, MFG, and IFG) for every task difficulty level (easy task and difficult task). This introduces complex correlations within individuals that need to be taken into account in the statistical model, in order to evaluate between-group differences in activation by task,

TABLE 3.5

Descriptive Statistics of Activation in fMRI Data Set by Task Difficulty Level, Region, and Working Memory Phase

Task Difficulty Level	Region	Phase	Mean	Standard Deviation
Easy	MFG	Encoding	0.35	0.17
Easy	MFG	Maintenance	0.01	0.16
Easy	MFG	Response	0.37	0.21
Easy	IFG	Encoding	0.32	0.16
Easy	IFG	Maintenance	0.04	0.16
Easy	IFG	Response	0.51	0.22
Easy	VIFG	Encoding	0.24	0.16
Easy	VIFG	Maintenance	0.02	0.15
Easy	VIFG	Response	0.30	0.16
Easy	SMFG	Encoding	0.35	0.25
Easy	SMFG	Maintenance	0.02	0.17
Easy	SMFG	Response	0.32	0.23
Hard	MFG	Encoding	0.49	0.23
Hard	MFG	Maintenance	0.04	0.21
Hard	MFG	Response	0.44	0.21
Hard	IFG	Encoding	0.42	0.25
Hard	IFG	Maintenance	0.05	0.19
Hard	IFG	Response	0.56	0.23
Hard	VIFG	Encoding	0.27	0.16
Hard	VIFG	Maintenance	0.02	0.16
Hard	VIFG	Response	0.32	0.15
Hard	SMFG	Encoding	0.44	0.32
Hard	SMFG	Maintenance	0.06	0.15
Hard	SMFG	Response	0.38	0.21

phase, and region. Furthermore, assessment of all possible interactions among the factors requires testing multifactor interactions (interactions involving two, three, or four factors).

We begin the exploration of these data by evaluating the sample variances and correlations between repeated observations on the same individual. Sample standard deviations by levels of the repeated measures factors are presented in Table 3.5. The range of the standard deviations is not very large (0.15–0.32) with the highest standard deviation (0.32) somewhat larger than the rest (the second largest standard deviation is 0.25). Correlations vary but are almost always positive (not shown but included in online materials). The raw data suggests that a structure based on a combination of random effects that imply positive correlations and equal variances may fit the data well, without the need to estimate a large number of distinct variances and correlations (i.e., not in combination with covariance patterns).

Table 3.6 presents the random effects models that we considered and the corresponding AIC and BIC, allowing us to compare different models. In all models the errors are assumed uncorrelated with equal variances. Models with combinations of random effects and structured variance–covariance matrices did not provide a better fit than the best model with random effects, and are not presented here. Furthermore, covariance pattern models without random effects did not converge, due to the large number of distinct variances and covariances that need to be estimated.

TABLE 3.6

Model Fit Criteria for the fMRI Study in Schizophrenia

Model	Random Effects	Fixed Effects	AIC	BIC
Model 1: Single-level random intercept	Intercept for subject	All main effects and interactions	−360.2	−357.7
Model 2: Two-level random intercept	Intercept for subject and for task within subject	All main effects and interactions	−362.2	−358.5
Model 3: Two-level random intercept	Intercept for subject and for phase within subject	All main effects and interactions	−401.2	−397.4
Model 4: Two-level random intercept	Intercept for subject and for region within subject	All main effects and interactions	−416.6	−412.9
Model 5: Variance components	**Random effects for subject, for task, phase, and region within subject**	**All main effects and interactions**	**−521.9**	**−515.6**
Model 6: Three-level random intercept	Intercept for subject, for task within subject and for region within subject by task	All main effects and interactions	−384.4	−379.3
Model 7: Three-level random intercept	Intercept for subject, for task within subject and for phase within subject by task	All main effects and interactions	−379.5	−374.4
Model 8: Variance components	**Random effects for subject, for task, phase, and region within subject**	**All main effects, group × phase, region × phase, task × phase, task × region**	**−607.9**	**−601.6**

Note: Model 5 is the model with all fixed effects and the best-fitting variance-covariance structure. Model 8 is the final model after backward elimination of the non-significant fixed effects.

In order to select the best-fitting variance–covariance structure, we first consider models with all possible fixed effects (i.e., the main effects of group, task difficulty level, region, and phase, and all possible interactions among them). This is necessary because the fixed effects explain some of the variance of the data. If we do not include all possible fixed effects, then we may end up selecting a variance–covariance structure that reflects some of the variance due to fixed effects. Once we select the best-fitting variance–covariance structure, we can drop non-significant fixed effects for the model, in order to achieve a more parsimonious model that describes the data well but is easier to interpret. The elimination of non-significant effects proceeds in a hierarchical fashion so that at each step the model is *hierarchically well-formulated*. This means that no lower order terms are omitted before higher order terms when these factors are dropped from the model. For example, we should not drop the main effects of factors when there are interactions involving these factors still in the model, and we should not drop two-way interactions among factors when three-way interactions involving these factors are present in the model. If the four-way interaction is significant, then we can't drop any of the lower order interactions or main effects from the model.

The elimination approach is as follows. We first consider the highest order interaction in the model and evaluate whether it is statistically significant at a pre-selected alpha level. If it is not statistically significant, we drop it, refit the model and evaluate the statistical significance of the highest order interactions in the new model. In the schizophrenia data, the highest order interaction involves four factors. If it is dropped from the model then we need to refit the model and evaluate the three-factor interactions. If at least one of these interactions is not significant at the pre-specified alpha level, then we drop the interaction with the largest p-value. Then the model is refit again and the least significant highest order interaction is dropped. This procedure continues until all highest order effects involving each factor in the model at the last stage are statistically significant. We now show how this is done on the schizophrenia data.

Of the considered models with all fixed effects in Table 3.6, model 5, which has a random intercept for subject, and for phase, region, and task difficulty level within subject, fits the data the best, according to both the AIC and BIC criteria. The random effects are all nested within subject and hence we call this model the *variance component model*, since it splits the total variance in parts due to the different factors within the subject. The exact model formulation for the random effects is as follows:

$$Y_{ijkl} = Mean_{ijkl} + b_i + b_{ij} + b_{ik} + b_{il} + \varepsilon_{ijk},$$

where:

- i denotes subject
- j denotes phase
- k denotes task difficulty level
- l denotes region

All random effects are assumed to be independent of one another and of the errors and normally distributed with different variances. This formulation results in equal variances across repeated occasions within the same subject but different correlations, depending on whether the observations are within the same task, phase, and/or region.

After selecting the best-fitting model, in terms of random effects and variance–covariance of the errors, we perform backward elimination in order to drop fixed effects that are not significant from the model. We drop the four-way interaction first, then all the three-way interactions in the following order (region × task × phase, group × region × phase, group × task × phase, group × task × region). Finally, the two-way interactions between group and region, and group and task are dropped. We are left with model 8, which has all main effects and four two-way interactions.

Table 3.7 presents the results from all overall tests of the effects in model 8. All two-way interactions involving phase are statistically significant, the interaction between task and region is

TABLE 3.7

Tests of Main Effects and Interactions from the Best-Fitting Mixed Model in the fMRI Study of Working Memory in Schizophrenia

Effect	Test Statistic	P-Value
Group	F(1,24) = 2.85	0.10
Difficulty level	**F(1,25.1) = 11.49**	**0.002**
Region	**F(3,74.7) = 8.00**	**0.0001**
Phase	**F(2,48) = 134.65**	**<0.0001**
Group × phase	**F(2,48) = 5.83**	**0.005**
Difficulty level × phase	**F(2,428) = 6.92**	**0.001**
Region × phase	**F(6,428) = 18.06**	**<0.0001**
Difficulty level × region	**F(3,430) = 2.77**	**0.04**

Note: Effects in bold are significant at 0.05 level.

also significant and the main effects of region, difficulty level, and phase are significant at 0.05 level. When interpreting significant effects in the models we focus on the highest order interactions that are significant. More information on the order of testing of effects in the model and different types of interactions (qualitative or quantitative) is provided in Chapter 6.

Table 3.8 presents the results from the tests of the simple effect of group within each phase. Similar tables can be produced for the other significant interactions in the model, however since the focus in this study is on identifying between-group differences we do not pursue post hoc analyses for the other significant effects in the model here. As seen from Table 3.8, there are significant differences in activation between groups during maintenance and response but not during encoding across regions and task difficulty levels. Estimated least square means and standard errors show that activation is lower in schizophrenic patients during maintenance and response compared to healthy controls. This indicates impaired performance during the maintenance and response phases of the working memory task across task difficulty levels and regions in the schizophrenia patients. Note that if adjustment for multiple testing of post hoc hypotheses is applied as if often needed in order to protect against committing a type II error (i.e., finding significant differences when there are in fact no differences), some of the significant p-values may become non-significant. Adjustment for multiple testing is considered in more detail in Chapter 6.

Figures 3.13 and 3.14 show plots of marginal and conditional studentized residuals, respectively, from the best-fitting model. The two sets of residuals differ in the following way. To obtain the marginal residual, the predicted value for each individual observation based only on the fixed-effects portion of the model is subtracted from the observed value. To obtain the conditional residual, the predicted value based on the fixed effects and the random effects portion of the model is subtracted from the observed value. Since there are

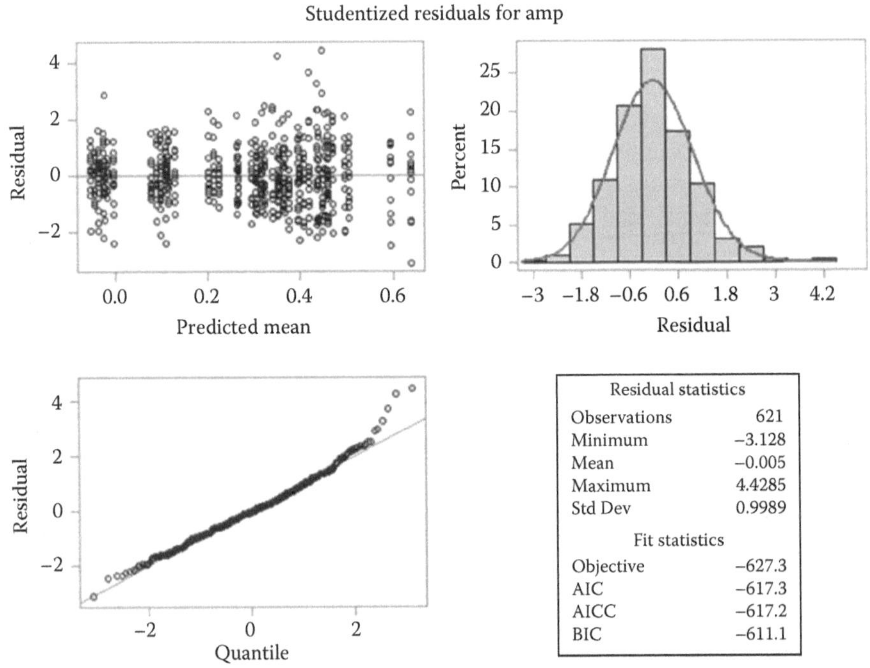

Residual statistics	
Observations	621
Minimum	−3.128
Mean	−0.005
Maximum	4.4285
Std Dev	0.9989
Fit statistics	
Objective	−627.3
AIC	−617.3
AICC	−617.2
BIC	−611.1

FIGURE 3.13
Plots of marginal studentized residuals for activation from the best-fitting model to the fMRI data set of working memory in schizophrenia.

TABLE 3.8

Tests of the Simple Effects of Group within Each Phase of the Working Memory Task in the fMRI Study in Schizophrenia

Effect	Simple Effect	At Level	LSM1 (SE1)	LSM2 (SE2)	Test Statistic	P-Value
Group × phase	schizophrenic vs. control	Encoding	0.36 (0.04)	0.35 (0.04)	$F(1,39.1) = 0.03$	0.86
Group × phase	schizophrenic vs. control	Maintenance	−0.03 (0.04)	0.11 (0.04)	$F(1,39.1) = 5.45$	0.025
Group × phase	schizophrenic vs. control	Response	0.34 (0.04)	0.47 (0.04)	$F(1,39.1) = 5.15$	0.029

Note: LSM, Least Square Mean; SE, Standard Error; 1, "schizophrenics"; 2, "controls."

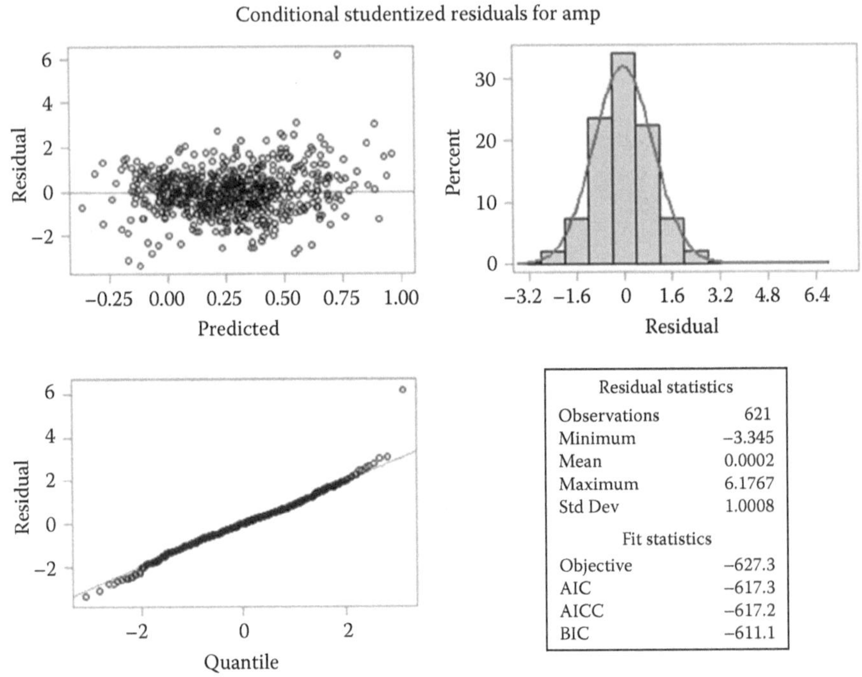

FIGURE 3.14
Plots of conditional studentized residuals for activation from the best-fitting model to the fMRI data set of working memory in schizophrenia.

several random effects, the predicted values are obtained by adding the mean prediction and the individual-specific estimates for the random effects obtained using the empirical Bayes method. Thus, the conditional residual adjusts for systematic individual-level variation from the mean due to random effects while the marginal residual does not.

In the upper-left plot of Figure 3.13, the marginal residuals are stacked in columns because there is a fixed number of different combinations of levels of the fixed effects. In contrast, in the corresponding plot in Figure 3.14 the residuals form a cloud with more randomness because in this case the predicted individual values have been obtained by adding the estimates of the random effects to the mean predictor. Both sets of residuals are approximately normally distributed with a few positive outliers. In particular, there is one large positive conditional residual as indicated in the lower left plot in Figure 3.14. Measures of influence can be used to ascertain whether these outliers are significantly affecting the results. A simple method of sensitivity analysis is to repeat the main analysis with and without the potential outliers. If the results do not change substantively, then the residuals are not influential. In this particular example, the results did not change substantively when the outlying observation was removed and hence the results can be considered to be robust.

3.8.4 Meta-Analysis of Clinical Trials in Schizophrenia

Mixed-effects models can also be used for joint analysis of data from different studies. Meta-analysis typically involves combining the results of studies of the effect of a particular medication or intervention so that an overall estimate of effect size can be obtained that succinctly summarizes the available empirical evidence in published and unpublished data. The individual observations in such an analysis are usually the effect sizes from different studies (e.g., standardized mean differences between the response on the experimental and the control treatment in each study) and a fixed effects or a random effects approach is used. The fixed-effects approach is focused on estimation of the overall effect where the study-specific effects are assumed to deviate randomly from the overall effect and are weighted according to their variability. The random effects approach incorporates additional random study-specific variability by introducing a random intercept in the model and thus allowing to account for heterogeneity in effects among the different studies. More information on statistical and other aspects of meta-analysis can be found in Normand (1999).

The *meta-analysis of clinical trials in schizophrenia* (Woods et al., 2005) introduced in Section 1.5.6 seeks to assess whether the degree of improvement with antipsychotic medication on active treatment depends on the type of design (i.e., whether the study includes an active, low dose or placebo control). To answer this question, the focus is on the average improvement on the outcome of interest in the active study arms rather than on the effect size comparing active to control groups. The response is the Brief Psychiatric Rating Scale (BPRS), with larger scores indicating worse symptoms, and the study-specific outcome measure is the change in BPRS scores from baseline to endpoint per treatment arm. Since multiple active arms per study are entered in this meta-analysis, it is imperative to include a random effect for study in order to account for both between-study heterogeneity and for correlations between outcomes in the different arms within study.

In this investigation (Woods et al., 2005), individual studies were categorized in one of three design types: placebo-controlled, low dose-controlled and active-controlled design. Each active dose arm in the studies was categorized in one of three dose ranges: effective doses that consistently separated from placebo, ineffective doses like those used as low dose controls and intermediate doses.

The random effects model we focus on includes fixed effects of drug (risperidone, olanzapine, quetiapine or ziprasidone), a combined dose/design variable (effective dose/placebo control, intermediate dose/placebo control, ineffective dose/placebo control, effective dose/low dose control, intermediate dose/low dose control, ineffective dose/low dose control, effective dose/active control), baseline BPRS mean and a random intercept. The response is mean BPRS change scores per treatment arm and the clusters are the different studies. The combined dose/design variable is needed because not all combinations of dose and design levels are possible and hence we should not simply include main effects of design and dose and their interaction. In particular, studies with active-control design designs do not have intermediate or ineffective doses as seen from Table 1.2 in Chapter 1, which gives descriptive statistics of the study-specific outcomes. The main hypothesis test of interest in the analysis, presented in the original publication and herein, is the test of the overall dose/design variable with post hoc contrasts to examine the effects of design within each level of dose. The analysis is performed in SAS using SAS PROC MIXED, the between-study variance is estimated together with the fixed effects and the standard errors of the change score means are held fixed at their reported values as is the common practice in meta-analyses. More details about the study and the analysis can be found in Woods et al. (2005) and the code to fit the models and estimate the effects is included in the online materials.

The overall test of the design/dose variable is statistically significant ($F(6,27)=15.93$, $p<0.0001$). Least square means and standard errors by design/dose level are shown in Figure 3.15. Post hoc mean comparisons of improvement in BPRS between different types of designs within dose range are included in Table 3.9. Average improvement on the BPRS at effective doses is significantly more in active-controlled designs than in either placebo-controlled or low dose-controlled designs. Improvement is also more substantial

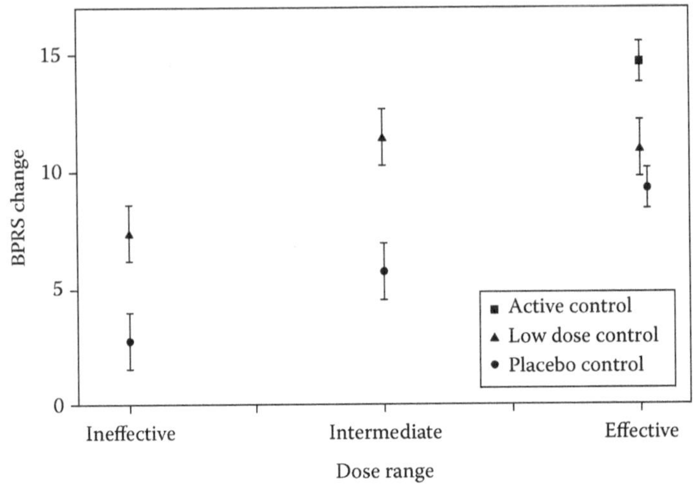

FIGURE 3.15
Model-based BPRS change mean and standard error estimates for the three different design types across dose ranges in the meta-analysis of clinical trials in schizophrenia.

TABLE 3.9
Tests of the Simple Effects of Design within Each dose Range in the Meta-Analysis of Clinical Trials in Schizophrenia

Effect	At Dose Range	LSM1 (SE1)	LSM2 (SE2)	P-Value	Least Square Mean Difference (95% CI)
Active control vs. placebo control	Effective	14.76 (0.76)	8.41 (0.87)	<0.001	6.35 (3.89, 8.82)
Active control vs. low dose control	Effective	14.76 (0.76)	10.18 (1.30)	0.005	4.58 (1.47, 7.69)
Low dose control vs. placebo control	Effective	10.18 (1.30)	8.41 (0.87)	0.27	1.77 (−1.43, 4.97)
Low dose control vs. placebo control	Intermediate	10.38 (1.42)	5.46 (0.97)	0.008	4.92 (1.38, 8.46)
Low dose control vs. placebo control	Ineffective	7.10 (1.36)	3.30 (1.24)	0.05	3.80 (0.03, 7.57)

Note: LSM, Least Square Mean; SE, Standard Error; 1, "schizophrenics"; 2, "controls."

at intermediate and ineffective doses but not at effective doses when low dose-controlled designs are compared to placebo-controlled designs.

This analysis demonstrates that magnitude of improvement in symptoms in clinical trials in schizophrenia depends on the type of design. In particular, in active-controlled trials the improvement on effective doses is nearly double (14.76 points on average) compared to the improvement in placebo-controlled trials (8.41 points on average). Multiple possible explanations for this result are possible. For example, there might be selection or expectancy bias as subjects who enroll in active-controlled trials may be different from subjects who enroll in placebo-controlled trials, or patients and providers may have different expectations and behavior in active vs. placebo-controlled trials. Detailed discussion of the results and their interpretation can be found in Woods et al. (2005). Herein, we focus on providing a different type of example of the application of mixed models in order to illustrate the flexibility and wide use of the approach.

3.8.5 Citalopram Effects on Depressive Symptom Clusters in the STAR*D Study

The first phase of the STAR*D clinical trial (described in more detail in Section 1.5.2), was a 12-week treatment with citalopram. Depression symptoms were assessed using the QIDS rating scale at several visits during the 12-week period with individuals deviating somewhat from the planned schedule of visits. In this analysis, we are interested in assessing the improvement in the average scores of the three clusters of depressive symptoms (core, sleep and atypical) and comparing the effects of citalopram on the different symptom clusters. Since individuals are assessed at different time points and hence the design is unbalanced, we need to use random effects rather than covariance-pattern models in order to take into account the correlations between repeated observations within individuals. We consider several random effects models of increasing complexity and compare the fit of these models as described below.

We analyze the three symptom clusters together, in order to be able to assess statistically whether the citalopram effects are similar or different across clusters. As in the augmentation study in depression example, for these data there is indication that the relationship between time and depression severity is curvilinear with larger initial improvement and then leveling off of the response on average. This seems to hold for each of the three clusters. Therefore, we again log-transform time and consider linear fixed effects in log time for each symptom cluster. Thus the fixed-effects portion of the model includes cluster (coded by two dummy variables), log time and the interactions between cluster and log time as shown in the model equation for the best model below. The interactions are needed to allow us to assess the differences in change over time for the three clusters.

We consider several random effects structures with increasing complexity. In particular, we start with a model with three random intercepts (one for each cluster) that are uncorrelated across the clusters, then consider a model with correlated random intercepts, then add on random slopes, first uncorrelated with the random intercepts and across clusters, then gradually build-in all possible correlations. Table 3.10 shows the model fit criteria for

TABLE 3.10

Model Fit Criteria for Mixed-Effects Models Fitted to the Depression Symptom Cluster Scores in the STAR*D Study

Model	Fixed Effects	AIC	BIC
Model 1: Uncorrelated random intercepts	Cluster Time Cluster × Time	78255.9	78281.1
Model 2: Correlated random intercepts	Cluster Time Cluster × Time	75290.8	75334.9
Model 3: Uncorrelated random intercepts and common random slope for all clusters	Cluster Time Cluster × Time	75234.9	75266.4
Model 4: Correlated random intercepts and common random slope for all clusters	Cluster Time Cluster × Time	72940.2	73009.5
Model 5: Random intercepts and slopes correlated only within cluster	Cluster Time Cluster × Time	75632.3	75689.0
Model 6: Correlated random intercepts and slopes	**Cluster Time Cluster × Time**	**71224.2**	**71362.7**

Note: Model 6 indicated in bold is the best-fitting model according to AIC and BIC.

these different models. The best-fitting model is the most general one with correlated random intercepts and slopes (Model 6).

Thus, the selected model is

$$Y_{ijk} = \beta_1 d_{j1} + \beta_2 d_{j2} + \beta_3 d_{j3} + \beta_4 d_{j1} \log t_{ik} + \beta_5 d_{j2} \log t_{ik} + \beta_6 d_{j3} \log t_{ik}$$

$$+ b_{i1} d_{j1} + b_{i2} d_{j2} + b_{i3} d_{j3} + b_{i4} d_{j1} \log t_{ik} + b_{i5} d_{j2} \log t_{ik} + b_{i6} d_{j3} \log t_{ik} + \varepsilon_{ijk}$$

where:

- i indicates individual
- j indicates cluster within individual
- k denotes time

The three dummy variables d_{j1}, d_{j2} and d_{j3} indicate the three different clusters. That is, for observations Y_{ijk} from the core cluster: $d_{j1}=1$, $d_{j2}=0$ and $d_{j3}=0$; from the atypical cluster: $d_{j1}=0$, $d_{j2}=1$ and $d_{j3}=0$; and from the sleep cluster: $d_{j1}=0$, $d_{j2}=0$ and $d_{j3}=1$. Since we are using as many dummy variables as there are clusters, we excluded the overall intercept and the main effect of time. This notation allows for a very simple interpretation of the coefficients in the model as intercepts and slopes in the appropriate clusters. By substituting the appropriate dummy codes, we get the following simple random intercept and slope models for each cluster:

Core cluster: $Y_{i1k} = \beta_1 + \beta_4 \log t_{ik} + b_{i1} + b_{i4} \log t_{ik} + \varepsilon_{i1k}$;

Atypical cluster: $Y_{i2k} = \beta_2 + \beta_5 \log t_{ik} + b_{i2} + b_{i5} \log t_{ik} + \varepsilon_{i2k}$;

Core cluster: $Y_{i3k} = \beta_3 + \beta_6 \log t_{ik} + b_{i3} + b_{i6} \log t_{ik} + \varepsilon_{i3k}$.

The reason we combined these in one model, is to take into account the correlations among observations on different clusters and to compare the fixed intercepts and slopes of the different clusters statistically. In the most general model from Table 3.10, the variances and covariances of the random effects are unrestricted.

All regression parameter estimates are highly statistically significant (p-values <0.0001) which is unsurprising given that the entire sample size is 4019 individuals with up to 27 observations per individual (up to 9 repeated observations on three clusters). Thus citalopram appears to significantly improve symptoms over time.

Figure 3.16 shows the estimated average cluster scores over time for the three clusters. Since the symptom scores on the three clusters have the same range (0–3) the values are directly comparable. From the differences in intercepts, we see that at baseline participants endorse more core and sleep symptoms than atypical symptoms. On the other hand, the improvement over time in core symptoms is most pronounced while sleep and atypical symptoms improve less and at a slower rate. To quantify these apparent differences, we refer to Table 3.11 which presents the estimated intercepts and slopes (in log time) and the comparisons among those with estimated 95% confidence intervals. The observations from the figure are confirmed by the estimates in this table with only the difference in intercepts between core and sleep clusters not statistically significant. Thus, we can conclude that citalopram has the most pronounced effect on core depressive symptoms with less of an effect on sleep symptoms and the least effect on atypical symptoms.

TABLE 3.11

Estimated Intercepts, Slopes, and Contrasts between Clusters with Associated 95% Confidence Intervals in the STAR*D Clinical Trial

Effect	Estimate (95% Confidence Interval)
Intercept for core cluster	1.76 (1.74, 1.78)
Intercept for atypical cluster	0.84 (0.82, 0.85)
Intercept for sleep cluster	1.74 (1.71, 1.76)
Difference in intercepts for core and atypical clusters	0.92 (0.91, 0.94)
Difference in intercepts for core and sleep clusters	0.02 (−0.01, 0.05)
Difference in intercepts for atypical and sleep clusters	−0.90 (−0.93, −0.87)
Slope for core cluster	−0.40 (−0.41, −0.39)
Slope for atypical cluster	−0.16 (−0.17, −0.16)
Slope for sleep cluster	−0.26 (−0.28, −0.25)
Difference in slopes for core and atypical clusters	−0.23 (−0.24, −0.22)
Difference in slopes for core and sleep clusters	−0.13 (−0.15, −0.12)
Difference in slopes for atypical and sleep clusters	0.10 (0.09, 0.11)

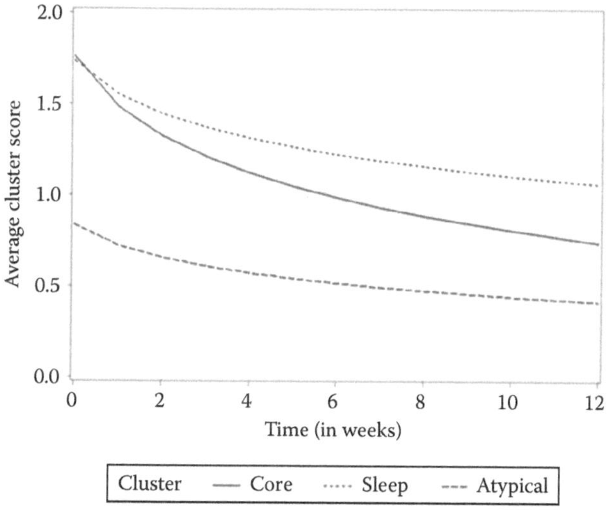

FIGURE 3.16
Predicted trajectories for average depression cluster symptom scores in the STRD*D clinical trial.

3.9 Summary

In this chapter, we introduced mixed-effects models for approximately normally distributed outcome measures and showed how correlations between repeated measures and data variability can be taken into account by random effects, structured variance–covariance matrices or combinations of the two. We focused on model definition, various error structures, selection of best-fitting model and briefly discussed model diagnostics. We also discussed interpretation and presented graphical methods for visualizing the results and checking of model assumptions. This is by no means a comprehensive treatment of this topic. We refer the interested reader to Brown and Prescott (2006) for information on different types of studies and how to fit models to such data using SAS, to Littell et al. (2000) for more on selection of the variance–covariance structure and to Weiss (2005), Hedeker and Gibbons (2006) and to Fitzmaurice et al. (2011) for more information on fitting trends over time.

Mixed-effects models are considered the gold standard method for the analysis of repeated measures data because they use all available data on individuals, are very flexible in accounting for variability across occasions and correlations between repeated measures in both balanced and unbalanced designs, and provide unbiased and efficient estimates under general assumptions for missing data. However, special attention needs to be paid to model formulation and interpretation. Since the selection of the best-fitting mixed model is not clear cut, there is potential for reaching different conclusions from different mixed models on the same data set. Additional topics related to mixed models such as effects of missing data and heterogeneous trajectories over time are considered in subsequent chapters. In particular, Chapter 7 discusses missing data in detail while Chapter 10 focuses on models that allow subgroups of the sample to follow categorically different trajectories over time. Chapter 4 shows how mixed models are extended for non-normally distributed outcomes, and Chapter 5 describes non-parametric alternatives. Chapter 12 mentions further extensions such as models for multiple repeatedly measured outcomes, non-parametric time modeling, intensive longitudinal data, non-linear and non-parametric models.

4

Linear Models for Non-Normal Outcomes

The linear mixed models (LMM), presented in the previous chapter, extend the classical linear models for non-correlated data to the analysis of clustered and longitudinal data when the outcome variable is quantitative and can be assumed to be approximately normally distributed. When the outcome is categorical or a count, or when its distribution is not normal and can't be transformed to normality, other models need to be considered. For example, very often treatment response in medical studies is measured by a categorical variable with two or more categories. Patients may be "responders" or "non-responders," showing a different degree of improvement ("very much improved," "improved," "not improved," or "deteriorated"), or diagnosed with different subtypes of a certain disease. Outcomes can also be non-negative counts: for example, the number of suicides per geographic area or the number of positive urine tests over a period. Other variables, such as number of drinks per drinking day, have distributions that are skewed and often can't be transformed to normality. A wider class of models than linear models, namely *generalized linear models* (GLM) (Nelder and Wedderburn, 1972), unite such outcomes under the same umbrella and allow statistical inference to be performed within the same theoretical framework. GLM are appropriate for cross-sectional data where there are no statistical associations among the observations, but extensions have been developed that allow incorporating statistical dependence between observations on the same individual or within a cluster.

GLM assume that the outcome variable has a distribution in the *exponential family* (McCullagh and Nelder, 1989). This family encompasses many distributions and includes the *Bernoulli* distribution for *binary data,* the *Poisson* distribution for *count data,* the *gamma* distribution for *skewed continuous data,* and the normal distribution for *bell-shaped continuous data.* GLM extensions are also available for dealing with categorical responses that may be *ordinal* (i.e., with ordered categories such as graded levels of improvement) or *nominal* (i.e., with categories that do not have natural ordering such as different disease types). In GLM, mathematically convenient functions relate the mean of the outcome to a linear combination of the predictors. This is necessary because the mean response is often restricted to be within a certain range, hence it is not appropriate to allow it to get outside of this range for some levels of the covariates. For example, the mean of dichotomous data is the same as the probability of the response of interest (e.g., treatment response or remission, usually coded as 1 with the opposite outcome coded as 0), which is restricted to be between 0 and 1. If we directly model the mean (probability) as a linear combination of the predictors, as is done in the linear model for normally distributed outcomes, then for some values of the predictors the estimated probability may be less than 0 or greater than 1. This is not reasonable and, therefore, for binary data, the effects of the predictors are often assessed on the logit (log odds) scale, as described in the next section. In the case of non-negative count data, the mean can't be negative because the counts can't be negative. Therefore, for count data, the log of the mean, rather than the mean itself, is related to the linear combination of the predictors. Interpretation of estimated coefficients in GLM is specific to the type of outcome and to the distributional and model assumptions.

In this chapter, we present two types of extensions of GLMs for longitudinal or clustered data: *marginal (population-averaged) models* that focus on estimation of the effects of predictor variables on the average response in the population and treat the association structure of the repeated measures as a nuisance, and *random effects (subject-specific) models* that focus on inference at the individual level and jointly estimate the parameters characterizing the mean and the association structure. Because of the non-linearity in the relationship between the predictors and the response with non-normal data, the population-averaged effect of a predictor is not the same as the subject-specific effect. For example, the odds ratio for the effect of a predictor within an individual is not the same as the odds ratio for the effect of the same predictor in the population. This distinction is explained in more detail further in this chapter.

The population-average approach presented herein is based on the classical *generalized estimating equations* (GEE) (Zeger et al., 1988) while the subject-specific approach is based on *generalized linear mixed models* (GLMM) (Clayton, 1992). These two classes of models are described in a fairly concise way without going into technical details and considering different extensions of the methodology. A multitude of publications has been dedicated to these approaches in recent years. Comprehensive textbooks are the works of Hardin and Hilbe (2013) and Ziegler (2011) for GEE, and of McCulloch and Searle (2001), Jiang (2007), and Stroup (2013) for GLMM. A fairly non-technical introduction for GEE is provided by Hanley et al. (2003), and for GLMM by Bolker et al. (2009).

While in LMM correlations between repeated measures are incorporated by assuming a certain pattern for the variances and covariances, and/or including random effects in the linear predictor, GEE and GLMM are different model extensions, depending on whether one specifies the variance–covariance structure directly or includes random effects. In GLMM statistical associations between repeated measures on the same individual are incorporated strictly by specifying random effects for individuals and/or clusters. GEE, on the other hand, do not include any random effects, consider the correlation structure of the repeated observations as a nuisance, and assume a working correlation structure that has minimal effect on the fixed-effects estimates, which are of primary interest. Figure 4.1 illustrates the relationship between these different classes of models and the underlying

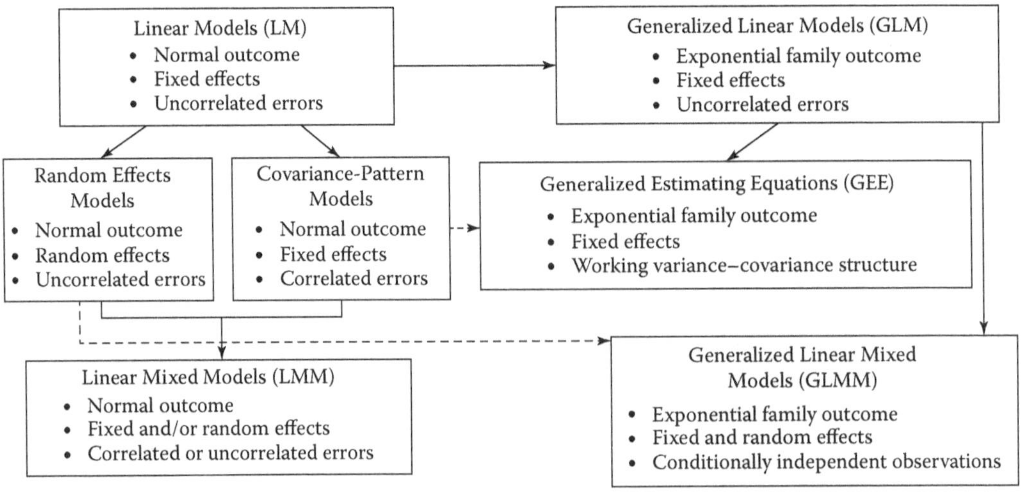

FIGURE 4.1
Relationship between different types of linear models.

assumptions for the outcomes, the presence or absence of random effects, and the statistical dependence of the observations. Note that GEE models can be regarded as extensions of covariance-pattern models while GLMM models can be regarded as extensions of random effects models for outcomes in the exponential family. When the outcome is not normally distributed, the two extensions of GLM can't be combined under the same umbrella, as was done for random effects models and covariance-pattern models in the LMM framework.

There are major differences in GLMM and GEE in model assumptions, estimation, and interpretation. While in LMM, the estimates of the fixed regression coefficients are interpreted exactly the same, regardless of whether the variance–covariance structure is directly modeled or implied by the use of random effects, in GEE and in GLMM the interpretation is different. In GEE, the focus is on estimation of *marginal effects*. That is, we estimate how the outcome in the population changes, on average, if the predictors are varied in the population. In contrast, in GLMM the focus is on individual-level response, and thus, the effects of the predictors have *subject-specific interpretation*. That is, we estimate how the outcome of an individual is expected to change if the predictors are varied for that individual. Thus, when interest lies in estimation of average effects in the population, one should use GEE, and when interest lies in estimation of the effects of predictors within individuals, one should use GLMM.

GEE and GLMM also differ in robustness of their inferences in the presence of missing data with GLMM, in general, providing valid results under a wider range of missing data assumptions. While GLMM models can handle unbalanced designs where individuals are observed at different occasions, GEE usually requires balanced designs. An exception is the *quasi-least squares* (QLS) approach for estimation of the correlation parameters in the framework of GEE (Shults and Hilbe, 2014). On the other hand, fewer assumptions are necessary for GEE models to provide valid inference, compared to GLMM, in situations when both can be used and missing data are not an issue (i.e., only the mean structure needs to be approximately correctly specified rather than both the mean and the variance structure).

In this chapter, we first provide a short introduction to GLM, which are the basis for both GEE and GLMM extensions. Particular attention is paid to binary, count, and ordinal outcomes. Separate sections are then devoted to GEE and GLMM. Data examples are used throughout for illustration and SAS code and output are available in the online materials. The chapter concludes with a summary and suggestions for further reading. Missing data issues are discussed in more detail in Chapter 7.

4.1 Generalized Linear Models (GLM)

GLM are extensions of linear models for outcomes with distributions in the *exponential family* (Harville, 1977; McCullagh and Nelder, 1989). This allows quantitative outcomes with approximately normal distributions and a wide range of other outcomes (binary, count, and quantitative outcomes with skewed distributions) to be considered within the same analytical framework. That is, the models can be constructed in a similar manner, the same estimation procedure can be used, and statistical inference is based on common theory. We first describe GLM by considering a couple of special cases (logistic regression for binary data, Poisson regression for count data) and show how these models are combined in the same framework. Note that in GLM the outcomes are assumed to be independent and hence GLM are not appropriate for clustered or longitudinal data. GLMM and GEE extensions for correlated data are presented in Sections 4.2 and 4.3.

4.1.1 Logistic Regression for Binary Data

Binary data are quite common in medical studies. For example, in substance abuse often the outcome is whether a subject is using a particular substance or not. Also, binary measures of treatment response and remission are of primary interest in many clinical trials. When a single binary measure is collected on each individual in a study, then *logistic regression* (Hosmer and Lemeshow, 1989) can be used to assess the effect of treatment, exposure, and/or covariates on the outcome. In logistic regression, we relate the log of the *odds* of the outcome of interest (e.g., response, remission; denoted by Y) to a linear function of predictors, as shown in Equation 4.1. As a reminder, the odds of an outcome are the ratio of the probability of that outcome and the probability of the opposite outcome. For example, the odds of remission are equal to the probability of remission divided by the probability of non-remission. If the probability of remission is one-half (1/2 or 0.5), then the odds of remission are 1 as both the probability of remission and the probability of non-remission are equal to one-half. If the probability of remission is one quarter (1/4 or 0.25), then the odds of remission are equal to one-third: $0.25/(1-0.25)=0.25/0.75=1/3$. It is important to keep in mind this difference between odds and probabilities, in order to interpret results from logistic regression models appropriately.

For simplicity, we define the basic logistic regression model in the context of an example. We consider the augmentation study in depression and treatment response (a score of 10 or less on the HDRS at endpoint) as a dichotomous outcome. The outcome Y_i is often coded as 1 or 0, where 1 denotes the event of interest. The unknown probability of the outcome (treatment response) for the ith subject is $P(Y_i=1)=p_i$. A simple logistic model that we can consider is as follows:

$$\log\left(\frac{p_i}{1-p_i}\right)=\beta_0+\beta_1 Group_i \tag{4.1}$$

That is, we hypothesize that the log odds of the outcome of interest (treatment response) are associated with group membership via the linear function in the beta regression coefficients on the right. The group is coded as 1 for individuals in the augmentation group, and as 0 for individuals in the control group. Thus the β_0 parameter is interpreted as the *log odds* (i.e., log-transformed odds) of response in the control group and the β_1 parameter is interpreted as the difference in the log odds of response in the augmentation group and in the control group. Since the difference of two logs is equal to the log of the ratio, the β_1 parameter is the *log odds ratio* of response in the augmentation group, compared to the control group. Exponentiating β_1 (i.e., taking $\exp(\beta_1)$) gives the odds ratio of the group effect (i.e., the odds ratio of response in the augmentation group compared to the control group). Exponentiating β_0 (i.e., taking $\exp(\beta_0)$) gives the odds of response in the control group, while exponentiating $\beta_0+\beta_1$ (i.e., taking $\exp(\beta_0+\beta_1)$) gives the odds of response in the augmentation group.

Note that $\beta_1>0$ corresponds to an odds ratio greater than 1 and a positive association between the group and the outcome (i.e., individuals have higher odds of the outcome in the treatment compared to the control group). On the other hand, $\beta_1 < 0$ corresponds to an odds ratio less than 1 and a negative association between the group and the outcome (i.e., individuals have lower odds of the outcome in the treatment group compared to the control group). $\beta_1 = 0$ corresponds to no association between group and the outcome, i.e., the odds of response are the same in both groups.

Based on the estimated odds of the outcome for each group, we can estimate the corresponding probabilities. If the odds are 1, then the probability is ½, if the odds are larger than 1 then the probability is greater than ½, and if the odds are smaller than 1 then the probability is smaller than ½.

In the depression data set, 17 out of 26 subjects (65.4%) in the augmentation group are responders at the end of the study, while 10 out of 24 subjects (41.7%) in the control group are responders. Thus the odds of response in the augmentation and control group are, respectively, 1.89 and 0.72. The odds ratio for the comparison between the augmentation and the control group is 2.64 (95% CI: 0.84, 8.31). This is interpreted as the odds of response in the augmentation group being more than two and a half times larger than in the control group. Since the confidence interval includes 1, the groups are not considered to be statistically significantly different in terms of their odds of achieving response.

Note that the coding of the outcomes and categorical predictor variables determines the interpretation of the odds ratio. If we switch the coding of the group variable so that the control group is coded as 1 and the augmentation group is coded as 0, the new parameter evaluating the group effect (let's call it β_1^*) is just the negative of $\beta_1 \left(\beta_1^* = -\beta_1\right)$ and corresponds to the log-odds ratio of response in the control group compared to the augmentation group. When we exponentiate to obtain the odds ratio for the comparison of the control group to the augmentation group, we get the inverse of the odds ratio when comparing the augmentation group to the control group: $\exp\left(\beta_1^*\right) = 1/\exp\left(\beta_1\right)$.

In the depression data the odds ratio for the comparison between the control and the augmentation group is 0.38 (95% CI: 0.12, 1.19) ($0.38 \approx 1/(2.67)$). Thus, the odds of response in the control group are less than 40% of the odds in the augmentation group.

As in linear models with normal outcomes, in logistic regression we usually have multiple predictors. For example, if there are more than 2 groups then several dummy variables are necessary to code all possible levels of the group factor and each dummy variable has its own beta coefficient. Depending on the coding, each beta coefficient corresponds to an odds ratio comparing a certain group to the reference group when keeping the rest of the predictors constant. There might also be additional continuous predictors, for example depression severity at baseline as shown in Equation 4.2.

$$\log\left(\frac{p_i}{1-p_i}\right) = \beta_0 + \beta_1 Group_i + \beta_2 BaselineHDRS_i \tag{4.2}$$

For continuous predictors, the regression coefficients are interpreted as the change in log odds of the outcome per unit change in the predictor when the other predictors are held constant. For example, the log odds of remission increases\decreases by β_2 (depending on the sign of β_2) for each unit increase in baseline HDRS score. Since there are no interactions in Equation 4.2 we assume that this change is the same in both groups. If we include an interaction between group and baseline HDRS score then we allow this effect to vary by group. Controlling for baseline covariates and interpreting main and interactive effects of baseline covariates and treatment is considered in more detail in Chapter 8.

To build up toward the GLM definition, we emphasize three aspects of the logistic regression model:

1. We assume that the binary outcomes Y_i are independent of one another and have *Bernoulli distribution* with the probability of the outcome of interest denoted by p_i. This means that the probability of the opposite outcome is $1-p_i$ The mean of the Bernoulli distribution is equal to p_i and the variance is equal to $p_i(1-p_i)$. Unlike the normal distribution, where the mean and the variance are entirely independent of one another, here the variance is related to the mean.
2. We describe the effects of covariates as a linear function in the parameters, as shown in the right-hand side expression of Equations 4.1 and 4.2. This expression is called the linear predictor and can be any linear combination of predictors (quantitative or categorical coded by dummy variables) including interactions.
3. We relate the mean of the response distribution (p_i) to the linear predictor via a mathematically convenient function. In logistic regression, we use the logit function, which is the log odds of the outcome of interest. This function takes a variable that is restricted to be between 0 and 1 and makes it unrestricted. This way, there is no problem with equating the log odds of the response to a linear predictor that is entirely unrestricted and can also take positive and negative values.

These three aspects are defined for each GLM model, as shown later in this chapter. We now turn attention to Poisson regression for count data.

4.1.2 Poisson Regression for Count Data

Counts are also frequently encountered as outcomes in a variety of studies. For example, the number of drinking days or number of drinks may be outcomes of interest in alcohol studies. The number of positive urine tests is often an outcome in substance use data sets. The number of symptoms or number of occurrences of certain side effects can also be of interest. Counts are positive integers or zero, and very often exhibit skewed distributions. Hence, using linear regression models for normally distributed outcomes is not appropriate. A commonly used distribution for count data is the Poisson distribution and *log-linear regression models* are used to assess the effects of predictors on average response.

To introduce the basic log-linear regression model for count data, we consider the COMBINE clinical trial, introduced in Chapter 1 (Section 1.5.3), which assessed the combined effects of three treatments in alcohol dependence on drinking measures over 16 weeks. The outcome of interest, herein, is the number of drinking days in the last four weeks (called month, for simplicity) of the study period. We chose this outcome because it allows us to illustrate several different GLM and extensions on the same data. Some of the considered models may not be entirely appropriate because assumptions may not be satisfied, but herein, we emphasize the mechanism of constructing such models. An overview of the different analyses and a recommendation for the preferred approach is provided toward the end of this chapter.

We denote the outcome for the ith subject as Y_i and assume that the outcome has a Poisson distribution with mean μ_i. Later on we describe why this assumption is not very reasonable. A simple log-linear model is as follows:

$$\log \mu_i = \beta_0 + \beta_1 Naltrexone_i + \beta_2 CBI_i + \beta_3 Naltrexone_i \times CBI_i \tag{4.3}$$

Here, $Naltrexone_i$ and CBI_i are indicator variables that are equal to 1 if the participant received active naltrexone or CBI, respectively, and 0 otherwise. For simplicity, we ignore whether individuals received the third randomized treatment in the study (acamprosate). The regression coefficients for the naltrexone and CBI effects are interpreted as logarithmically transformed ratios of means. More commonly the coefficients are interpreted as logarithmically transformed ratios of rates since the Poisson distribution is often used in situations when subjects are followed up for different amounts of time or when rare events are modeled (e.g., suicide rates in a population).

In the COMBINE study, some subjects have missing data in the last four weeks of treatment, therefore, for them there are fewer days over which the counts of heavy drinking data can be accumulated. If τ_i corresponds to the actual number of days for which information on the ith subject is available, the model can be modified as follows:

$$\log\left(\frac{\mu_i}{\tau_i}\right) = \beta_0^* + \beta_1^* Naltrexone_i + \beta_2^* CBI_i + \beta_3^* Naltrexone_i \times CBI_i \quad (4.4)$$

or equivalently

$$\log \mu_i = \log \tau_i + \beta_0^* + \beta_1^* Naltrexone_i + \beta_2^* CBI_i + \beta_3^* Naltrexone_i \times CBI_i \quad (4.5)$$

where $\log \tau_i$ is called the offset.

In this new formulation, the regression parameters are in general different and the offset can't be combined with the intercept because subjects have different follow-up times. The beta star parameters of the group effects are interpreted as logarithmically transformed mean (or rate) ratios of drinking adjusted for the actual lengths of follow-up for the different subjects. For simplicity, from here on we refer to these as rate ratios although sometimes it may be better to interpret in terms of mean ratios.

Exponentiating the regression coefficients provides the rate ratios, which are of primary interest. In particular, $\exp(\beta_1)$ is the rate ratio for the comparison of the naltrexone only group to the control group who did not get either naltrexone or CBI, $\exp(\beta_2)$ is the rate ratio for the comparison of the CBI only group to the control group, $\exp(\beta_1+\beta_3)$ is the rate ratio for the comparison of the active naltrexone+CBI group to the CBI only group, and $\exp(\beta_2+\beta_3)$ is the rate ratio for the comparison of the active naltrexone+CBI group to the naltrexone only group.

Testing whether β_3 is different from 0 is a test of the interaction between the two treatments. $\beta_3=0$ implies that there is no interaction between the two treatments while $\beta_3>0$ corresponds to a rate ratio greater than 1 and $\beta_3<0$ corresponds to a rate ratio less than 1 If, in addition, there are continuous predictors then the coefficients for these predictors are interpreted as rate ratios corresponding to unit change in the predictor when the other predictors are held constant.

When the Poisson log-linear model is fitted to the number of drinking days in the last month of the COMBINE study, all estimated beta coefficients are statistically significantly different from 0 ($p<0.0001$). The estimated means for the four groups together with 95% confidence intervals are provided in the third column of Table 4.1. The means are slightly different than the raw (unadjusted) means, since they adjust for the length of follow-up. The second column in Table 4.2 shows the corresponding rate ratios for all possible

TABLE 4.1

Raw and Model-Based Means of Number of Drinking Days in the Last Month of Treatment in the COMBINE Study

Treatment Group	Unadjusted Mean (SD)	Poisson Model Mean 95% CI	Poisson Model with Overdispersion Mean 95% CI	Negative Binomial Model Mean95% CI	Binomial Model95% CI	Binomial Model with Overdispersion95% CI
Naltrexone and CBI	6.55 (8.82)	6.55 (6.27, 6.86)	6.55 (5.63, 7.63)	6.55 (5.38, 7.98)	6.55 (6.30, 6.82)	6.55 (5.54, 7.69)
Naltrexone	6.28 (8.95)	6.34 (6.06, 6.65)	6.34 (5.42, 7.42)	6.34 (5.19, 7.74)	6.34 (6.09, 6.61)	6.34 (5.33, 7.49)
CBI	6.76 (8.87)	6.79 (6.50, 7.10)	6.79 (5.85, 7.89)	6.78 (5.57, 8.26)	6.79 (6.53, 7.06)	6.79 (5.76, 7.94)
Neither	8.75 (9.80)	8.80 (8.46, 9.15)	8.80 (7.71, 10.04)	8.78 (7.21, 10.69)	8.80 (8.52, 9.09)	8.80 (7.66, 10.03)

TABLE 4.2

Rate Ratios, Odds Ratios, and Associated 95% Confidence Intervals for Number of Drinking Days in the Last Month of the Treatment Period for all Pairwise Comparisons between the Treatment Groups in the COMBINE Study

Treatment Group	Comparison Treatment Group	Poisson Model	Poisson Model with Overdispersion	Negative Binomial Model	Binomial Model	Binomial Model with Overdispersion
		Rate Ratio (95% CI)	Rate Ratio (95% CI)	Rate Ratio (95% CI)	Odds Ratio (95% CI)	Odds Ratio (95% CI)
Naltrexone and CBI	Naltrexone	1.03 (0.97, 1.10)	1.03 (0.83, 1.29)	1.03 (0.78, 1.37)	1.04 (0.97, 1.12)	1.04 (0.77, 1.42)
Naltrexone and CBI	CBI	0.96 (0.91, 1.03)	0.96 (0.78, 1.19)	0.97 (0.73, 1.28)	0.95 (0.89, 1.03)	0.95 (0.71, 1.29)
Naltrexone and CBI	Neither	0.74 (0.70, 0.79)	0.74 (0.61, 0.91)	0.75 (0.57, 0.99)	0.67 (0.62, 0.72)	0.67 (0.50, 0.89)
Naltrexone	CBI	0.93 (0.88, 1.00)	0.93 (0.75, 1.16)	0.94 (0.71, 1.24)	0.91 (0.85, 0.98)	0.91 (0.67, 1.24)
Naltrexone	Neither	0.72 (0.68, 0.77)	0.72 (0.59, 0.89)	0.72 (0.55, 0.96)	0.64 (0.60, 0.69)	0.64 (0.48, 0.86)
CBI	Neither	0.77 (0.73, 0.82)	0.77 (0.63, 0.94)	0.77 (0.58, 1.02)	0.70 (0.65, 0.75)	0.70 (0.52, 0.93)

pairwise comparisons between the treatments with associated 95% confidence intervals for this model. Compared to the control group, all three active groups have significantly lower rates of drinking. That is, because all three rate ratios are significantly less than 1 as the associated 95% confidence intervals are entirely below 1. This indicates that naltrexone and CBI, whether together or alone, appear to reduce the rate of drinking in the last month of treatment.

We now highlight the parallelism between the logistic regression model definition and the log-linear models for count data:

1. We assume that the count outcomes Y_i are independent of one another and have *Poisson distributions* with means μ_i.
2. We describe the effects of covariates as a linear function in the parameters, as shown in the right-hand side expression of Equations 4.3 and 4.5. This expression is called the linear predictor and can be any linear combination of predictors (quantitative or categorical coded by dummy variables) including interactions.
3. We relate the mean of the response distribution (μ_i) to the linear predictor via a mathematically convenient function. In Poisson regression, we use the log function.

We see that both logistic regression for binary data and log-linear models for count data are described completely by specifying each of the three components above. We are now ready to introduce the class of generalized linear models.

4.1.3 Generalized Linear Models

4.1.3.1 Model Definition and Most Commonly Used Specifications

GLM extend linear models for normal outcomes so that a larger class of outcomes can be considered. To define a GLM, three components need to be specified: a *random component*, a *systematic component* and a *link function*. The random component is the distribution of the independent observations on the outcome variable. In GLM the distribution needs to be from the exponential family. The Bernoulli distribution, the Poisson distribution, and the normal distribution are all exponential family distributions. The second column of Table 4.3 shows the most commonly used distributions in this family. The systematic component is the linear function of the predictor variables that are hypothesized to be related to the mean of the outcome most commonly referred to as the linear predictor (denoted in the technical literature as η, herein we use *lp*). The link is a mathematically convenient function that links the random and systematic components. There are multiple link options for the different distributions but for each distribution there is a preferable function (called *canonical link*) that makes estimation and interpretation easier. Table 4.3 provides information on the most commonly used functions for each distribution.

In the previous two subsections, we showed how the three GLM components are defined in logistic regression for binary data and in Poisson regression for count data. The special case in which the random component is a normal distribution, corresponds to the linear model introduced in Chapter 1. In this case, the mean response is directly equated to the linear predictor and hence the link function is the identity. The regression coefficients in linear models with normal outcomes are interpreted as the mean change in the outcome per unit change in a continuous predictor or as the mean difference in the outcome at a

TABLE 4.3

Commonly Used Distributions in the Exponential Family with Corresponding Link Functions

Type of Outcome	Random Component	Link Function	Interpretation of Coefficients
Continuous	Normal distribution: $N(\mu_i, \sigma^2)$	Identity: $\mu_i = lp_i$	Mean differences
Binary or number of "successes" out of n_i independent trials with a dichotomous outcome	Binomial distribution: $\text{Bin}(n_i, p_i)$	Logit: $log\left(\frac{p_i}{1-p_i}\right) = lp_i$	Log-transformed odds-ratios
Count	Poisson distribution: $Po(\mu_i)$	Log: $\log(\mu_i) = lp_i$	Log-transformed mean ratios (rate ratios)
Count	Negative binomial distribution: $NegBin(k, \mu_i)$	Log: $\log(\mu_i) = lp_i$	Log-transformed mean ratios
Positive continuous	Gamma distribution: Gamma (μ_i, v)	Reciprocal: $\frac{1}{\mu_i} = lp_i$ or log: $\log(\mu_i) = lp_i$	Depends on link

certain level of a categorical predictor, compared to a reference level when the rest of the predictors are held constant.

Logistic regression is used when the outcome is a single binary variable (e.g., 1 versus 0, "success" versus "failure") or a number of successes out of a certain number of independent trials. In the depression example, the single binary outcome we considered was the response to treatment and it was assessed at the last available time point for each individual in the study. In other applications, the outcome can be number of "successes" out of a certain number of "trials."

In the COMBINE study, the 28 days at the end of treatment, during which we previously considered the number of drinking days, might be regarded as 28 different trials with a dichotomous outcome (drinking or not drinking) for each subject on each test day. If we assume for a moment that the observations on different days within the same subject are independent of one another (which is not the case and hence we will need to modify the model later on), and that the probability of drinking does not vary by day, then the total number of drinking days in this period for an individual can be regarded as a number of "successes" in a binomial experiment. Thus, we can fit a binomial distribution to these data and estimate how the odds of drinking on a particular day vary by treatment group. The sixth column of Table 4.2 provides the corresponding odds ratio estimates and 95% confidence intervals for each group. The sixth column of Table 4.1 shows the estimated mean number of drinking days and the corresponding 95% confidence intervals. Similar to the conclusions from the Poisson model, based on the estimates from these two tables, we can conclude that all three active treatments compared to the control have significantly lower odds of drinking. Note that the effects in this case are represented as odds ratios rather than as rate ratios. Also, the naltrexone group has significantly lower odds of drinking than the CBI group. We continue the discussion of these results and focus on the issues of model selection later in this chapter, following the introduction of the additional models considered in these two tables.

The logit link function is the most commonly used function for binary/binomial data. The choice of this function is not unique. Another relatively frequently used possibility for binary data is the probit function (Agresti, 2002), which is very similar to the logit but does not provide as simple interpretation for the fixed-effects coefficients. However, for correlated data it has certain advantages over the logit link as it generalizes more easily from the case of independent to dependent observations.

Poisson and negative binomial GLMs are used when the outcomes are counts. For example, the number of heavy drinking days in a period is a non-negative count. The Poisson distribution has a very restrictive feature that the mean and the variance of the observations need to be the same. In reality, this restriction is rarely satisfied with count data as the variance is often several times larger than the mean. For example, the average number of drinking days in the last month in the treatment period in COMBINE is 7.1 while the variance is 83.9. Within treatment group, the ratio is very similar as can be inferred from the means and standard deviations (the variance is the square of the standard deviation) in the second column of Table 4.1. This situation is referred to as *overdispersion* and is discussed in the next subsection. The negative binomial distribution seamlessly accommodates overdispersion in the data and hence is often preferred to the Poisson distribution in such situations.

The gamma distribution is also part of the exponential family and is useful for modeling positive continuous variables with skewed distributions. It has two parameters that determine the mean and the variance and hence has more flexibility to fit observed data than distributions with only one parameter. In general, the variance is proportional to the square of the mean, which makes it well suited for positively skewed data. The mathematically most convenient link function for the gamma is the inverse. However, the log link is most often used. The effects of covariates are estimated on the log-mean scale. In COMBINE, the number of drinks per drinking day can be modeled using gamma distribution as the values are positive with right-skewed distribution.

4.1.3.2 Overdispersion

In many of the GLM, the variance is a function of the mean but data may exhibit more variability than predicted by the theoretical model. As mentioned above, the Poisson distribution assumes that the variance is equal to the mean, which rarely corresponds to reality. This situation is referred to as *overdispersion* and can be handled by estimating an additional parameter ϕ so that the variance of the Poisson outcome is equal to $\phi\mu_i$, rather than to μ_i. However, this is a rather artificial fix to the problem as the overdispersed Poisson is not a proper statistical distribution.

Note that some apparent overdispersion may result when important fixed effects are omitted from the linear predictor. Hence, before fitting an overdispersed model, one needs to make sure that all important variables are included in the linear predictor. With the additional parameter ϕ the variance is allowed to be higher than the mean. Since ϕ is not restricted (except to be positive), one can also model underdispersion (variance smaller than the mean), although this situation is encountered much less frequently in practice.

The negative binomial distribution is directly applicable to overdispersed data because its variance is equal to $\mu_i + \mu_i^2/k$ for some positive number k and hence is larger than the mean. Estimating the extra parameter k allows us to determine the degree of overdispersion. As k gets larger and larger, the negative binomial distribution gets closer and closer to the Poisson distribution. The negative binomial distribution is preferable to the overdispersed Poisson distribution, except in situations when there might be underdispersion, because it is a proper statistical distribution.

Overdispersion can also be present with binomial data where the variance is also determined by the mean. For the binomial distribution, the variance is equal to $n_i p_i(1-p_i)$ and it is quite possible that the observed variance relative to the observed mean does not follow this pattern. Similar to the case with the Poisson distribution, an extra overdispersion parameter can be estimated in order to deal with this situation. In general, any GLM where the variance is related to the mean can be augmented by an extra dispersion parameter so that overdispersion can be handled seamlessly within the GLM framework.

Tables 4.1 and 4.2 provide the mean estimates and rate ratios with 95% confidence intervals for the overdispersed Poisson model and the negative binomial model, and also the mean estimates and odds ratios with 95% confidence intervals for the overdispersed binomial model. This allows for direct comparison of the results from the overdispersed Poisson and the negative binomial models to the results from the Poisson model without overdispersion. Similarly, the results from the overdispersed binomial model can be compared to the results from the regular binomial model.

We first focus on the Poisson and negative binomial models. The mean estimates in the two Poisson models (without and with overdispersion), and hence also the rate ratio estimates are exactly the same. The corresponding estimates from the negative binomial model are also very close. However, the confidence intervals are markedly wider in the overdispersed models (when an additional overdispersion parameter is estimated) because the standard errors are adjusted and are appropriately larger. This leads to fewer comparisons being declared statistically significant in the models that allow for overdispersion compared to the classical Poisson and binomial models.

4.1.3.3 Estimation and Assessment of Model Fit

Maximum likelihood estimates for the model parameters are obtained using an iterative procedure, as shown in McCullagh and Nelder (1989). To determine whether there is substantial overdispersion, one needs to assess the goodness of fit of the corresponding model (the Poisson or the binomial, in this case). This is done by examining goodness-of-fit measures such as the *deviance* or the *generalized Pearson's Chi-square statistic*. The deviance of a model is defined as two times the difference of the log-likelihood for the maximum achievable model (i.e., when there is a separate parameter for each subject's response and the response serves as a unique estimate of the corresponding parameter), and the log-likelihood under the fitted model. If the deviance is about equal to the residual degrees of freedom of the model then there is no evidence of overdispersion or underdispersion. If the deviance is noticeably larger (i.e., by 50% or more) than the corresponding degrees of freedom, then there is substantial overdispersion. If the deviance is much smaller than the degrees of freedom, then there is underdispersion.

Similarly, the Pearson's Chi-square statistic, which is defined as the sum of squared differences between observed and expected outcomes properly standardized by the corresponding variances, can be compared to the residual degrees of freedom. The difference in the deviance and degrees of freedom of two nested models can be used in likelihood ratio chi-square tests for model comparison. More details about tests involving deviance, can be found in McCullagh and Nelder (1989) and Agresti (2002), for example.

In the COMBINE data set, when the Poisson model without overdispersion is fit to the number of drinking days at the end of the treatment, the deviance is 12979.1 on 1143 degrees of freedom, which results in a ratio of 11.4 approximately, that is, the deviance is more than 11 times larger than the corresponding degrees of freedom and hence the data are undoubtedly overdispersed. Similarly, the Pearson's Chi-square statistic is 13409.1 on 1143 degrees of freedom for a ratio of about 11.7. Thus, it is imperative to take into account this extra variability. For the negative binomial model, the deviance is 1213.1 on 1143 degrees of freedom, which results in a ratio of 1.06 approximately, and hence the variability in the data is properly absorbed by the negative binomial distribution.

Similarly, when the binomial model without overdispersion is fit to the data, the deviance is 19773.2 on 1143 degrees of freedom, that is, the deviance is more than 17 times larger than the corresponding degrees of freedom and the data are overdispersed with respect to the binomial distribution too. The Pearson's Chi-square statistic is 17984 on 1143 degrees of freedom, that is, more than 15 times larger than the corresponding degrees of freedom. Thus, if a binomial model is selected to fit the data, then an extra parameter needs to be estimated to account for overdispersion.

Note that in many situations, overdispersion results from dependencies between the individual observations that violate the basic assumptions of the model. In particular, in COMBINE and in similar studies the 28 days at the end of the treatment are not independent of one another. If a subject drinks on a particular day, he or she is arguably more likely to drink on the next day too and the reverse may also be true (if a subject abstains on a particular day, they are more likely to abstain on the next day). Thus, the total number of drinking days when there is dependence will have a more dispersed distribution than predicted by the binomial distribution. If the days are independent of one another and the probabilities of drinking are not extreme (very close to 0 or very close to 1), the probabilities of 0 drinking days or 28 drinking days will be very low so there should be virtually no people with such data in the sample. Yet, by the end of the treatment period, some subjects drink on all days and others don't drink at all and there are more subjects with counts close to the two extremes than predicted by the binomial distribution. Thus, overdispersion is expected with such data and by itself should not preclude the corresponding distribution to be used to fit the data if an extra parameter is estimated to account for the increased variance.

Which distribution to use for the data, depends largely on the goals of the analysis and how well the model describes the data. Measures such as AIC and BIC can't be used to compare models with different response distributions since the formulae for the likelihoods are different and the information criteria are based on the likelihoods. In the COMBINE data example, the main difference in the conclusions from the models considering three different possible distributions in the exponential family (binomial, Poisson, and negative binomial) is in the interpretation of the results. From the binomial model odds ratios are estimated and interpreted, while from the Poisson and negative binomial models mean (or rate) ratios are estimated. Arguably, rate ratios are easier to interpret than odds ratios so on this basis (and also because it seamlessly handles overdispersion) the negative binomial model may be preferred. Note that, in some cases, even the linear model for normal data may fit count data well and this model is the easiest to interpret. Residual plots can be used to assess how well the models fit the data.

4.1.3.4 Zero-Inflated and Hurdle Models

Count data can also exhibit floor effect with a larger number of zeros than predicted by either the Poisson or the negative binomial distributions. In such a case, the extra zeros can be accommodated using *zero-inflated models* or *hurdle* versions of the Poisson and negative binomial models: see, for example, Heilbron (1994), Lambert (1992), or Min and Agresti (2005). In zero-inflated models, the zeros are assumed to be generated either from the Poisson or negative binomial distribution, or to be "real" zeros (e.g., subjects who don't drink at all). The probabilities of extra zeros are modeled using logistic regression and may or may not depend on covariates. In *hurdle models*, the zeros occur only in the logistic regression part of the model. The rest of the observations (i.e., the positive counts) come from zero-truncated censored Poisson or negative binomial distribution. We do not consider such models in this chapter, but examples with repeated measures data can be found in Hedeker and Gibbons (2006), Hu et al. (2011), and Min and Agresti (2005).

4.1.3.5 GLM Summary

Uniting different models under the same framework allows common methods to be used to obtain estimates and to perform statistical inference. GLM covers many useful models for continuous and discrete outcomes. The models are fitted using iteratively reweighted least squares procedure for maximum likelihood estimation. Model selection is performed using likelihood ratio tests and deviance statistics. Residual plots can be used to assess model assumptions. McCullagh and Nelder (1989) and Agresti (2015) provide detailed information about GLMs.

4.1.4 GLM Extensions for Ordinal and Nominal Data

When the outcome of interest is a categorical variable with more than two levels, GLM extensions can be used to model the effects of predictors on the outcome. Different models are appropriate for ordinal (categories are ordered) and for nominal (categories are not ordered) categorical variables. For example, in the augmentation depression study, one of the outcomes of interest is the Clinical Global Impressions (CGI) score, which is an ordinal measure with values from 1 to 7, 1 indicating "normal, not at all ill," and 7 indicating "among the most severely ill patients." The intermediate categories are 2 = "borderline mentally ill," 3 = "mildly ill," 4 = "moderately ill," 5 = "markedly ill," 6 = "severely ill." Another example of an ordinal measure is self-rated health in the Health and Retirement Study with possible values: 1 = "excellent," 2 = "very good," 3 = "good," 4 = "fair," and 5 = "poor."

Nominal measures are often collected when individuals are asked to choose among different alternatives. For example, smokers may be asked to choose between e-cigarettes, regular cigarettes, or neither. Dropout in clinical trials can be due to a variety of reasons (inefficacy, side effects, or unrelated to treatment). Diseases can be classified into different subtypes.

Generalizations of logistic regression are often used to model ordinal and nominal data. We focus first on ordinal data which are frequently encountered in medical research.

4.1.4.1 Cumulative Logit Model for Ordinal Data

The most commonly used model for ordinal data is the *proportional odds cumulative logit model,* in which the probability of observations in lower (or higher) categories is related to the linear predictor with logit transformation. The random component of this model is the *multinomial distribution,* which is a multivariate generalization of the binomial distribution with more than two possible outcome categories. The systematic component is the linear predictor which is constructed in a similar way as for other GLM. The link function is the *cumulative logit link,* which is the log of the odds of observation in lower categories versus higher categories, also known as *cumulative odds.*

To illustrate, we consider the augmentation depression study. The ordinal CGI outcome at the end of the treatment for the ith subject is denoted as Y_i, with possible values of 1 through 7. In reality, only categories 1 through 4 are observed at endpoint as all completers improve at least slightly. $P(Y_i \le k)$ denotes the probability that the CGI score is in the lower k categories and corresponds to a better clinical outcome than the opposite event (i.e., outcome in a higher than the kth category). A simple cumulative logit model is defined as follows:

$$\log\left(\frac{P(Y_i \leq k)}{P(Y_i > k)}\right) = \beta_{0k} + \beta_1 Group_i \tag{4.6}$$

This is the same as $\log\left(\frac{P(Y_i \leq k)}{1 - P(Y_i \leq k)}\right) = \beta_{0k} + \beta_1 Group_i$.

On the left-hand sides of these equations are the cumulative logits for a response in lower categories, since $P(Y_i \leq k) = P(Y_i = 1) + P(Y_i = 2) + \ldots P(Y_i = k)$. Note that the parameters β_{0k} (intercepts, also called thresholds) are different depending on k (i.e., the category where we draw the line for the comparison of lower versus higher categories). Necessarily, $\beta_{01} < \beta_{02} < \ldots < \beta_{0,k-1}$ because the cumulative odds can't decrease and we need to be able to distinguish between categories.

The thresholds β_{0k} correspond to the log of the cumulative odds of response in the kth or lower category in the control group. Exponentiating the parameter (i.e., taking $\exp(\beta_{0k})$) gives the corresponding cumulative odds in the control group. To obtain the cumulative odds in the augmentation group, we add β_1 to the thresholds and then exponentiate. Thus, the log of the cumulative odds of response in the kth or lower category in the augmentation group is $\beta_{0k} + \beta_1$ and the cumulative odds are $\exp(\beta_{0k} + \beta_1)$. To assess whether there is a difference between the augmentation and control group, we test whether β_1 is equal to 0. If $\beta_1 = 0$, then the cumulative odds in the two groups are the same, if $\beta_1 > 0$, then the log cumulative odds in the augmentation group are higher than in the control group, and if $\beta_1 < 0$, then the log cumulative odds in the augmentation group are lower than in the control group.

$\text{Exp}(\beta_1)$ is the *cumulative odds ratio* between the two groups. When $\beta_1 = 0$ the odds ratio is 1. $\beta_1 > 0$ corresponds to $\exp(\beta_1) > 1$, and hence an odds ratio greater than 1. $\beta_1 < 0$ corresponds to $\exp(\beta_1) < 1$, and hence an odds ratio less than 1. Unlike the intercepts, which are in general different for different k, β_1 is the same for each k. This means that the cumulative odds ratios are the same whether we compare the first category versus the rest, the first two categories versus the rest, or all the categories except the last one versus the last one. This is often referred to as the *proportional odds assumption* and may or may not be satisfied in a particular data set.

In the augmentation depression study, β_{0k} are the log odds of being less ill in the control group, $\beta_{0k} + \beta_1$ are the log odds of being less ill in the augmentation group, and β_1 is the log odds ratio for the comparison of the augmentation and control groups, which is assumed to be the same for all possible cutoffs for severity. If this assumption does not seem to be reasonable, then different beta parameters can be estimated for each split by replacing β_1 with β_{1k} and interpreting different odds ratios for each cutoff.

Based on the estimated betas in the augmentation study, we calculate the odds of response in lower categories, shown in Table 4.4, and the cumulative odds ratio for the comparison of the augmentation and control groups. The estimates are based only on the sample of completers in the study and, since at the end of treatment there are no subjects with CGI scores in categories 5 through 7 (markedly ill, severely ill, or among the most ill patients), not all possible comparisons are represented in Table 4.4. Because the odds are ratios of two complementary probabilities, odds less than 1 imply that the probability in the numerator is lower than the probability in the denominator, and odds greater than 1

TABLE 4.4

Cumulative Odds of Better Response and Cumulative Odds Ratio for the Comparison of the Augmentation and Control Groups in the Augmentation Study in Depression

Comparisons	Cumulative Odds or Odds Ratio	95% CI
Odds for "normal, not at all ill" versus "borderline ill," "mildly ill," or "moderately ill" in the control group	0.21	(0.07, 0.59)
Odds for "normal, not at all ill" or "borderline ill" versus "mildly ill" or "moderately ill" in the control group	1.44	(0.60, 3.41)
Odds for "normal, not at all ill," "borderline ill," or "mildly ill" versus "moderately ill" in the control group	3.05	(1.19, 7.85)
Odds for "normal, not at all ill" versus "borderline ill," "mildly ill," or "moderately ill" in the augmentation group	0.53	(0.22, 1.27)
Odds for "normal, not at all ill" or "borderline ill" versus "mildly ill" or "moderately ill" in the augmentation group	3.60	(1.34, 9.66)
Odds for "normal, not at all ill," "borderline ill," or "mildly ill" versus "moderately ill" in the augmentation group	7.66	(2.48, 23.62)
Cumulative odds ratio for less severe illness in augmentation versus control group	2.51	(0.75, 8.43)

imply that the probability in the numerator is higher than the probability in the denominator. For example, the estimated probability of "normal, not at all ill" is significantly lower compared to the cumulative probabilities in the rest of the categories in the control group, because the entire confidence interval for the odds is below 1 (OR = 0.21, 95% CI: (0.07, 0.59)). This is not the case for the augmentation group where the confidence interval includes 1.

The common odds ratio for the comparison of the odds of better outcome in the augmentation and control group is not significantly different from 1, since the confidence interval includes 1 (OR = 2.51, 95% CI: (0.75, 8.43)). Thus, we don't have sufficient evidence in this small sample to conclude that severity at the end of treatment is significantly different between the augmentation and the control groups.

Table 4.5 shows the correspondence between raw proportions and estimated probabilities in each outcome category. The estimated probabilities are obtained from the estimated cumulative odds in each group by first calculating the cumulative probabilities (cumulative probability = cumulative odds/(1 + cumulative odds) and then taking the differences between successive cumulative probabilities. The estimated probabilities in the first and fourth category are fairly close, but the model estimates lower probability of "borderline ill"

TABLE 4.5

Proportions and Estimated Probabilities by Category in the Augmentation Study in Depression

Treatment Group		Normal, not at all ill	Borderline ill	Mildly ill	Moderately ill
Augmentation	Sample proportion	0.32	0.53	0	0.16
	Estimated probability	0.35	0.44	0.10	0.12
Control	Sample proportion	0.21	0.32	0.26	0.21
	Estimated probability	0.17	0.42	0.16	0.25

in the augmentation group, compared to the proportion in the raw data, and higher probability of "borderline ill" in the control group, compared to the proportion in the raw data. This is compensated by the estimated probabilities in the next category, "mildly ill." Since this is a small sample, we can't say that this is a large discrepancy but it is some indication that the proportional odds assumption may not be satisfied in this data set.

The cumulative odds model is not the only option to consider for ordinal data but is the most commonly used due to the relative ease of interpretation. Other models are also available for ordinal data. One such example is the *adjacent-category logit* model where the odds of response in category k versus in category $k+1$ are modeled. Also, probit versions of all logit models are also available and, in some cases (e.g., when data are correlated), may be preferable. More information on the cumulative logit model and other alternatives can be found in Agresti (2002).

4.1.4.2 Baseline Category Logit Model for Nominal Data

When the outcome is nominal (i.e., the categories are unordered), the most commonly used GLM model is the *baseline category logit* model, which is also known as the *generalized logit model*. The random component is again the multinomial distribution, the systematic component is the linear predictor, and we use a *baseline category logit link* function, as shown below. If we suppose for a moment that the categories of CGI are unordered and the last one (K) is the reference category, then the baseline category logit model is defined as follows:

$$\log\left(\frac{P(Y_i = k)}{P(Y_i = K)}\right) = \beta_{0k} + \beta_{1k} Group_i \tag{4.7}$$

Here, the intercept β_{0k} is the log of the ratio of the probability for response in category k and the probability for response in the reference category for the control group. The corresponding log ratio in the augmentation group is $\beta_{0k}+\beta_{1k}$. Note that there are separate β_{1k} parameters for each non-reference category and hence, the difference between the log ratios in the augmentation and control group varies depending on which category we compare to the reference. Thus, the baseline category logit model does not make a proportionality assumption the way the cumulative logit model does.

By exponentiating β_{0k}, one obtains estimates of the ratios of probabilities in each category and the probability in the reference category in the control group and by exponentiating $\beta_{0k}+\beta_{1k}$ one obtains the corresponding ratios of probabilities in the treatment group. Based on these estimates, one also obtains estimates of the probabilities of response in each category. Testing whether all β_{1k} are different from 0 allows one to assess whether there are significant differences between the augmentation and control groups. In this simple situation, this is equivalent to performing the ordinary χ^2 test of independence in a two-way table. For more information on baseline category logit models consult Agresti (2002).

4.2 Generalized Estimating Equations (GEE)

It is very common for categorical, count, or other non-normal outcomes to be observed repeatedly over the time. For example, in the augmentation study in depression, CGI was assessed every week for the duration of the study. In the Health and Retirement Study, the ordinal measure of self-rated health was collected every two years. In the COMBINE Study, drinking data were collected daily during the double-blind treatment phase. In all these situations, it is likely that there are correlations between repeated observations on the same individual. These correlations need to be taken into account in the statistical analysis. When the focus of statistical inference is on the estimation of population level effects (i.e., average effects of treatment and/or covariates in the population), the correlation structure is considered a nuisance and the design is balanced in longitudinal studies (i.e., the observations on all individuals are taken at the same set of fixed time points), one can use the classical Generalized Estimating Equations (GEE) approach. This is known as the *marginal approach* of repeated measures analysis, as it requires that the marginal means and variances at each repeated occasion are specified and the marginal means are related to predictors via an appropriate link function. A working correlation structure is assumed between the repeated observations to take into account the dependence among them.

4.2.1 Modeling the Mean

Any exponential family distribution can be considered to generate the data at each occasion and thus imply some structure for the means and variances of the repeated observations. The link function that relates the mean of the response to the predictors, is chosen based on the options for the particular exponential family distribution as described in the GLM section of this chapter.

The type of marginal distribution at each time point and the link function are selected to match the data. Table 4.3 can be used as a guide for the most commonly encountered data types, distributions, and link functions. In particular, for dichotomous data the Bernoulli distribution (or the binomial if dichotomous data are aggregated) with a logit link function could be selected, for count data either the Poisson or negative binomial with log link might be chosen; for positively skewed data the gamma distribution with inverse or log link may be appropriate. Note that GEE can also be used with normally distributed data, in which case, the normal distribution with identity link is selected.

To illustrate the definition for the mean structure of the model, we consider several examples, some of which are described in more detail further in this chapter. Correlation structure considerations follow immediately after the examples.

In the augmentation depression study, we can formulate a GEE model to assess whether there are between-group differences in the probability of achieving treatment response over the six study weeks. The outcome, in this case, is treatment response (1 = yes, 0 = no) which is measured weekly for the duration of the study for each subject (we use Y_{ij} to denote this outcome where, as usual, i denotes subject and j denotes time point). Because the outcome is binary, it is logical to consider the Bernoulli distribution at each time point and to relate the probability of treatment response p_{ij} via the logit link to the linear predictor which should include the effects of treatment group, time, and the interaction of group and time. Thus, we can specify the marginal model as follows:

$$\log\left(\frac{p_{ij}}{1-p_{ij}}\right) = \beta_0 + \beta_1 Group_i + \beta_2 Time_j + \beta_3 Group_i Time_j \tag{4.8}$$

We consider time as a continuous predictor just for simplicity of the expression. We can use dummy coding to specify time as a categorical predictor since this is a balanced design. If the observation times were unique for different individuals, the only possible choice would be to treat time as a continuous predictor.

In the COMBINE study, we can formulate a GEE model to assess whether there are between-group differences in the average number of drinking days or average number of drinks per drinking day (i.e., day on which the subject drank) per month during the treatment period. For the number of drinking days, it is convenient to consider either a Poisson or a negative binomial distribution while for drinks per drinking day a gamma distribution is appropriate, as shown in the previous section. For both outcomes and all distribution choices, the main focus is on the mean (i.e., the average number of drinking days or the average number of drinks per drinking day) and the log link provides a nice interpretation of the regression coefficients. Thus, to complete the marginal specification in each interval we define:

$$\log \mu_{ij} = \beta_0 + \beta_1 N_i + \beta_2 CBI_i + \beta_3 t_j + \beta_4 N_i CBI_i + \beta_5 N_i t_j + \beta_6 CBI_i t_j + \beta_7 N_i CBI_i t_j \tag{4.9}$$

where:

N_i and CBI_i are indicators for naltrexone and CBI treatment (1 corresponds to active treatment, 0 to placebo or no treatment)
t_j denotes month (1 through 4)
μ_{ij} denotes the mean response for subject i at time j

Again, time is shown here as a continuous predictor but can be categorized using dummy variables.

In the Health and Retirement Study from Section 1.5.4, we are interested in assessing change in self-rated health over time and how it relates to gender and smoking status at baseline. For the ordinal measure of self-rated health (higher category corresponds to poorer health), we consider the multinomial distribution and assume a cumulative logit model, which allows to assess the effect of predictors on the cumulative odds of poorer self-rated health. The model can be formulated as follows.

$$\log\left(\frac{P(Y_{ij} \geq k)}{P(Y_{ij} < k)}\right) = \beta_{0k} + \beta_1 F_i + \beta_2 S_i + \beta_3 W_j + \beta_4 F_i S_i + \beta_5 F_i W_j + \beta_6 S_i W_j + \beta_7 S_i F_i W_j \tag{4.10}$$

where:

F_i = 1 for female sex and 0 otherwise
S_i = 1 if smoker at baseline and 0 otherwise
W_j corresponds to wave with values of 1 through 7

Note that in this model we are accumulating the categories from the highest to the lowest one (5–1). This is because we want to model the cumulative odds of poorer rather than better health.

4.2.2 Specifying the Working Correlation Structure

To fully specify the GEE model, in addition to the model for the mean or probability at each occasion, we need to specify a working correlation structure between the outcomes on repeated occasions. The most popular choices of working correlation structures are independent, exchangeable, first-order auto regressive, and unstructured. We show them here in the case of four repeated occasions.

$$\text{Independent: } \begin{pmatrix} 1 & 0 & 0 & 0 \\ 0 & 1 & 0 & 0 \\ 0 & 0 & 1 & 0 \\ 0 & 0 & 0 & 1 \end{pmatrix}$$

$$\text{Exchangeable: } \begin{pmatrix} 1 & \rho & \rho & \rho \\ \rho & 1 & \rho & \rho \\ \rho & \rho & 1 & \rho \\ \rho & \rho & \rho & 1 \end{pmatrix}$$

$$\text{Autoregressive: } \begin{pmatrix} 1 & \rho & \rho^2 & \rho^3 \\ \rho & 1 & \rho & \rho^2 \\ \rho^2 & \rho & 1 & \rho \\ \rho^3 & \rho^2 & \rho & 1 \end{pmatrix}$$

$$\text{Unstructured: } \begin{pmatrix} 1 & \rho_{12} & \rho_{13} & \rho_{14} \\ \rho_{12} & 1 & \rho_{23} & \rho_{24} \\ \rho_{13} & \rho_{23} & 1 & \rho_{34} \\ \rho_{14} & \rho_{24} & \rho_{34} & 1 \end{pmatrix}$$

These structures correspond to the independent, compound symmetry, first-order autoregressive, and unstructured variance–covariance structures in linear mixed models, introduced in Chapter 3. In general, most variance–covariance structures used in linear mixed models have corresponding correlation structures for GEE but note that in GEE we focus on the correlation rather than the covariance since the variances on each repeated occasion depend on the mean according to the relationship implied by the assumed exponential family distribution. Extra parameters can be introduced (e.g., to deal with overdispersion) but there is still an underlying relationship between the variance and the mean for most exponential family distributions. For some distributions (e.g., the multinomial), the choice of working correlation structures in software packages may be restricted. For binary or ordinal outcomes, an alternative method to account for the associations among the measurements is based on log odds ratios between pairs of responses. Details about this alternating logistic regressions (ALR) algorithm can be found in Carey et al. (1993) and Heagerty and Zeger (1996).

The selection of the correlation structure should be based on substantive considerations or, in the absence of such, on a modification of the AIC criterion for correlated data developed by Pan (2001), namely the *quasi-likelihood under the independence model criterion* (QIC). Other criteria are also available for selecting the working correlation structure for GEE (see Section 8.1 in Shults and Hilbe, 2014). Similar to the AIC and BIC measures, we can't compare the QIC measures of different types of models (i.e., models that assume different outcome distributions). The selection of the marginal model needs to be based on substantive considerations (e.g., interpretation) and how well the fitted data correspond to the observed data.

4.2.3 Estimation Process and Properties

Based on the choice of the marginal GLM model, and the assumed working correlation structure, parameter estimates are obtained by solving a set of estimating equations. Note that this approach does not require the joint distribution of all repeated observations to be completely specified as, in general, this is a very complicated task for non-normally distributed data. As long as the marginal distributions on each repeated occasion (i.e., the distribution of the data when each time point is considered separately) and the GLM model relating the mean of the response to the predictors match the data reasonably well, even if the correlation structure is miss-specified (e.g., a compound symmetry structure is assumed while the true structure is autoregressive), the estimates of the parameters in the mean model are consistent (i.e., converge to the true value as the sample size increases). Note, though, that the estimates of the covariance matrix may fail to be consistent when the working correlation structure is incorrect (Sutradhar and Das, 2000), in particular, when the estimator of the correlation parameter is not consistent. Thus, although the regression parameters are consistent, the associated p-values and standard errors may not be valid. Furthermore, the regression estimates are fully efficient (i.e., have the smallest variance) only if the correlation structure is correctly specified but efficiency loss is often quite small when the correlation structure is miss-specified and decreases with increasing sample size. Thus, care should be taken in selecting the working correlation structure.

The technical aspects of GEE estimation are not presented in this book. The interested reader can consult Hardin and Hilbe (2013) or Ziegler (2011). Herein, we consider several examples to illustrate how this approach works and how the results are interpreted.

4.2.4 GEE Analysis of Count Data: Number of Drinking Days in the COMBINE Study

The active treatment period in COMBINE was approximately four months (16 weeks to be precise). In the previous section, we used GLM in order to model the number of drinking days in the last four weeks of the study period (loosely referred to as the last month). However, these analyses do not provide information about the change in drinking behavior over time. In particular, we are interested in the change in the number of drinking days per month from randomization until the end of double-blind treatment. We consider several different GEE models to assess trends over time and see whether these trends differ by treatment. In particular, we fit GEE models with Poisson and negative binomial outcome distributions, respectively, log links, linear predictors as the one specified in Equation 4.9, but with time treated as a categorical predictor (i.e., dummy-coded with three dichotomous 0–1 variables) and different working correlation structures. The actual number of days used to calculate the outcome for each individual is included as an offset. We also fit GEE models with binomial outcome distribution, logit link, the same linear predictor as in the Poisson and negative binomial models, and the same set of working correlation structures. The considered working correlation structures are independent, exchangeable, autoregressive of first order, and unstructured.

Table 4.6 includes the QIC values of the different models that we consider. All of them have fixed effects of naltrexone, CBI, and time, and all possible interactions among these factors. Both the Poisson and binomial marginal formulations include an extra overdispersion parameter although this parameter has no effect on the value of the QIC statistic.

From Table 4.6 we see that the QIC is the smallest when the independence structure is assumed with the binomial marginal model and when the unstructured working

TABLE 4.6

Assessment of Model Fit as Measured by the Quasi-Likelihood under the Independence Model Criterion for Different GEE Models

Working Correlation Structure	Binomial	Poisson	Negative Binomial
Independence	391.7	−5226.5	−152712.3
Exchangeable	392.3	−5246.9	−154124.3
Autoregressive	392.3	−5242.3	−153977.6
Unstructured	394.4	−5248.5	−154124.0

correlation matrix is assumed with the Poisson and negative binomial marginal models. Since the independence structure may be over-selected in some settings (Shults and Hilbe, 2014), and since we expect positive correlations among repeated measures, in the binomial setting we can choose one of the working correlation structures based on substantive considerations. However, because the negative binomial model allows for overdispersion and provides a fairly easy interpretation of the estimated regression coefficients, we focus on this model and use the unstructured working correlation pattern. Note that the results are very similar if we consider other working correlation structures, so, in this example, the choice of structure does not matter much. In smaller samples the differences can be more dramatic.

The overall tests of main and interactive effects in all models (not shown) indicate that there is a significant time effect, a significant naltrexone by CBI interaction, and a significant CBI by time interaction. The test statistics and corresponding p-values for these in the negative binomial model are as follows: $\chi^2(1)=4.78$, $p=0.03$ for the naltrexone by CBI interaction; $\chi^2(3)=50.05$, $p<0.0001$ for the main effect of time (time is considered as a categorical predictor) and $\chi^2(3)=8.45$, $p=0.04$ for the CBI by time interaction. Figure 4.2 shows the raw and estimated marginal means by treatment group and time. The two sets of means are almost the same because all predictors in the model are categorical and the model-based means are expected to match the raw means if every individual has complete data. Since there are some missing data, an offset is specified and there are slight differences between the model-based means and the raw means.

Figure 4.2 shows that the control group that does not receive either active naltrexone or CBI has a sizeable increase in average number of drinking days from the first to the fourth month during treatment. The other three groups also show a slight increase, which occurs mainly between the first and the second month. Since the three-way interaction between naltrexone, CBI, and time is not significant we proceed with interpretation of the significant two-way interactions. While it is possible to do this in the context of the complete model, sometimes it is simpler to refit the model after dropping the non-significant three-way interaction and interpret the significant two-way interactions.

Table 4.7 presents rate ratios for the significant effects in the model that help explain the effects. The estimates for the naltrexone by CBI interaction are averaged over time, the estimates for the CBI by time interaction are averaged over naltrexone, and the estimates for the time effect are averaged over naltrexone and CBI. Of all possible pairwise comparisons among the four treatment groups averaged over time (first four rows), only the rate ratios for naltrexone versus control and for CBI versus control are significantly below 1. Thus, either the medication therapy or the behavioral therapy is associated with a lower rate of drinking than the control condition. The decrease is about 23% for naltrexone alone and 18% for CBI alone.

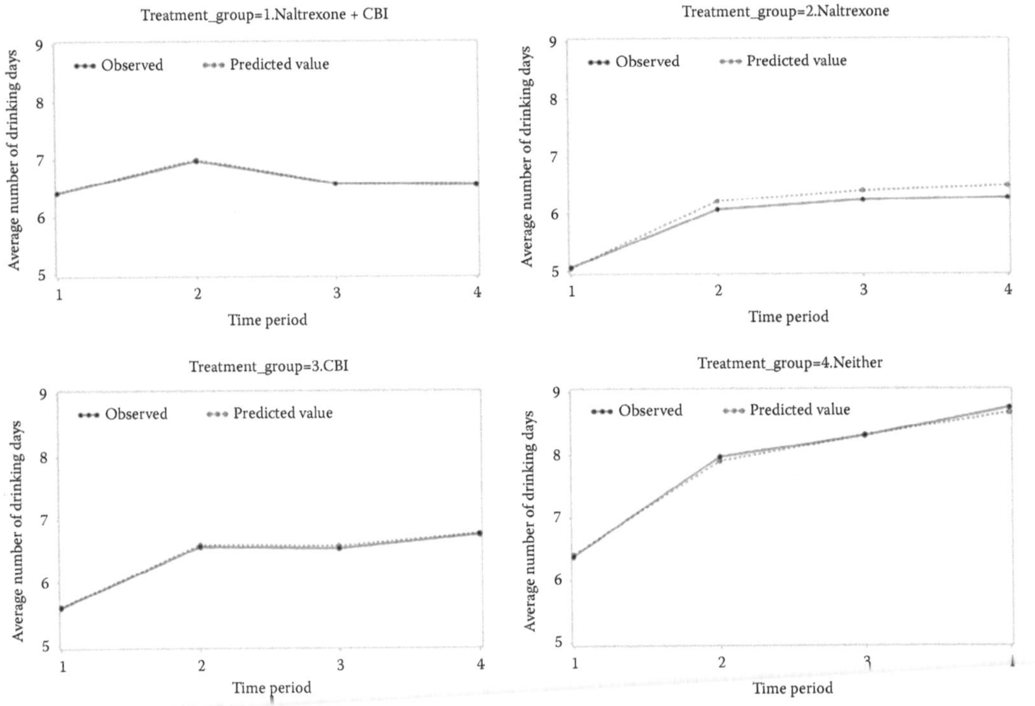

FIGURE 4.2
Raw means and model-based means from the GEE model with negative binominal distribution and log link for number of drinking days per month during treatment in the COMBINE study.

TABLE 4.7
Rate Ratios for the Significant Effects in the Negative Binomial GEE Model with Log Link Fitted to Number of Drinking Days in the COMBINE Study Assuming Unstructured Working Correlation Matrix

Effect	Level	Comparison Level	Rate Ratio (95% CI)
Naltrexone × CBI Interaction	Naltrexone and CBI	Naltrexone	1.10 (0.91, 1.33)
	Naltrexone and CBI	CBI	1.04 (0.86, 1.25)
	Naltrexone and CBI	Neither	0.85 (0.71, 1.02)
	Naltrexone	CBI	0.95 (0.78, 1.15)
	Naltrexone	Neither	0.77 (0.64, 0.93)
	CBI	Neither	0.82 (0.68, 0.98)
CBI × Time	CBI in period 1	No CBI in period 1	1.06 (0.91, 1.22)
	CBI in period 2	No CBI in period 2	0.96 (0.83, 1.11)
	CBI in period 3	No CBI in period 3	0.90 (0.78, 1.04)
	CBI in period 4	No CBI in period 4	0.88 (0.76, 1.02)
Main Effect of Time	Period 1	Period 2	0.85 (0.82, 0.89)
	Period 1	Period 3	0.85 (0.80, 0.90)
	Period 1	Period 4	0.83 (0.79, 0.89)
	Period 2	Period 3	1.00 (0.96, 1.04)
	Period 2	Period 4	0.98 (0.93, 1.03)
	Period 3	Period 4	0.98 (0.95, 1.02)

The rate ratios for the comparisons between CBI and no CBI are not significant at any of the time points (since all confidence intervals contain 1) but they are steadily decreasing over time so that, during the first month, participants on CBI have on average a higher number of drinking days, but during the later months the direction of the effect is reversed and in the fourth month participants on CBI have more than 10% lower rates of drinking than participants in the control group. This trend is consistent with how CBI is expected to work. As a behavioral treatment, it takes time to see its effects but the benefit may be longer lasting than the benefits of medication treatment. The post hoc comparisons for the main effect of time show that averaged across treatments, the rates of drinking increase over time.

The estimated working correlation matrix of the data is as follows:

$$\begin{pmatrix} 1 & 0.82 & 0.71 & 0.67 \\ 0.82 & 1 & 0.85 & 0.79 \\ 0.71 & 0.85 & 1 & 0.90 \\ 0.67 & 0.79 & 0.90 & 1 \end{pmatrix}$$

There are high correlations across time points but they are slightly decreasing with increasing time lag.

Note that by selecting the negative binomial marginal model we took into account the overdispersion in the data. Another aspect of distribution violations observed with this and other data sets is the presence of extra zeros. GEE zero-inflated models are not yet available in SAS software and are not considered here. Recent research shows how such models can be defined and fit (Kong et al., 2015).

4.2.5 GEE Analysis of Ordinal Data: Self-Rated Health in the Health and Retirement Study

To illustrate GEE analysis of ordinal data, we consider the data set from the Health and Retirement Study, introduced in Section 1.5.4, which assesses a number of measures on individuals in their transition from work to retirement biennially over 14 years. Our focus here is to assess the association between smoking and self-rated health and to see whether the association varies by gender. For the marginal response at each wave, we consider the cumulative logit model specified in Equation 4.10. Time is considered as a continuous predictor with a linear trend, which appears to be a reasonable assumption for these data.

We also include the individual's age at wave 1 (centered at the mean age of the sample at wave 1) in the linear predictor of the model but, since controlling for covariates is not considered until later in this book, we do not elaborate on this effect. Herein, we just emphasize that the effects of the other factors in the model are adjusted for age. Consideration of covariate effects is considered in more detail in Chapter 8.

Note that self-rated health is an ordinal variable with 5 categories: 1= "excellent," 2="very good," 3="good," 4="fair," and 5="poor," and we focus on the cumulative odds of poorer health. That is, we model the odds of "poor" versus the rest of the categories; "poor" or "fair" versus the rest of the categories; "poor," "fair," or "good" versus "very good" or "excellent," and "poor," "fair," "good," or "very good" versus "excellent." The proportional odds assumption in this case means that the cumulative odds ratios for the effects of gender, smoking status, and time, are the same for all these comparisons.

To formulate the GEE model fully, we specify the distribution of the data and the working correlation structure. Since there are five different categories of self-rated health, the distribution is multinomial. For this distribution, the only working correlation structure that can currently be specified in SAS PROC GENMOD is the independence structure. Note that although the estimates are obtained under no correlation, the standard errors are based on an empirical sandwich estimate and take into account the correlations in the data. We use the cumulative logit link as shown in Equation 4.10.

The results from the overall tests of interactions and main effects show significant two-way interactions between gender and smoking ($\chi^2(1) = 4.21$, $p = 0.04$) and between wave and smoking ($\chi^2(1) = 4.73$, $p = 0.03$); and also, significant main effects of smoking ($\chi^2(1) = 174.38$, $p < 0.0001$) and wave ($\chi^2(1) = 459.54$, $p < 0.0001$).

Post hoc analyses (estimation of slopes and tests of differences) are performed to explain the significant interactions in the models. The estimated slope over time for non-smokers (averaged across gender) is 0.08 (SE = 0.004) and for smokers is 0.10 (SE = 0.007). The interpretation of the two slope estimates is that the log cumulative odds of poorer self-rated health increase by 0.08 per wave (two-year period) in non-smokers and by 0.10 in smokers. The difference in slopes is −0.02 (SE = 0.008), showing that the log cumulative odds of poorer health in non-smokers increase slightly slower than in smokers. Since it is not convenient to interpret odds and odds ratios on the log scale, we exponentiate the corresponding estimates. The cumulative odds ratio comparing the effect of time in non-smokers to smokers is 0.98 (95% CI: (0.97, 1.00), Table 4.8), indicating that the rate of increase in the odds of poorer health over time is lower by about 2% in non-smokers compared to smokers.

Figure 4.3 shows the estimated cumulative odds over time of "poor," "fair," or "good" self-reported health versus "very good" or "excellent" self-rated health by gender and baseline smoking status. These are obtained by exponentiation of the corresponding combinations of regression coefficients and thus, show some curvature. The change in cumulative odds over time for the other cutoffs (e.g., "poor" versus the rest of the categories; "poor" or "fair" versus the rest of the categories), are very similar in terms of shape but the cumulative odds themselves change since there is a different intercept in the model for each possible comparison

TABLE 4.8

Cumulative Odds Ratios for the Significant Effects in the Cumulative Logit GEE Model Fit to Self-Rated Health in the Health and Retirement Study

Effect	Level	Comparison Level	Cumulative Odds Ratio (95% CI)
Main effect of time	Next wave	Previous wave	1.10 (1.09, 1.11)
Effect of smoking (evaluated at wave 1)	Non-smoker	Smoker	0.57 (0.53, 0.62)
Gender × smoking interaction (evaluated at wave 1)	Female non-smoker	Female non-smoker	0.63 (0.56, 0.70)
	Male non-smoker	Male non-smoker	0.53 (0.47, 0.59)
	Male non-smoker	Female non-smoker	0.92 (0.85, 1.00)
	Male non-smoker	Female non-smoker	1.10 (0.96, 1.25)
Time × smoking interaction	Next wave non-smoker	Previous wave non-smoker	1.09 (1.08, 1.10)
	Next wave non-smoker	Previous wave non-smoker	1.11 (1.09, 1.12)
	Next wave versus previous wave × Non-smoker versus smoker		0.98 (0.97, 1.00)

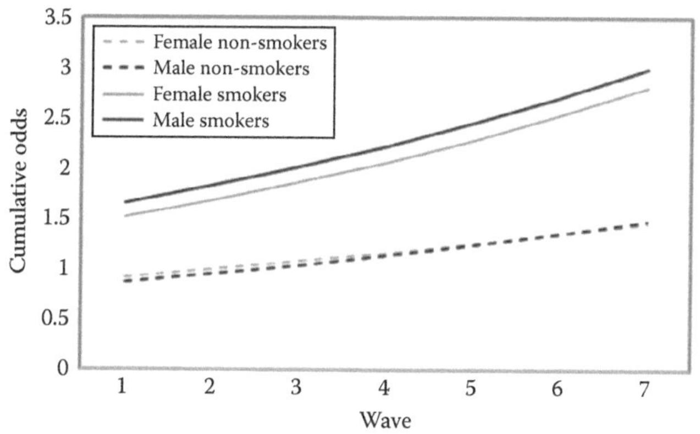

FIGURE 4.3
Cumulative odds of "poor," "fair," or "good" versus "very good" or "excellent" self-reported health over time by gender and baseline smoking status in the Health and Retirement Study.

to reflect the different cumulative probabilities. Figure 4.3 shows steeper increase in cumulative odds of poorer health for smokers of both genders and also shows that there are substantial differences in the cumulative odds at wave 1 between smokers and non-smokers. The change seems to be more sizeable for males than for females. Post hoc pairwise cumulative odds ratios at wave 1 confirm that non-smokers of both genders have significantly lower odds of acknowledging poorer health than smokers (see Table 4.8). Substantively, the same results are obtained if one evaluates these post hoc comparisons at other waves.

In summary, smokers have lower self-rated health at baseline than non-smokers with the difference slightly more pronounced in males. Deterioration in self-rated health proceeds at a slower rate in non-smokers than in smokers over time. The actual regression estimates are population-averaged, which means they are interpreted as average changes in the population.

To estimate how much the response for a particular individual is expected to change if we could change the predictors for this individual, it is better to consider models that allow for subject-specific interpretation of the regression coefficients such as random effects models which we now introduce.

4.3 Generalized Linear Mixed Models (GLMM)

An alternative to direct specification of the correlation structure is to include random effects in the model formulation in order to account for correlations within the individual or cluster. This approach has a simple intuitive interpretation as individuals are allowed to vary randomly around the group averages and thus, between-subject heterogeneity is directly modeled. As shown in the previous chapter, in the context of linear models, individuals in longitudinal studies can start higher or lower than the average and can have a faster or slower rate of change. Also, clusters can vary randomly from one another in their response and individuals/observations within each cluster are correlated. Generalized linear mixed models (GLMM) are natural extensions of LMM that allow us to consider any distribution in the exponential family. Thus, binary, count, skewed continuous data can be modeled within the same framework.

4.3.1 Modeling the Mean

The difference in formulating GLMM compared to GLM and to GEE is that the linear predictor specifying the effects of predictors on the outcome includes random effects (usually assumed to be normally distributed) and that conditional on these random effects, the repeatedly measured outcomes are assumed to be independent of one another. To illustrate, we consider the same three examples used to explain the GEE approach.

In the augmentation depression data, we formulate a GLMM by specifying

$$\log\left(\frac{p_{ij}}{1-p_{ij}}\right) = \beta_0 + \beta_1 Group_i + \beta_2 Time_j + \beta_3 Group_i Time_j + b_{i0} + b_{i1} Time_j \tag{4.11}$$

where:

b_{i0} is a random intercept
b_{i1} is a random slope

Both are assumed to be normally distributed with zero means and unknown variances and, in general, are correlated with one another.

Thus, for each individual the log odds of treatment response are allowed to vary randomly from the average log odds associated with the particular treatment and time point, and to deviate from those in a linear fashion over time. Conditional on these random effects (i.e., assuming that we know what the random effects are), the usual assumptions of a GLM are made. That is, the responses are assumed to be Bernoulli distributed with probability of the outcome of interest on a particular occasion for a particular individual p_{ij} related to the linear predictors, as shown in Equation 4.11. The individual observations are assumed to be independent, conditional on the random effects. This does not mean that repeated measurements on the same subject are uncorrelated since the random effects are shared within subject. Rather, it means that all statistical associations that exist between the repeated observations on the same subject are due to the shared random effects.

Note that in GLMM the regression coefficients have a subject-specific interpretation. This means that they show how much the outcome (in this case the log odds of treatment response) of a particular individual changes if we change the predictor for this individual. For example, the β_3 regression coefficient shows how much the log odds of treatment response are expected to change per week if a subject received the augmentation treatment versus the control treatment. Note that this is somewhat of an extrapolation as we have no data on individuals who change their treatment assignment. While the subject-specific interpretation of the time effect is reasonable in GLMM, because all subjects have repeated measures over time, the interpretation of the group by time interaction is not as intuitive.

In contrast to GLMM models, in the GEE models, the regression coefficients have population-averaged interpretations. In particular, the regression coefficient for the group by time effect in the corresponding GEE model for the augmentation depression data (β_3 in Equation 4.8) shows how much the log odds of treatment response in the population who (could) receive active treatment change per week, when compared to the log odds of treatment response in the population who (could) receive control treatment. The subject-specific and population-averaged effects are not the same unless the outcome is normally distributed and the identity link is used. Often subject-specific effects are larger in magnitude than the corresponding population-averaged effects, especially with binary and ordinal data. Subject-specific and population-averaged effects are similar when the variability due to individual/cluster is low.

In the COMBINE data, we formulate a GLMM for the number of drinking days or drinks per drinking day, by specifying

$$\log \mu_{ij} = \beta_0 + \beta_1 N_i + \beta_2 CBI_i + \beta_3 t_j + \beta_4 N_i CBI_i + \beta_5 N_i t_j + \beta_6 CBI_i t_j + \beta_7 N_i CBI_i t_j + b_{i0} \quad (4.12)$$

where b_{i0} is a random intercept, which is assumed to be normally distributed with zero mean and unknown variance

We choose to use a random intercept only in order to show a different random effect structure than the one used in the previous example. Conditional on the random intercept, the outcomes can be assumed to have Poisson, negative binomial (for number of drinking days), or gamma distribution (for drinks per drinking day) and repeated observations on the same subject are conditionally independent. Individuals are also assumed to be independent of one another.

Since there is only a random intercept in this model, the correlations between repeated observations on the same individual are the same regardless of how far apart the observations are. If we also include a random slope in the model, the strength of the correlations depends on the time lag between observations. Multiple level random effects can also be added, for example, we can add a random effect for the clinical center and specify that individual-level random effects are nested within the center. This allows to account for positive correlations of the observations on different individuals within the center.

The interpretation of the regression coefficients is subject-specific. That is, the regression coefficients show how much the outcome is expected to change for a particular individual when the corresponding covariate is changed by 1 unit for a continuous predictor and when a particular category of a categorical predictor is compared to the reference category. As in the case of binary data, the subject-specific effects are not the same as the population-averaged effects.

Similarly, in the Health and Retirement Study, we can modify Equation 4.10 to include random effects. Conditional on the random effects, we assume a multinomial distribution for the ordinal measure of self-rated health and relate the cumulative logit of poorer health self-assessment to the linear predictor augmented with the random effects. The repeated observations within the individual are assumed to be independent, conditional on the random effects, and individuals are assumed to be independent of one another. As in the other GLMM examples, the regression parameters have subject-specific interpretations.

Thus, to summarize, we define a GLMM by the following:

1. Specify a linear predictor with fixed and random effects.
2. Assume that conditional on the random effects, the repeated observations within the individual/cluster are independent with a distribution in the exponential family.
3. Choose an appropriate link to relate the mean of the exponential family distribution to the linear predictor.

4.3.2 Implied Variance–Covariance Structure

In GLMM the individual observations are assumed to be independent, conditional on the random effects. As explained above, this means that all statistical associations that exist between the repeated observations on the same individual or within the cluster are due to the shared random effects. Thus, there are equal associations when there is only a random intercept in the model and more complicated structures when there are random slopes and other configurations of random effects. The variances of individual observations are a combination of the residual variances, according to the specific GLM that is chosen, and the variances of random effects. Herein, we just consider random effects that are normally distributed but other distributions of the random effects could be chosen (e.g., t-distributions, discrete distributions). This complicates model fitting and there is limited software for such models, but it is possible.

4.3.3 Estimation, Model Fit, and Interpretation

Due to the complicated form of the likelihood function of GLMM, model fitting requires that analytical, stochastic, or numerical approximations are used. Nowadays, many software packages include modules for fitting such models. In particular, we use the GLIMMIX procedure in SAS in order to fit GLMM models to the data examples.

Model selection among models with different fixed and random effects (but the same response distribution and fitted to the same data) are based on information criteria such as the AIC and the BIC. Smaller values of these criteria are indicative of a better fit. Likelihood ratio tests can also be used to compare nested models with different numbers of fixed effects.

The estimated parameters of the fixed effects in the GLMMs have subject-specific interpretation as described above. Empirical Bayes estimates of the random effects indicate how a particular subject's responses deviate from the expected response of an average individual (i.e., individual with random effects set to 0) and, based on these estimates and the estimates of the fixed effects, individualized predictions of the outcome can be performed.

Model diagnostics for GLMMs also have been recently developed that allow an evaluation of the fit of the model to the data. Details about GLMMs are provided in McCulloch and Searle (2001), Jiang (2007), and Stroup (2013).

4.3.4 GLMM for Count Data: Number of Drinking Days in the COMBINE Study

In parallel to the GEE analyses considered in the previous section, we fit a GLMM with a negative binomial distribution to the number of drinking days per month during the double-blind treatment phase of the study. We could also consider Poisson, binomial, or even normal GLMM, but as discussed before, the negative binomial model has the advantage of seamlessly taking into account the overdispersion in the data and has intuitive interpretation in terms of percent change, so we focus on this model. We consider the same fixed effects in the linear predictor as before (i.e., main effects of naltrexone, CBI, time, and all possible interactions). Note that unlike the GEE approach, where we treated time as a categorical predictor, herein, we consider time as a continuous predictor as this is more natural in the context of models with random effects where individual trends over time are the focus, and we are interested in describing these parsimoniously. We present two different random effects models (a random intercept, and a random intercept and slope model) in order to illustrate the implications of random structure assumptions and to compare and contrast the GLMM and GEE approaches. In terms of model fit, the random intercept and slope model fits significantly better than the random intercept model (AIC = 22937.5 compared to AIC = 23241.7) so this would be the chosen final GLMM model. The decision between the GEE or GLMM approach is based on the goals of the analysis (i.e., whether population-averaged or subject-specific effects are of interest) and can't be based on model fit statistics.

4.3.4.1 Random Intercept Model

The estimated variance of the random intercept is large compared to its standard error (variance of 3.86 with a standard error of 0.21) suggesting that there is significant between-subject variability in overall drinking frequency. The first two columns with results from Table 4.9 present the subject-specific slope estimates and the rate ratios from the GLMM negative binomial models for the significant effects in the model: a significant naltrexone by time interaction ($F(1,3488)=5.84$, $p=0.02$) and a significant CBI by time interaction ($F(1,3488)=8.44$, $p=0.004$). There is also a statistically significant main effect of time ($F(1,3488)=12.02$, $p=0.0005$). Since there are only random intercepts in the model, individuals are expected to start higher or lower than the average but their rate of change is expected to be the same. Thus, the fixed slope estimates show the rate of change for a random individual. For example, the rate ratio estimate in the first row is 1.01 which means that the rate of drinking increases by 1% per month for a random subject on naltrexone. Similarly, from the second row the rate of drinking increases by 7% for a random subject on placebo.

Note that the difference between the estimated fixed slopes on naltrexone and on placebo estimates the magnitude of the naltrexone by time interaction. This difference is estimated to be 0.05 with a corresponding rate ratio exp(0.05) or 1.05 (95% CI: 1.01, 1.10). The interpretation is as follows: if we consider any specific individual and could change his treatment assignment from naltrexone to placebo, we expect the rate of drinking to jump up by about 5% in a month. The estimated interaction between CBI and time is of a similar magnitude.

However, the subject-specific interpretation of this interaction is problematic since individuals do not switch treatments in this study. Thus, we are de facto performing extrapolation from the data. It is more natural to consider population-averaged estimates of the treatment by time effects from GEE. In GEE, the naltrexone by time effect is interpreted as the ratio of drinking frequency per month when comparing subjects on naltrexone and on placebo (we can think of comparing an average subject on naltrexone to an average subject on placebo). Often, the two sets of estimates are quite close. Note that the interpretation

TABLE 4.9

Fixed Slope Estimates and Rate Ratios for the Significant Effects in the Negative Binomial GLMM with Log Link Applied to Number of Drinking Days in the COMBINE Study

Fixed Slope of the Time Effect	Random Intercept Model		Random Intercept and Slope Model	
	Estimate (95% CI)	**Rate Ratio (95% CI)**	**Estimate (95% CI)**	**Rate Ratio (95% CI)**
For subjects on naltrexone	0.01 (−0.02, 0.04)	1.01 (0.98, 1.04)	−0.06 (−0.11, −0.01)	0.94 (0.89, 0.99)
For subjects on placebo	0.06 (0.03, 0.09)	1.07 (1.04, 1.10)	0.01 (−0.04, 0.06)	1.01 (0.96, 1.06)
For subjects on CBI	0.01 (−0.02, 0.04)	1.01 (0.98, 1.04)	−0.06 (−0.11, −0.01)	0.94 (0.90, 0.99)
For subjects not on CBI	0.07 (0.04, 0.10)	1.07 (1.04, 1.10)	0.01 (−0.04, 0.06)	1.01 (0.96, 1.06)

of the within-subject effect of time from GLMM is quite natural and not at all problematic since all subjects have repeated measures over time. However, the random intercept model is limited in terms of what it tells us about the individual change over time since it forces all individuals in a group to have the same slope. We now consider the random intercept and slope model which is more flexible in addition to fitting the data better.

4.3.4.2 Random Intercept and Slope Model

The estimated variances of the random intercept and slope are fairly large compared to their standard errors (variance of 3.89 with a standard error of 0.29 for the random intercept and variance of 0.13 with a standard error of 0.01 for the random slope) suggesting that there is significant between-subject variability in overall drinking frequency and rate of change over time. The intercept and slope are also negatively correlated (covariance = −0.13 with a standard error of 0.05).

The last two columns of Table 4.9 present the subject-specific slope estimates and the rate ratios from the GLMM negative binomial models for the significant effects in the model: A significant naltrexone by time interaction ($F(1,2310) = 5.22$, $p = 0.02$) and a significant CBI by time interaction ($F(1,2310) = 4.73$, $p = 0.03$). Since there are random intercepts and slopes in the model, the fixed slope estimates show the rate of change for an individual who is in the middle of the corresponding treatment group, in terms of rate of change, that is, who has a random slope of 0. We call this individual a "middle" individual (in contrast to an average individual, which is sometimes used in the context of population-averaged models). The rate ratios are obtained by exponentiating the fixed slope estimates and can be interpreted as the percent change per month for such a "middle" individual. Thus, we estimate that the "middle" individual on naltrexone has a 6% decrease in the number of drinking days per month (since the rate ratio is 0.94 and we compare it to 1), while the "middle" individual on placebo has a 1% increase per month. The estimated effect for CBI is very similar (almost identical within rounding error).

However, other individuals in the group are estimated to have different rates of change which are obtained by adding the fixed slope estimate and the predicted random slope for the particular individual. For example, an individual on naltrexone with a random slope one standard deviation above the "middle" individual's random slope of 0 has an estimated slope equal to −0.06 + 0.36 (−0.06 is the fixed slope and 0.36 is the estimated standard deviation of the random slope, obtained as the square root of the variance) or 0.30 and thus, is estimated to increase (rather than decrease) his drinking days exp(0.30) = 1.35 times per month (i.e., by 35%). Similarly, an individual on naltrexone with an estimated random slope one standard deviation below the slope of the "middle" individual has an estimated slope of −0.06–0.36 = −0.42 and thus decreases her drinking days exp(−0.42) = 0.66 times (i.e., by 34%). The difference in rate of change over time, when considering two individuals, one with a random slope two standard deviations above, and one with a random slope two standard deviations below 0, is even more dramatic: an increase of 93% versus a decrease of 54%.

Like in the random intercept model, in the random intercept and slope model, conditional on the random effects, the difference between the estimated fixed slopes on naltrexone and on placebo is the same (−0.06 to 0.01 = −0.07) and the corresponding rate ratio (exp(−0.07) = 0.93) is the same. Thus, if we consider any specific individual and could change their treatment assignment from placebo to naltrexone, we expect the rate of change over time to decrease by about 7%. This estimated decrease is the same regardless of which individual we consider (i.e., whether they have higher or lower rate of change over time, and whether they start higher or lower than the average individual). However, this interpretation is problematic, as we already pointed out, because individuals do not switch between treatments during the period we consider. Thus, although technically we can estimate subject-specific effects of between-subject factors, such as treatment, we need to be cautious when interpreting those. In contrast, the subject-specific slope estimates for time are perfectly interpretable because all subjects have repeated observations over time.

Note that there are sizeable differences between the estimates for the fixed portion of the slopes from the random intercept model, and from the random intercept and slope model. This is not always the case but it demonstrates that the estimates for the fixed portion of the GLMM can be affected by the assumptions about the random effects.

Figure 4.4 shows the predicted number of drinking days for individuals by treatment group, based on the GLMM. Due to the different intercepts and slopes, there is a wide variety of predicted responses. While most individuals have zero or few drinking days throughout the study (judging by the denseness of the lines at the lower end of the scale), there are some who drink intensively and show substantial increase over time. The variety of individual predictions comes in contrast to what one sees in a GEE, where each individual's predicted response is equal to the estimated average response for the group to which the individual belongs.

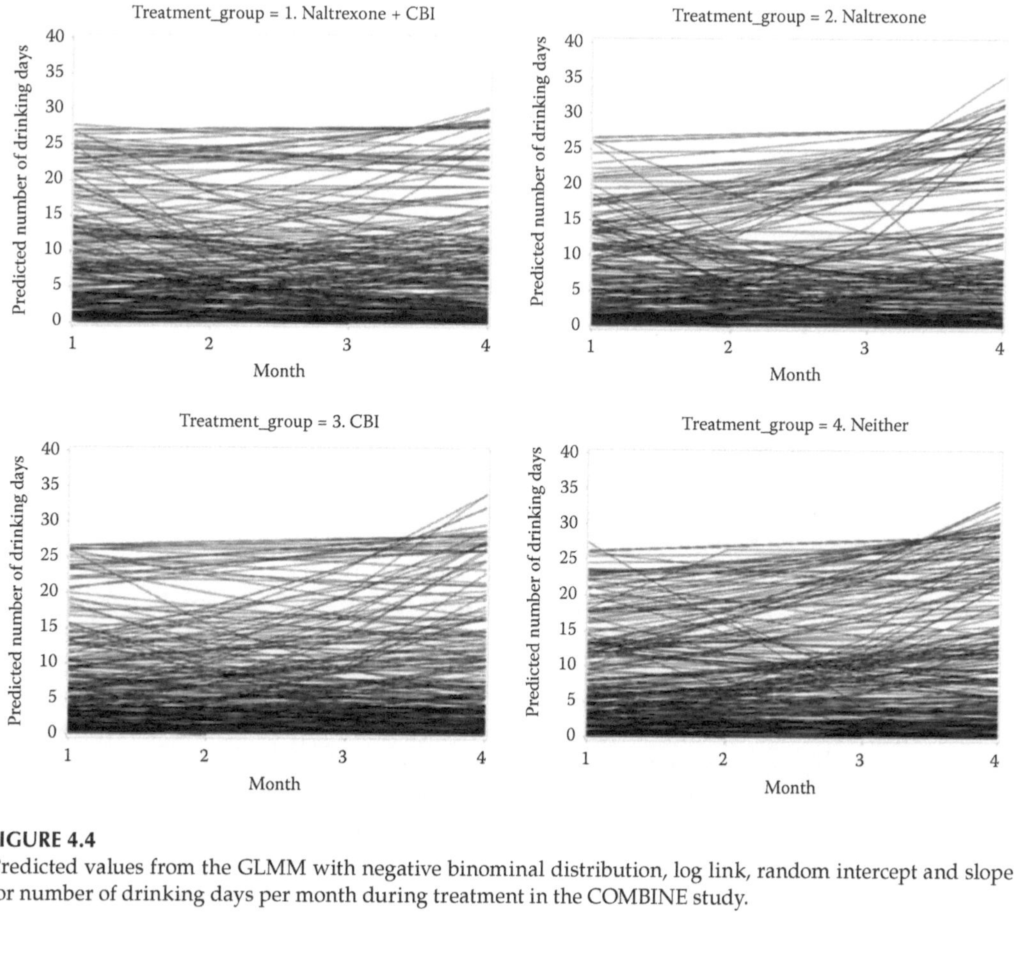

FIGURE 4.4
Predicted values from the GLMM with negative binominal distribution, log link, random intercept and slope for number of drinking days per month during treatment in the COMBINE study.

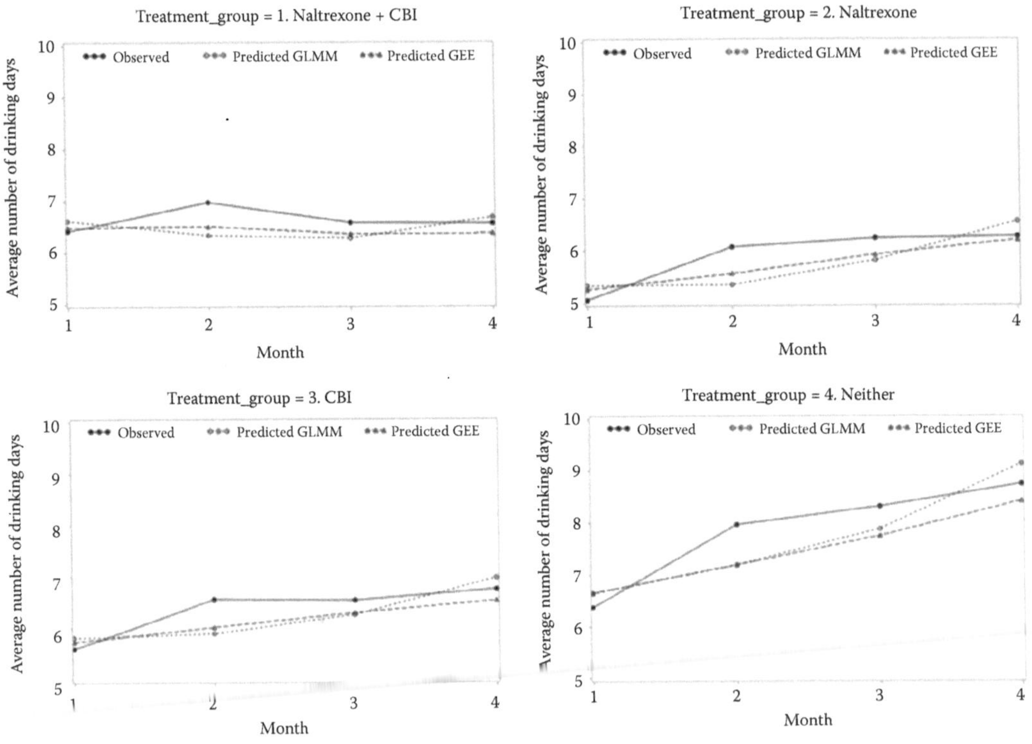

FIGURE 4.5
Raw means, average predicted values from the GLMM, and model-based means from the GEE model, with negative binominal distribution and log link for number of drinking days per month during treatment in the COMBINE study.

Figure 4.5 shows the averages of the predicted values per treatment group, based on the GLMM, the population-averaged estimates from the corresponding GEE (i.e., a GEE with the same fixed portion of the linear predictor, response distribution and link function, and unstructured working correlation matrix), together with the raw means of the observed number of drinking days per month. Note that the estimated trajectories from the GEE are the same for all individuals, while the estimated trajectories from the GLMM are averages of the lines from Figure 4.4. Both the GLMM and the GEE provide a similar fit to the raw means with more noticeable curvature in the estimates from the GLMM. Interestingly, although we have only linear time effects, the estimated means show a curvilinear change over time as we are averaging the predictions for subjects with different intercepts and slopes (in the GLMM) and are using a non-linear function (log) to relate the response to the predictors (in both models). Compared to the GEE with categorical time, here the match of the means from both the GLMM and GEE models with continuous time to the raw means is not as good because we are using linear time effects, which describe the longitudinal trends more parsimoniously but fail to capture some of the curvature in the data.

The fixed slope and rate ratio estimates from GEE models with different working correlation structures are shown in Table 4.10. We focus on the results from the GEE model with unstructured working correlation shown in the last two columns in Table 4.10.

TABLE 4.10

Slope Estimates and Rate Ratios for the Naltrexone by Time and CBI by Time Effects from the GEE Negative Binomial Model with Log Link Applied to Number of Drinking Days in the COMBINE Study

	Exchangeable Working Correlation		Unstructured Working Correlation	
Fixed Slope of the Time Effect	**Estimate (95% CI)**	**Rate Ratio (95% CI)**	**Estimate (95% CI)**	**Rate Ratio (95% CI)**
For subjects on naltrexone	0.04 (0.01, 0.07)	1.04 (1.01, 1.07)	0.02 (−0.01, 0.05)	1.02 (0.99, 1.05)
For subjects on placebo	0.07 (0.05, 0.10)	1.08 (1.05, 1.11)	0.06 (0.03, 0.09)	1.06 (1.03, 1.09)
For subjects on CBI	0.02 (−0.00, 0.05)	1.02 (1.00, 1.05)	0.01 (−0.02, 0.04)	1.01 (0.98, 1.05)
For subjects not on CBI	0.08 (0.06, 0.11)	1.09 (1.06, 1.12)	0.07 (0.04, 0.09)	1.07 (1.04, 1.10)

In contrast to the GLMM, with random intercept and slope, where the estimated subject-specific slope estimates for the "middle" individual on naltrexone or on CBI are negative, the population-average slope estimates in the GEE are positive with the slopes on active treatment much closer to 0, while the slopes not on active treatment are significantly larger than 0. This may appear contradictory to the results from the GLMM but it is not, since the two types of models are estimating different parameters (population-averaged in GEE versus subject-specific in GLMM). As illustrated above, in the random intercept and slope GLMM, the estimated slope and rate ratios for time vary depending on which individual we consider. The rate ratio describing change over time for the "middle" individual is not the same as the average of the rate ratios of all individuals in the same group because of the non-linearity of the link function. However, although the fixed slope estimates over time are different in the two random effects models and in the GEE model, the differences between treatment groups are very similar. Indeed, the population-average analysis suggests that in the absence of treatment there is significant worsening of outcome over time, and treatment ameliorates that, while the subject-specific analysis suggests that for a "middle" individual there is slight but not significant deterioration in the absence of treatment, and treatment significantly improves the outcome. Both analyses find a substantial advantage of either naltrexone or CBI, but not of the combination.

We should note that if the focus is on the treatment group by time effect, the GEE approach is preferable since treatment is a between-subject factor and the treatment by time effect has more intuitive population-averaged interpretation. However, the GLMM approach is more flexible in describing subject-specific trends over time and hence, when the focus is on estimating individual-level change over time, the GLMM approach is preferable. Also, GLMM is more flexible in terms of modeling change over time and can seamlessly be used with any unbalanced designs.

Of note, inclusion of random effects allows us to account for some degree of overdispersion in the data. Sometimes a random intercept can be added just with this purpose in mind. Fitting other appropriate models for count data, such as the generalized Poisson model, which allows us to account for overdispersion, zero-inflated and hurdle mixed models which allow us to account for extra zeros is described in Littell (2006).

4.3.5 GLMM Analysis of Ordinal Data: Self-Rated Health in the Health and Retirement Study

In parallel to the GEE analysis of these data, we consider a cumulative logit model with the same fixed effects as in the GEE model, but also including a random intercept and a random slope. Thus, the GLMM is specified by the following equation:

$$\log\left(\frac{P(Y_{ij} \geq k)}{P(Y_{ij} < k)}\right) = \beta_{0k} + \beta_1 F_i + \beta_2 S_i + \beta_3 W_j + \beta_4 F_i S_i + \beta_5 F_i W_j + \beta_6 S_i W_j + \beta_7 S_i F_i W_j + b_{i0} + b_{i1} W_j$$

where the random effects b_{i0} and b_{i1} are assumed to be normally distributed and, in general, correlated.

The observations on the same individual are conditionally independent, given these random effects, and have a multinomial distribution. The inclusion of the random effects allows the cumulative odds of poorer self-rated health for each individual to deviate systematically from the cumulative odds associated with the particular combination of fixed predictors. Individual-level odds can be larger or smaller than predicted by the fixed effects and the rate of change in these odds over time may be faster or slower than the rate predicted by the fixed effects. We also include subject's age at wave 1 (centered at the mean age of the sample at wave 1) in the linear predictor of the model.

As in the GEE model, in the GLMM self-rated health is an ordinal variable with 5 categories: 1 = excellent, 2 = very good, 3 = good, 4 = fair, and 5 = poor, and we focus on the cumulative odds of poorer health self-assessment. That is, we model the odds of "poor" versus the rest of the categories; "poor" or "fair" versus the rest of the categories; "poor," "fair," or "good" versus "very good" or "excellent," and "poor," "fair," "good," or "very good" versus "excellent."

We first report the significant results from the tests of the fixed effects in the model (interactions and main effects). There are significant two-way interactions between gender and smoking ($F(1,36682) = 6.72$, $p = 0.01$), between wave and smoking ($F(1,36682) = 29.25$, $p<0.0001$), and between wave and gender ($F(1,36682) = 7.22$, $p = 0.01$); and also significant main effects of smoking ($F(1,36682) = 205.19$, $p < 0.0001$) and wave ($F(1,9113) = 1333.44$, $p<0.0001$).

Post hoc analyses (estimation of slopes) are performed to explain the significant effects in the models. The estimated slope over time for a "middle" non-smoking individual (i.e., the random intercept and slope are both 0) is 0.20 (SE = 0.006) and for an "average" smoking individual is 0.27 (SE = 0.01). The interpretation of the two slope estimates is that the log cumulative odds of poorer self-rated health increase by 0.20 per wave (two-year period) in a "middle" non-smoking individual and by 0.27 in a "middle" smoking individual. The difference in slopes is −0.07 (SE = 0.01) showing that the log cumulative odds of poorer health in "middle" non-smoking individuals increase at a slower rate than in "middle" smoking individuals. Exponentiating this estimate gives a cumulative odds ratio of poorer health of 0.93 (95% CI: 0.91, 0.96) or we estimate that not smoking is associated with about 7% slower rate of decrease in a particular individual. The difference due to smoking is the same in all individuals and does not depend on whether they start higher or lower than the average or have higher or lower rate of change over time.

Similarly, the estimated slope for a "middle" female is 0.22 (SE = 0.009) and for a "middle" male is 0.25 (SE = 0.009), with a difference of 0.03 (SE = 0.01). Exponentiating gives us a cumulative odds ratio of poorer health of 1.03 (95% CI: 1.01, 1.06) or an approximate 3% difference in the rate of change over time with faster deterioration in males than in females. Note, though, that it is difficult to conceptualize this as a subject-specific effect as individuals don't change their gender during the study. Rather, one could think of this effect as comparing a male and female individual with the same values of their random effects.

Note that these estimates are larger in absolute value than the corresponding estimates from the population-averaged GEE model, which reflect the average effects in the population rather than the effects within individual or "middle" individuals. This is often the case when comparing subject-specific and population-averaged estimates. Individuals have steeper or flatter rates of change than the "middle" individual, depending on their random effect estimates. They also start lower or higher than the "middle" individual.

Figure 4.6 shows the estimated cumulative odds over time of "poor," "fair," or "good" versus "very good" or "excellent" self-rated health for a "middle" individual in each of the four groups (non-smoking females, non-smoking males, smoking females, and smoking males). These are obtained by exponentiation of the corresponding combinations of regression coefficients and thus, show some curvature. The change in cumulative odds over time for the other cutoffs (e.g., "poor" versus the rest of the categories, or "poor" or "fair" versus the rest of the categories) is very similar in terms of shape, but the cumulative odds themselves change, since there is a different intercept in the model for each possible comparison. Figure 4.6 shows steeper increase in cumulative odds of poorer health for smokers of both genders and also shows that there are substantial differences in the cumulative odds at wave 1 due to smoking. Post hoc pairwise cumulative odds ratios at wave 1 confirm that "middle" non-smokers of both genders have significantly lower odds (about 60%–70% lower) of acknowledging poorer health than "middle" smokers (see Table 4.11). The effect is more pronounced for males than for females: cumulative odds ratio = 0.29, 95% CI: (0.23, 0.35) compared to cumulative odds ratio = 0.42, 95% CI: (0.34, 0.52). Substantively, the same results are obtained if one evaluates these post hoc comparisons at other waves.

Figure 4.7 shows the estimated odds of poorer health over time in individuals by gender and smoking status at baseline. The individual-level variability is evident in this plot with larger spread of the values among smoking males and females. Unlike the GEE model,

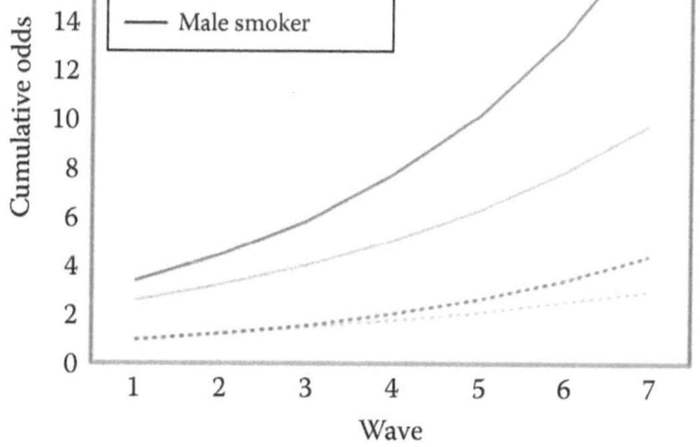

FIGURE 4.6
Cumulative odds of "poor," "fair," or "good" versus "very good" or "excellent" self-rated health estimated from the cumulative logit GLMM fitted to the Health and Retirement Study data.

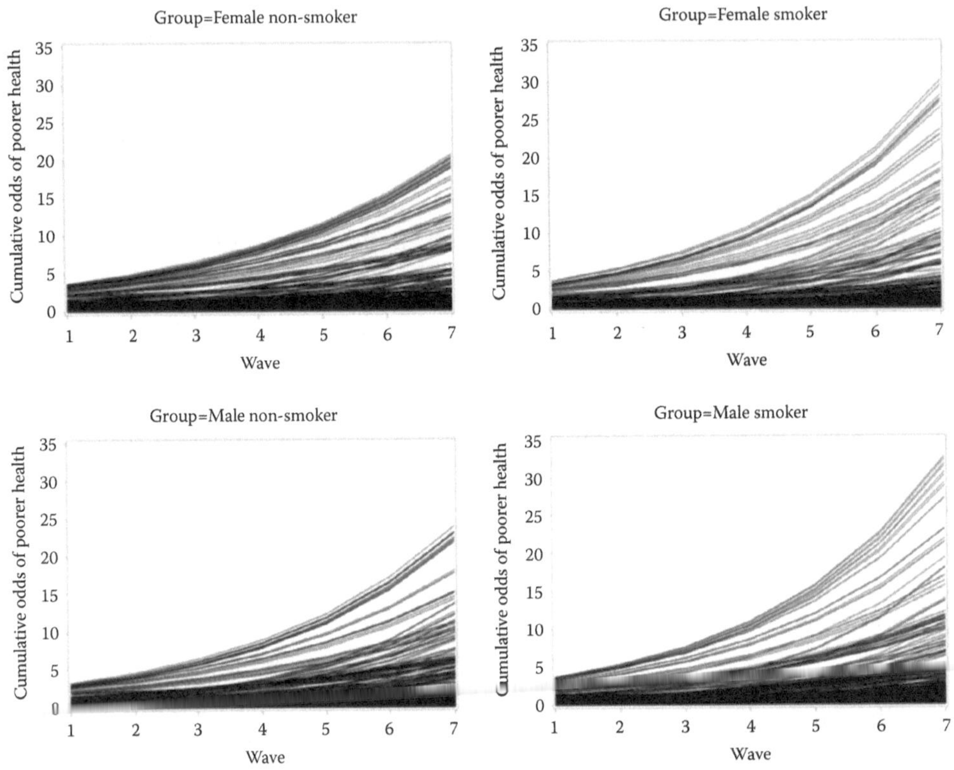

FIGURE 4.7
Predicted individual odds of "poor" health based on the cumulative logit GLMM applied to the Health and Retirement Study data.

which implies the same estimated cumulative odds of individuals with the same levels of the predictors (gender and smoking status), here each individual has their own estimated trajectory. Even individuals with missing data have complete estimated trajectories. The magnitude of the variability is due to the variance in the intercept in slope. In the GLMM, the estimated variance of the random intercept is 7.98 (SE = 0.17), while the variance of the random slope is estimated to be 0.07 (SE = 0.004). Both random effects are necessary to be included in the model as evidenced by the AIC of the model with random intercept and slope (AIC = 132297.7) compared to the AIC of the model just with a random intercept (AIC = 132804.9) and the model without any random effects (AIC = 164909.7).

In summary, smokers have lower self-rated health at baseline than non-smokers with the difference more pronounced in males, and deterioration in self-rated health proceeds at a slower rate in non-smokers over time than in smokers. The actual regression estimates are subject-specific, which means that this is the expected change for a particular subject if we could change the predictors for this individual. In the case of time, this is very reasonable, as time is a within-subject effect in the model. Smoking status could also potentially be changed, although in this example, we used smoking status at baseline. However, gender is arguably not changeable and hence the gender differences can't be interpreted as subject-specific. Rather, one can think of comparing males and females with the same values of their random effects. In general, subject-specific estimates are larger in absolute value than population-averaged estimates. However, this is not always the case, especially when odds or rate ratios are close to 1.

TABLE 4.11

Cumulative Odds Ratios for the Significant Effects in the Cumulative Logit GLMM Fit to Self-Rated Health in the Health and Retirement Study

Effect	Level	Comparison Level	Cumulative Odds Ratio (95% CI)
Main effect of time	Next wave	Previous wave	1.26 (1.25, 1.28)
Effect of smoking (evaluated at wave 1)	Not smoking	Smoking	0.35 (0.30, 0.40)
Effect of gender (evaluated at wave 1)	Female	Male	0.98 (0.85, 1.14)
Gender × smoking interaction (evaluated at wave 1)	Female not smoking	Female smoking	0.42 (0.34, 0.52)
	Male not smoking	Male smoking	0.29 (0.23, 0.35)
	Male not smoking	Female not smoking	0.84 (0.72, 0.98)
	Male smoking	Female smoking	1.23 (0.96, 1.58)
Time × gender interaction	Next wave female	Previous wave female	1.24 (1.22, 1.26)
	Next wave male	Previous wave male	1.28 (1.26, 1.31)
	Next wave versus previous wave × Female versus male		1.03 (1.01, 1.06)
Time × smoking interaction	Next wave not smoking	Previous wave not smoking	1.22 (1.21, 1.24)
	Next wave smoking	Previous wave smoking	1.31 (1.28, 1.33)
	Next wave versus previous wave × Not smoking versus smoking		0.93 (0.91, 0.96)

4.4 Summary

In this chapter, we introduced two classes of models (GEE and GLMM) that can be used to assess the effects of predictors on non-normally distributed outcomes in studies, with repeated measures and presented data analyses from clinical trials and observational studies as illustration. We focused on binary, ordinal, and count data, since these are the most commonly encountered types of non-normally distributed data in medical studies, and showed how these outcomes fit in the same statistical framework, which simplifies model fitting and inference. Nevertheless, each type of outcome requires specific interpretation of the effects (e.g., effects are expressed as odds ratios for binary data, cumulative odds ratios for ordinal data, and rate ratios for count data). Moreover, depending on how the correlation between repeated measures is accounted for (i.e., by assuming a working correlation structure or by incorporating random effects in the linear predictor), estimates have either population-averaged (in GEE models) or subject-specific (in GLMM) interpretation. Hence, deciding which model to use is much more challenging than in linear mixed models when the outcome is normally distributed.

In general, when interest lies in predicting the outcome of individual subjects, the design is unbalanced (i.e., observations are not taken at the same time points for all subjects), and/or there is substantial proportion of missing data, GLMM would be the preferred approach. On the other hand, when interest lies in estimation of average effects in the population, the correlations are not of particular interest in themselves, and missing data are not a particular concern, GEE would be the preferred approach. Once a particular approach and an appropriate outcome distribution are chosen, model selection between models with different correlation structures and fixed effects can be based on information criteria. Interpretation of estimated fixed (and random) effects is based on the choice of the model.

Although GLMM and GEE are more complicated than the LMM they extend, they provide much needed flexibility in modeling non-normal outcomes. Nevertheless, even these models may not be appropriate for some types of data that do not conform well to distributions in the exponential family. In such situations, an entirely non-parametric approach to repeated measures data can be considered. We focus on such an approach in Chapter 5.

5

Non-Parametric Methods for the Analysis of Repeatedly Measured Data

In the previous two chapters, *parametric models* for different types of repeatedly measured outcomes were presented. These models require that the distribution of the response closely resembles one of a set of pre-specified distributions (e.g., normal for continuous data, Poisson for count data). While these models cover a wide variety of scenarios, there are situations where none of the distributions provide a very good fit to the data and transformations are not very useful in bringing the data in line with theoretical expectations. For example, most mathematically convenient distributions do not accommodate data that show floor or ceiling effects (i.e., when there is a substantial number of observations at the end of the distribution range). In Chapter 4, we encountered such a scenario with the number of drinking days in the COMBINE study, which had many more zeros than predicted by the theoretical distributions we considered. Although in this particular case, one might fit hurdle or zero-inflated models, an alternative is to use a *non-parametric approach*, which does not require that a specific distribution for the data be assumed.

Another example that we presented in Chapter 1, is the *human laboratory study of menthol's effects on nicotine reinforcement in smokers*. Rewarding effects of nicotine in this small cross-over trial under different menthol and nicotine conditions were assessed using the drug effects questionnaire. Observed scores were mostly 0 at baseline and, depending on the dose of nicotine, had small or large variability post-baseline but with a substantial number of observed zeros. None of the parametric models presented so far fit these data well because of limited or no variability at baseline, floor effects, and the different variances at different levels of the predictors.

Covariance patterns are also hard to fit with such types of data. In situations when hypotheses testing is the main focus of analysis and the design is balanced (i.e., individuals are evaluated at the same time points), a non-parametric approach that does not assume a particular shape or form for the outcome and structure of the variances and covariances is more appropriate. It allows to test for main and interactive effects of the factors and provides appropriately conservative tests of study hypotheses. However, since balanced design is required, this approach can't be applied to situations when individuals are measured at different time points.

In the first section of this chapter, we briefly mention some classical non-parametric procedures in order to introduce non-parametric methods and outline their advantages and disadvantages. In the second section, we include a brief presentation and discussion of the first non-parametric test used for repeated measures data, namely Friedman's test. The major emphasis in this chapter is on the general approach for longitudinal data in factorial experiments presented at a non-technical level in the third section. The overall idea is to rank the data (from smallest to largest observation) and then run a linear mixed model on the ranks with special options selected for the estimation of the variances and covariances, and for approximation of the test statistics. This method can be used in a variety of repeated measures situations and is described in detail in Brunner, Domhof, and Langer

(2002). We use two of the data examples introduced in Chapter 1 for illustration. SAS programs and output files are available in the online materials.

The non-parametric methods discussed here should be distinguished from non-parametric modeling of time trends in longitudinal studies, known as non-parametric regression smoothing. Smoothing methods are usually applied to intensive longitudinal data when no *a priori* assumptions of the form or shape of time trends over time are made, and it is of interest to estimate the trajectory of change over time. This is a very different situation from the one we focus on here, where we have relatively few repeated occasions and a non-parametric approach is needed because response distributions and/or variance structures do not correspond to mathematically convenient choices provided by parametric models. Readers interested in the topic of non-parametric regression smoothing are referred to Wu and Zhang (2006), Lin and Carroll (2009), or Lin and Pan (2013).

5.1 Classical Non-Parametric Methods for Independent Samples

Non-parametric procedures are statistical procedures that are valid under mild assumptions. In particular, they are distribution-free and, as such, they enjoy several advantages over parametric methods. They require fewer assumptions, are not as sensitive to outliers, can be used in situations when parametric methods are not appropriate, and are, in general, easy to implement. However, they are focused on hypothesis testing, effect sizes provided by non-parametric tests may not be as interpretable, and non-parametric alternatives, in general, are less powerful when assumptions for parametric procedures are satisfied.

Non-parametric procedures use *ranks* rather than actual observed values of the dependent variables. That is, observations are ranked from the smallest to the largest, with the smallest observation assigned a rank of 1 and the largest observation assigned a rank equal to the number of observations that are ranked.

A simple example is presented below with 10 observations in total and two sets of tied observations (*ties*, observations with the same value).

Values	3	7	3	10	−1	−1	3	5.5	2	33
Ranks	5	8	5	9	1.5	1.5	5	7	3	10

When the 10 observations are ranked (−1, −1, 2, 3, 3, 3, 5.5, 7, 10, 33), the smallest in value is assigned a rank of 1, the second smallest is assigned a rank of 2, and ranking continues until the largest in value is assigned a rank of 10. However, when there are ties, they are assigned the mid-rank. In the example, the smallest value is −1 and there are two observations with this value. Hence, they are assigned the mid-rank of 1 and 2 which is 1.5. The next smallest value is 2 and it is assigned a rank of 3 since there are two observations with smaller values. Then comes 3 which represents a three-way tie, hence, each of these observations is assigned a rank of 5 (the mid-rank of 4, 5, and 6). Ranking continues until the largest observation is assigned a rank of 10 because there are 10 observations. Once ranks are assigned, test statistics are calculated based on these ranks.

Some of the simplest and most commonly used non-parametric procedures are *Spearman's rank correlation coefficient*, for assessing the relationship between two variables, *Mann–Whitney's U test*, for evaluating whether two sets of observations come from the same distribution, *Kruskal–Wallis's test*, which extends the Mann–Whitney procedure for more than two samples, and *Wilcoxon's signed-rank test* for matched pairs. Each of these procedures is based on ranks and is used when the corresponding parametric test can't be applied because its assumptions are not satisfied. Non-parametric tests are also often preferred in very small samples (e.g., sample sizes less than 10), although they have very low power in these situations.

Spearman's rank correlation coefficient is calculated as the Pearson's correlation between the ranks of the observations on two variables with the observations on each variable ranked separately. It can be used to assess the association of continuous or discrete (including ordinal) data, in particular, to determine whether larger values on one variable correspond to larger/smaller values on the other variable. Spearman's rank correlation coefficient is the non-parametric alternative of Pearson's correlation for two continuous variables and it assesses whether the ranks, rather than the actual values, are linearly related.

Mann–Whitney's U test is the non-parametric equivalent of the two-sample t-test for normally distributed data, and is used to assess whether there are differences in location between the distributions of the two groups that are compared. The null hypothesis is that the continuous distributions of the populations from which the two samples are obtained are the same (i.e., that all observations come from the same distribution) while the alternative is that one distribution is shifted toward larger or smaller values. To test this hypothesis, all observations from both samples are ranked together, the ranks of the observations in each sample are summed, and a test statistic based on the sums of the ranks in one of the samples is calculated. An exact distribution of the test statistic is used to obtain p-values in small samples, while in large samples approximations are used.

Kruskal–Wallis's test is the non-parametric alternative to one-way analysis of variance and is used to compare the distributions of two or more groups. Similar to Mann–Whitney's U test, all observations are ranked together as if they come from the same continuous distribution. The test statistic is then very similar to the test statistic of treatment effects in one-way ANOVA, with the only difference that the ranks of the observations are used as response values, rather than the actual values. That is, the between-group variability of the ranks is compared to the within-group variability of the ranks and if the former is much larger than the latter, then it is concluded that the distribution of at least one of the groups is shifted with respect to the other distributions.

Details of these simple procedures, and a wide variety of other non-parametric tests, can be found in the comprehensive text of Hollander and Wolfe (1999). The common theme in all such tests is that the observations are ranked and a test statistic based on the ranks is calculated. Usually in these tests, it is assumed that the data come from a continuous distribution and hence, ties are not expected. When ties are present, the test statistics require some adjustments but these are automatically handled by software programs.

Since emphasis herein is on correlated data, we focus on non-parametric tests for repeated measures data of increasing complexity. We start with Wilcoxon's signed-rank test and Friedman's test, and continue with the general approach of non-parametric analysis of data with repeated measures.

5.2 Simple Non-Parametric Tests for Repeated Measures Data

Wilcoxon's signed rank-test is the non-parametric equivalent to a paired t-test and, as such, is the simplest non-parametric test that can be used for repeated measures data. If there are only two repeated occasions, and it is of interest to test whether there is significant change from one occasion to the other, then Wilcoxon's signed-rank test can be used. The test involves calculating the absolute differences between paired observations (i.e., observations on the same individual) and the signs of these differences (positive or negative). The absolute differences are then ranked and the test statistic is the sum of the signed ranks (hence, the name of the test). Extreme values of the test statistic are supportive of the hypothesis of change from occasion 1 to occasion 2. For small samples, the p-values are calculated based on the exact distribution of the test statistic, while for large values an approximation is used.

Friedman's test is the non-parametric equivalent of analysis of variance in complete block designs. In the context of repeated measures data, it can be applied when each subject is observed at the same set of repeated occasions and the goal is to assess whether there are differences in distributions across occasions (i.e., whether the values on some occasions are systematically larger or smaller than the values on other occasions). Friedman's test involves ranking the repeated observations within the same subject (cluster, block), calculating the average ranks per occasion and looking at the variability of these average ranks. Large values of the test statistic indicate differences in the distributions on repeated occasions. Details about the test statistic, its distribution, and the effect of ties can be found in Hollander and Wolfe (1999).

Friedman's test can also be performed by first ranking the data within the subject, performing two-way ANOVA analysis on the ranked data with the subject and occasion as factors (without interactions between them), and assessing the significance of the occasion effect. In the case of data without ties, this approach results exactly in Friedman's test statistic. When there are ties, adjustment to the test statistic is necessary and it is better to use specialized procedures for such analysis. In the online materials, we show how to apply Friedman's test in SAS directly, and using ANOVA, on the ranks for the example considered next.

In the COMBINE data set, it is of interest to assess whether there is an overall increase in drinking over time. To illustrate how Friedman's test can be used to test this hypothesis, we focus on the number of drinking days during double-blind treatment in a subsample of COMBINE subjects. Since non-parametric methods are often used in small samples where it is not possible to verify the assumptions of normality, we consider only 10 subjects and show how the data are ranked in Table 5.1.

As seen from the table, in this subsample of 10 subjects, the average ranks (and hence, the number of drinking days) increase with time. The test statistic for Friedman's test is 7.8 with a borderline significant p-value of 0.05. This indicates that there are statistically significant differences among the occasions. However, the average ranks do not provide information about how large the increase is and which occasions are significantly different from one another. While the first shortcoming is typical of non-parametric tests, pairwise comparisons among the repeated occasions can pinpoint where the differences are and address the second issue. To compare each pair of occasions we use Wilcoxon's signed-rank tests.

The results are shown in Table 5.2. There are significant differences between periods 1 and 3, periods 2 and 3, and periods 1 and 4, at 0.05 significance level. From the average ranks, we see that there is significant increase in ranks from periods 1 and 2 to period 3, and then slight (non-significant) decrease from period 3 to period 4. Overall the ranks in period 3 are the highest. Note that this is a small subsample of the entire sample that we used for illustration of the test in order to show how the data are ranked. In general, the significance of the effects is largely dependent on sample size and in small sample

TABLE 5.1

Number of Drinking Days (NDD) per Month for 10 Individuals in the COMBINE Study with Corresponding within-Subject Ranks and Result from Friedman's Test of Change in Drinking over Time

Individual	NDD_1	NDD_2	NDD_3	NDD_4	Rank_1	Rank_2	Rank_3	Rank_4
I1	1	9	10	14	1	2	3	4
I2	1	4	6	13	1	2	3	4
I3	10	8	11	7	3	2	4	1
I4	23	17	20	22	4	1	2	3
I5	13	14	28	24	1	2	4	3
I6	4	13	9	10	1	4	2	3
I7	3	8	12	28	1	2	3	4
I8	11	19	26	22	1	2	4	3
I9	8	6	7	3	4	2	3	1
I10	5	7	17	9	1	2	4	3
Average					1.8	2.1	3.2	2.9
Test statistic and p-value	TS=7.8, p=0.05							

TABLE 5.2

Pairwise Comparisons between Months based on Wilcoxon's Signed-Rank Tests in the Subsample of 10 Subjects from the COMBINE Study

	Period 2	Period 3	Period 4
Period 1	TS=−14.5, p=0.16	TS=−23, p=0.02	TS=−20.5, p=0.04
Period 2		TS=−21, p=0.03	TS=−18.5, p=0.06
Period 3			TS=1.5, p=0.93

sizes it is quite possible to miss actual effects. Also, in general, corrections for multiple testing need to be applied for post hoc tests, which can also change the significance of the results (considered in detail in Chapter 6).

Friedman's test and Wilcoxon's signed-rank comparisons on the entire sample show significant differences across time points (Friedman's TS = 10.4, $p = 0.02$) but only the first month is statistically significantly different from the rest (p-values $< .0001$).

Friedman's test is useful for hypothesis testing in balanced repeated measures designs with only one repeated measures factor. However, as illustrated in the example data sets in Chapter 1, usually longitudinal and clustered data studies have more than one repeated measures factor and hence, more complicated statistical procedures are needed to evaluate such scenarios. We next present the general approach to repeated measures analysis in studies with balanced repeated measures designs (Brunner et al., 2002).

5.3 Non-Parametric Analysis of Repeated Measures Data in Factorial Designs

A commonly used but potentially misleading approach to the non-parametric analysis of repeatedly measured data is to rank all observations in the data set and then perform mixed model analysis on the ranked data, as usual. With simple designs without repeated measures, such as one-way ANOVA, this often works well, however, with repeated measures designs with more factors, this method can lead to widely differing variances within the different groups or on repeated occasions. Failure to account for the heterogeneity in variances can result in conclusions that are not supported by the data. Brunner, Munzel, and Puri (1999) and Brunner and Puri (2001) provide a technical description of the issues and develop appropriate procedures for the non-parametric analysis of repeatedly measured data. The basic idea is still based on ranking the observations, but once the data are ranked, special options need to be used when fitting linear mixed models (LMM) to the ranks, in order to estimate the variances correctly and to have valid tests of the effects in the model. In the mean portion of the LMM, all predictors are treated as categorical and all main effects and interactions are included in the model. In the variance portion of the model, the variances and covariances of the repeated observations within individuals are unrestricted and different unstructured variance–covariance matrices must be estimated within each combination of levels of the between-subject factors. The technical details are beyond the scope of this book but the main options that need to be selected for proper inferences are provided here.

In particular, variances and covariances must be obtained using moment-based rather than maximum likelihood or restricted maximum likelihood methods. *Moment-based methods* match the expected powers of the outcome (*theoretical moments,* e.g., the mean, the mean of squares) to the *sample moments* (e.g., the sample mean, the average of the squared observations), and solve the resulting equations to obtain estimates of the parameters of interest. Furthermore, special *ANOVA-type statistics* (ATS), based on the moment-based variance estimates, must be used for hypothesis testing. The ATS are similar to F-test statistics for the effects in the model but use the correct variance estimates and have only one associated set of degrees of freedom (unlike F-test statistics, where there are numerator and denominator degrees of freedom). They are requested by specifying a special option in SAS PROC MIXED.

The resulting algorithm performs well in large and small samples, with data that have floor/ceiling effects and are continuous or discrete. This is in contrast to other non-parametric procedures that require that distributions be continuous and require special handling of ties. Ties do not present a problem for the approach described herein. Also, the approach can seamlessly handle missing data at pre-specified occasions in a balanced design. *Relative marginal effects* can be plotted to compare the magnitudes of average ranks at different combinations of levels of the between-subject and within-subject factors and thus indicate direction and magnitude of effects, albeit not on the original scale. However, the non-parametric method is problematic to use if there are too many repeated occasions and can't be used at all when individuals are observed at different time points.

Theoretical details and discussion of advantages and disadvantages of this approach are described in the book of Brunner et al. (2002). In summary, the advantages include accommodating an outcome with any distribution, designs with multiple within-subject and between-subject factors, allowance for missing data, and unbiased tests of all the main and interactive effects. The disadvantages are that the approach requires a balanced design (i.e., individuals are measured on the same occasions), is not as powerful as a parametric approach when distributional assumptions are satisfied, and that it does not provide very meaningful effect size measures. The non-parametric approach is easily applied in SAS PROC MIXED, where all necessary options are available. SAS code is included for all examples considered in this chapter.

TABLE 5.3

Number of Drinking Days (NDD) per Month for 10 Individuals in the COMBINE Study with Corresponding Ranks, Hypothesis Testing Results, and Relative Marginal Effects from the Non-Parametric Analysis of Repeated Measured in Factorial Designs Approach

Individual	NDD_1	NDD_2	NDD_3	NDD_4	Rank_1	Rank_2	Rank_3	Rank_4
I1	1	9	10	14	1.5	17	20	28.5
I2	1	4	6	13	1.5	5.5	8.5	26
I3	10	8	11	7	20	14	22.5	11
I4	23	17	20	22	36	30.5	33	34.5
I5	13	14	28	24	26	28.5	39.5	37
I6	4	13	9	10	5.5	26	17	20
I7	3	8	12	28	3.5	14	24	39.5
I8	11	19	26	22	22.5	32	38	34.5
I9	8	6	7	3	14	8.5	11	3.5
I10	5	7	17	9	7	11	30.5	17
Average ranks					13.75	18.70	24.4	25.15
Relative marginal effects					0.33	0.46	0.60	0.62
Test statistic and p-value	ATS(1.92) = 5.01, p = 0.007							

We now illustrate how to apply this approach on the subsample of the COMBINE study considered earlier in this chapter, and gradually increase the complexity of the models that we consider. We start with the repeated measures design with only one within-subject factor. In the COMBINE subsample of 10 individuals, we are interested in testing whether there is a significant change over time in frequency of drinking, regardless of treatment. Table 5.3 shows the number of drinking days per month for the 10 individuals and the corresponding ranks when data are ranked according to the general non-parametric approach. Unlike Friedman's test, where data are ranked within the individual, here all observations (whether from the same individual or from different individuals) are ranked together. The lowest value in the sample is 1, as before, but it gets a rank of 1.5 since two subjects report one drinking day per period in this subsample. The largest value is 28, corresponding to drinking on all possible days since each period consists of 28 days and it gets a rank of 39.5, since this value occurs twice among the observations on the 10 subjects. The average ranks per period are increasing over time from 13.75 in month 1 to 25.15 in month 4. Since the actual numbers are heavily dependent on the number of values that are being ranked, it is better to consider the relative marginal effects. The relative marginal effects are obtained from the average ranks on each occasion by subtracting 0.5 and dividing by the total number of observations that are ranked (40 in this example). Relative marginal effects can also be plotted in order to better understand the effects, especially in more complicated designs. Since there is only one factor here, it is easy to compare the magnitudes of the relative marginal effects from the table.

To obtain the estimates of the main effect of time and post hoc comparisons, a LMM is fit to the ranked data with time as a within-subject categorical factor and unstructured variance–covariance matrix of the repeated measurements. Options to use moment-based estimates of the variance components and to calculate ANOVA-type statistics are specified (see online materials for SAS code). The ANOVA-type statistic (ATS) for the test of the main effect of time is ATS(1.92) = 5.01, p = 0.007 (i.e., the value of the test statistic is

TABLE 5.4

Pairwise Comparisons between Months Based on Pairwise Comparisons with ANOVA-Type Statistics in the Subsample of 10 Subjects from the COMBINE Study

	Period 2	Period 3	Period 4
Period 1	ATS(1) = 2.94, p = 0.09	ATS(1) = 12.63, p = 0.0004	ATS(1) = 5.58, p = 0.02
Period 2		ATS(1) = 5.89, p = 0.02	ATS(1) = 3.79, p = 0.05
Period 3			ATS(1) = 0.05, p = 0.82

5.01, the associated degrees of freedom are 1.92, and the corresponding p-value is quite small at 0.007). Therefore, there is a statistically significant change over time. This confirms the substantive results from Friedman's test. However, the p-value of the ANOVA-type statistic is much smaller than the p-value of Friedman's test (p = 0.007 vs. p = 0.05). In small samples, it is common for different results to occur depending on which test is used. The ANOVA-type statistic is recommended for small samples since it protects the error rates better than statistics relying on large sample approximations. For large samples the Wald-type statistic can also be used. However, a very large sample may be needed for this statistic to be well-behaved. Therefore, Brunner and Puri (2001) recommend using the ANOVA-type statistic in general.

Post hoc comparison between time points is also performed with the ANOVA-type statistic for contrasts within the LMM. Results are shown in Table 5.4. There are significant differences between periods 1 and 3, periods 2 and 3, and periods 1 and 4, which leads to the same substantive conclusions as performing pairwise Wilcoxon's signed-rank tests, except that the difference between periods 2 and 4 is borderline significant (p = 0.05). From the relative marginal effects, we see that there is significant increase in frequency of drinking from periods 1 and 2, to period 3, and then leveling off for period 3 and period 4.

Four different variances (one for each occasion) and six different covariances are estimated, based on the method of moments in the mixed procedure (not shown).

In the subsample of 10 subjects, there are three subjects who were randomized to active naltrexone and seven subjects who were randomized to placebo naltrexone. Next, we illustrate how to use the non-parametric approach with one between-subject and one within-subject factor, by taking into account treatment assignment and testing the interaction between naltrexone in addition to the main effects of naltrexone and time.

The ranking of the data is performed exactly as shown in Table 5.3. The average ranks and the relative marginal effects per occasion are also exactly the same. However, we also need to calculate average ranks and relative marginal effects for each treatment level, and for each combination of treatment level and occasion, in order to be able to test the naltrexone main effect and the interaction between naltrexone and time. Subjects I3, I4, and I5 from Table 5.3 are the ones who received active naltrexone. The rest of the subjects received placebo. We calculate the average of all ranks for subjects on naltrexone and the average of all ranks for subjects on placebo. We also calculate the averages of the ranks for subjects on active naltrexone and the averages of the ranks for subjects on placebo at each repeated occasion. Relative marginal effects are then calculated by subtracting 0.5 from the average ranks and dividing by the number of ranked observations. Table 5.5 shows all average ranks and Figure 5.1 shows the relative marginal effects.

TABLE 5.5
Average Ranks by Naltrexone Group and Time in the Subsample of 10 Subjects from the COMBINE Study

	Period 1	Period 2	Period 3	Period 4	Average
Active naltrexone	27.33	24.33	31.67	27.50	27.71
Placebo naltrexone	7.93	16.29	21.29	24.14	17.41
Average	13.75	18.70	24.40	25.15	20.5

Average ranks increase in the placebo naltrexone group and stay level (but higher) in the active naltrexone group. In this particular subsample, the average ranks on active naltrexone are higher than the average ranks on placebo naltrexone, but this is not representative of the entire study sample. The relative marginal effects show the same pattern (Figure 5.1) and can be used for visualization of the effects.

To test statistically the significance of the interaction between naltrexone and time, and the main effects of naltrexone and time, a LMM is fit to the ranked data with naltrexone, time, and their interaction as categorical predictors, unstructured variance–covariance matrix for the repeated measures over time, and specifying the methods-of-moments estimation option, and the ANOVA-type statistics option (see online materials for SAS code).

The interaction between naltrexone and time is not statistically significant (ATS(1.96) = 2.69, $p = 0.07$) and neither is the main effect of naltrexone (ATS(1) = 2.84, $p = 0.09$). Only the main effect of time is statistically significant (ATS(1.96) = 4.37, $p = 0.01$). Post hoc pairwise comparisons show significant differences between periods 1 and 3 ($p = 0.003$), periods 1 and 4 ($p = 0.04$), and periods 2 and 3 ($p = 0.003$), and a marginally significant difference between periods 2 and 4 ($p = 0.05$). Note that while Figure 5.1 nicely illustrates on which occasions the observations have on average larger values, the absolute differences in relative marginal effects do not provide information about how large the differences are. Other descriptive statistics (e.g., medians and interquartile ranges) can be calculated in order to get a better idea of the magnitude of effects.

We next focus on the complete factorial design of the study with three between-subject factors (naltrexone, acamprosate, and CBI), and one within-subject factor (time), and test

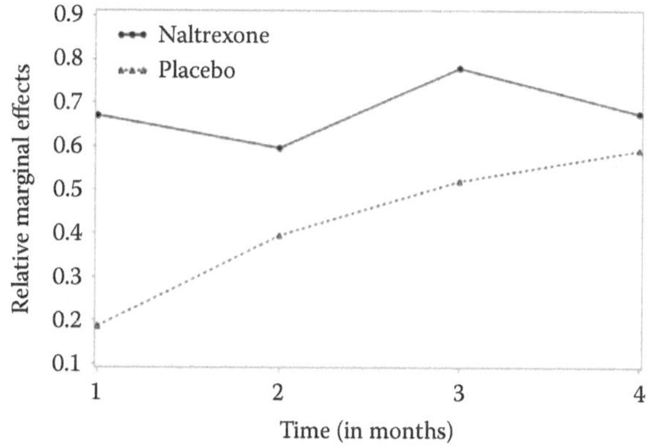

FIGURE 5.1
Relative marginal effects by naltrexone treatment and month in the subsample of 10 individuals from the COMBINE study.

all possible interactions and main effects in the entire sample. Another example is also included in the following section.

5.4 Data Examples

5.4.1 COMBINE Study

Participants in the COMBINE study of treatments for alcohol dependence were randomized to all possible combinations of naltrexone (active versus placebo), acamprosate (active versus placebo), and CBI (CBI versus no CBI), in addition to medication management in order to assess the main and interactive effects of the three treatments over 16 weeks of treatment (considered as four monthly periods). We apply the non-parametric approach to assess the effects of treatments on the number of drinking days by ranking all observations together and then fitting a LMM to the ranks with fixed effects of naltrexone, acamprosate, CBI, and all possible interactions, and the unstructured variance–covariance matrix over time. Moment-based estimators of eight different unstructured variance–covariance structures over time for the eight different combinations of between-subject factors are obtained. Although this leads to a large number of variance–covariance parameters (80 total, four variances and six covariances for each of the eight treatment combinations), this is seamlessly handled by the algorithm. All available data on each subject are used in the analysis.

ANOVA-type statistics are calculated for all possible main and interactive effects. Table 5.6 shows the statistics and the associated p-values. There are significant interactions between naltrexone and CBI (ATS(1) = 4.21, p = 0.04), and between naltrexone and time (ATS(2.41) = 2.98, p = 0.04), and also significant main effects of naltrexone (ATS(1) = 5.32, p = 0.02) and time (ATS(2.41) = 5.40, p = 0.003). Figure 5.2 shows all relative marginal effects.

TABLE 5.6

Non-Parametric Tests of Main and Interactive Effects of Treatments and Time on Number of Drinking Days per Month in the COMBINE Study

Effects	ANOVA-Type Statistics	p-Value
Main effect of naltrexone	ATS(1) = 5.32	0.02
Main effect of acamprosate	ATS(1) = 0.11	0.74
Main effect of CBI	ATS(1) = 0.31	0.58
Naltrexone*acamprosate	ATS(1) = 0.06	0.80
Naltrexone*CBI	ATS(1) = 4.21	0.04
Acamprosate*CBI	ATS(1) = 0.27	0.60
Naltrexone*acamprosate*CBI	ATS(1) = 1.76	0.18
Main effect of time	ATS(2.41) = 5.40	0.003
Naltrexone × time	ATS(2.41) = 2.98	0.04
Acamprosate × time	ATS(2.41) = 0.06	0.97
CBI × time	ATS(2.41) = 1.92	0.14
Naltrexone × acamprosate × time	ATS(2.41) = 0.33	0.76
Naltrexone × CBI × time	ATS(2.41) = 0.14	0.90
Acamprosate × CBI × time	ATS(2.41) = 0.46	0.67
Naltrexone × acamprosate × CBI × time	ATS(2.41) = 0.31	0.78

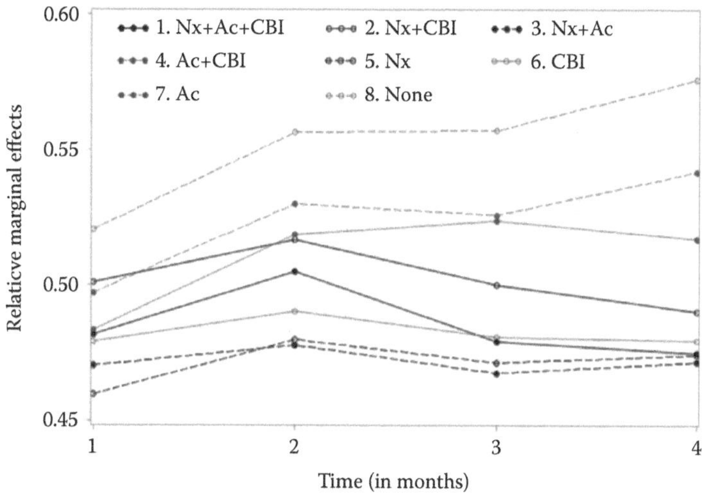

FIGURE 5.2
Relative marginal effects for the number of drinking days by naltrexone, acamprosate, and CBI treatment over time in the COMBINE study. Nx = naltrexone, Ac = acamprosate, CBI = Combined Behavioral Intervention.

Since there are no significant acamprosate effects, we averaged the relative marginal effects of the active and placebo acamprosate groups and Figure 5.3 shows these averaged relative marginal effects.

It is clear from Figure 5.3 that subjects who did not receive either naltrexone or CBI increased the number of drinking days over time. Subjects who received naltrexone had the lowest relative marginal effects, while subjects on the combination of naltrexone and CBI, or on CBI alone, were in the middle. Table 5.7 provides the test statistics and p-values for the post hoc comparisons to explain the significant effects in the model. Consistent with results from the alternative analyses reported in Chapter 4 for this data set, the group receiving naltrexone by itself appears have fewer drinking days compared to the group that did not receive naltrexone or CBI ($p = 0.002$). The combination of naltrexone

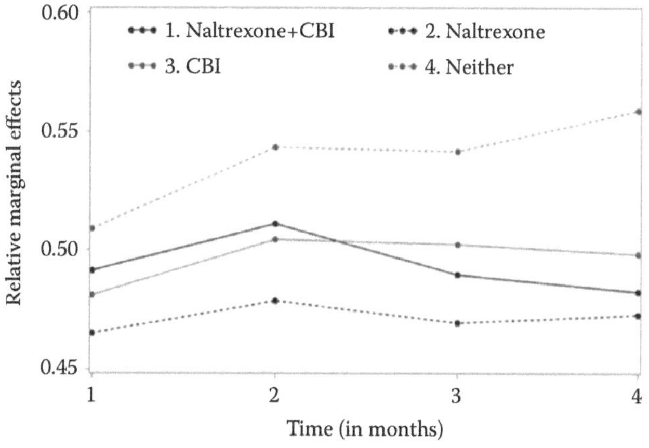

FIGURE 5.3
Relative marginal effects for the number of drinking days by naltrexone and CBI treatment over time in the COMBINE study.

TABLE 5.7

ANOVA-Type Statistics for the Post Hoc Comparisons for the Significant Effects in the Non-Parametric Mixed Model Fitted to Number of Drinking Days per Month in the COMBINE Study

Effect	Level	Comparison Level	ANOVA-Type Statistic	p-Value
Naltrexone × CBI interaction	Naltrexone and CBI	Naltrexone	ATS(1) = 1.13	p = 0.29
	Naltrexone and CBI	CBI	ATS(1) = 0.03	p = 0.86
	Naltrexone and CBI	Neither	ATS(1) = 3.93	p = 0.05
	Naltrexone	CBI	ATS(1) = 1.60	p = 0.21
	Naltrexone	Neither	ATS(1) = 9.32	p = 0.002
	CBI	Neither	ATS(1) = 3.36	p = 0.07
Naltrexone × month	Naltrexone at month 1	Placebo at month 1	ATS(1) = 1.28	p = 0.26
	Naltrexone at month 2	Placebo at month 2	ATS(1) = 3.31	p = 0.07
	Naltrexone at month 3	Placebo at month 3	ATS(1) = 5.88	p = 0.02
	Naltrexone at month 4	Placebo at month 4	ATS(1) = 8.45	p = 0.004
Main effect of time	Month 1	Month 2	ATS(1) = 20.56	p < .0001
	Month 1	Month 3	ATS(1) = 4.65	p = 0.03
	Month 1	Month 4	ATS(1) = 4.77	p = 0.03
	Month 2	Month 3	ATS(1) = 3.29	p = 0.07
	Month 2	Month 4	ATS(1) = 1.51	p = 0.22
	Month 3	Month 4	ATS(1) = 0.10	p = 0.76

and CBI is also associated with fewer drinking days compared to placebo naltrexone and no CBI ($p = 0.05$), but is not significantly more advantageous than the monotherapies. CBI is not associated with a significant improvement compared to no CBI. Comparisons of subjects on active naltrexone versus placebo naltrexone are statistically significant in the last two months ($p = 0.02$ and 0.004, respectively), but not in the first two months. The ranks during the first month are, on average, significantly lower than the ranks during the other months.

Note that there are some differences between these results and the results from the GEE and random effects analyses in Chapter 4. In particular, there is a significant CBI by time interaction in the parametric analyses, but in the non-parametric analysis the naltrexone by time interaction, rather than the CBI by time interaction, is statistically significant. In general, discrepancies between non-parametric and parametric analyses are possible, especially when assumptions of parametric procedures are not satisfied. While the results from the non-parametric approach are valid under a wider range of assumptions, a definite disadvantage is that this approach does not provide effect size estimates on the original scale. Thus, we can conclude that there are significant effects but their magnitudes are harder to quantify.

5.4.2 Human Laboratory Study of Menthol's Effects on Nicotine Reinforcement in Smokers

This study, introduced in Section 1.5.7, used a two-level cross-over experimental design to examine whether menthol at different doses, compared to placebo, alters nicotine reinforcement in young adult smokers. The two-level cross-over design of the study with three menthol doses (high dose, low dose, and no menthol) administered on three separate days

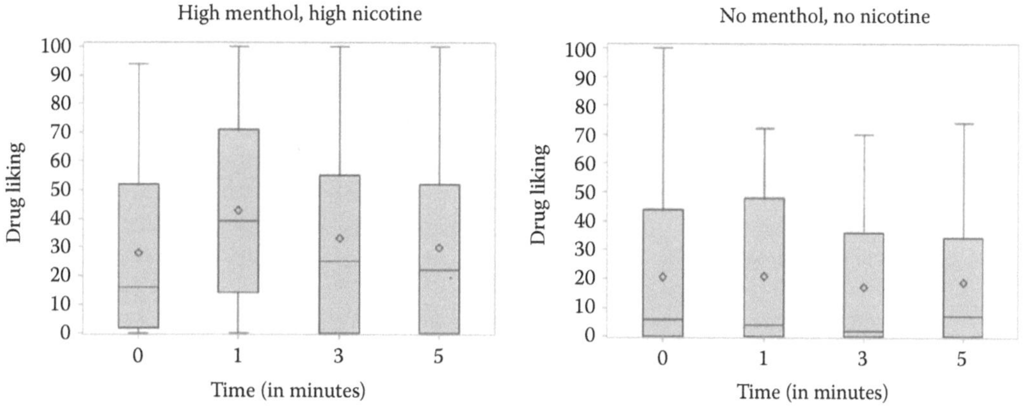

FIGURE 5.4
Box plots of "drug liking" effects of nicotine at two experimental conditions.

and three nicotine doses (saline, 5 μg/kg, 10 μg/kg), infused in random order on each test day, is shown in Figure 1.12. The main outcome of interest is the rewarding effect of nicotine measured by the Drug Effects Questionnaire (DEQ). We focus on the item measuring how much subjects liked the perceived nicotine effects during the first 5 minutes of the infusion. Four separate ratings were collected during this time period within each infusion on each test day.

The hypothesis is that concurrent menthol and nicotine administration, as compared to nicotine and control flavor, or saline and control flavor, enhances the rewarding effects of nicotine. Since, in this data set, there are correlations within subject between repeated observations on the same test day and on different test days, we need to use a method for repeated measures analysis in order to take these correlations into account. However, as illustrated by the box plots in Figure 5.4 for two of the conditions, the data are skewed, exhibit floor effects, and the variability differs by time point, nicotine, and menthol dose. Hence, this data set is particularly suited to be analyzed with the non-parametric approach to repeated measures.

We fit a LMM with menthol, nicotine, time, and all possible interactions on the ranked data, with the unstructured variance–covariance matrix and the required options for proper estimates. This allows us to test the hypotheses of main and interactive effects, according to the non-parametric approach.

The first part of Table 5.8 shows the ANOVA-type statistics and the associated p-values for the main and interactive effects in the model. There is a statistically significant interaction between nicotine and time ($ATS(5.69) = 3.83$, $p = 0.001$). There are also significant main effects of nicotine ($ATS(1.80) = 22.21$, $p < .0001$) and time ($ATS(2.52) = 10.93$, $p < .0001$). Post hoc comparisons among the three nicotine doses are then performed at each time point, in order to explain the significant interaction in the model. These comparisons show that at minutes 1, 3, and 5, there are significant differences among all three nicotine doses with the high dose associated with the highest liking rating and saline associated with lowest rating. Figure 5.5 illustrates this effect with a plot of the relative marginal effects. When high dose nicotine is infused, there is a sizeable increase in the drug liking effect, with subsequent decrease to baseline levels. When low dose nicotine is infused, there is a small change upward but responses go down after the first minute. When saline is infused, there is no increase and drug liking effects decrease. Detailed tests for these

TABLE 5.8

Non-Parametric Tests of the Effects of Menthol, Nicotine, and Time in the Human Laboratory Study of Nicotine Reinforcement in Smokers

Effects	ANOVA-Type Statistics	p-Value
Main effect of nicotine	ATS(1.80) = 22.21	< 0.0001
Main effect of menthol	ATS(1.67) = 1.65	0.20
Main effect of time	ATS(2.52) = 10.93	< .0001
Nicotine × menthol	ATS(3.84) = 0.94	0.44
Nicotine × time	ATS(5.69) = 3.83	0.001
Menthol × time	ATS(5.28) = 0.63	0.69
Nicotine × menthol × time	ATS(10.6) = 0.58	0.84
Post hoc tests:		
High dose versus low dose nicotine at time 0	ATS(1) = 0.00	0.96
Low dose nicotine versus saline at time 0	ATS(1) = 0.51	0.48
High dose nicotine versus saline at time 0	ATS(1) = 0.47	0.49
High dose versus low dose nicotine at time 1	ATS(1) = 9.98	0.002
Low dose nicotine versus saline at time 1	ATS(1) = 9.49	0.002
High dose nicotine versus saline at time 1	ATS(1) = 28.83	< .0001
High dose versus low dose nicotine at time 3	ATS(1) = 5.63	0.02
Low dose nicotine versus saline at time 3	ATS(1) = 6.35	0.01
High dose nicotine versus saline at time 3	ATS(1) = 18.61	< .0001
High dose versus low dose nicotine at time 5	ATS(1) = 5.92	0.02
Low dose nicotine versus saline at time 5	ATS(1) = 4.66	0.03
High dose nicotine versus saline at time 5	ATS(1) = 17.13	< .0001

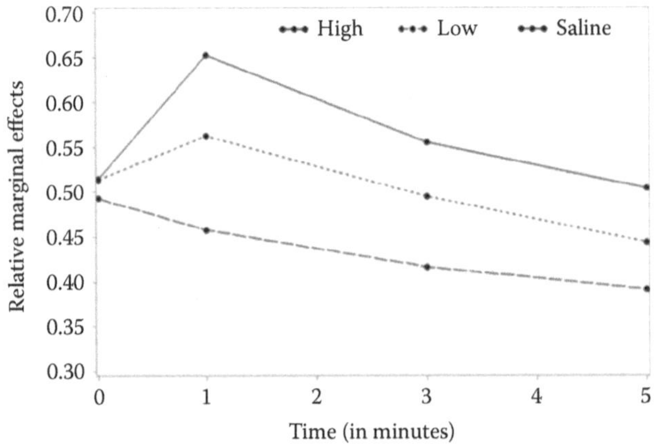

FIGURE 5.5
Relative marginal effects for drug liking by nicotine dose over time in the human laboratory study of nicotine reinforcement.

effects are provided in the online materials. In conclusion, this analysis confirms that individual studies respond to nicotine infusions with an increase in liking but there is no evidence that menthol modifies this effect.

5.5 Summary

In this chapter, we introduced non-parametric methods for the analysis of repeated measures data and focused on the approach described by Brunner et al. (2002) for factorial experiments. This approach can be used in a variety of situations with longitudinal and clustered data when data do not conform to normality or other distributions in the exponential family. The basic idea of ranking the observations, and performing mixed model analysis on the ranks, is simple but special options must be used in order to estimate the variances correctly and to have valid tests of the effects in the model.

Advantages of the approach are that it can be applied to discrete and continuous data with all kinds of distributions, in large and in small samples, and that the method is not substantially affected by missing data. Disadvantages are that this approach is limited to balanced designs and that the focus is on hypothesis testing, rather than effect size estimation. The relative marginal effects do provide effect size measures but they are not in the metric of the original observations and hence, are not as useful. Power may also be diminished, compared to parametric models, when parametric models can be used. Further information on the non-parametric approach can be found in Brunner et al. (2002), Brunner et al. (1999), and Brunner and Puri (2001).

6

Post Hoc Analysis and Adjustments for Multiple Comparisons

In the previous three chapters, we showed that analysis of repeated measures data with at least two factors usually involves testing of main effects and interactions, followed by multiple individual comparisons (whether pre-planned or post hoc), in order to explain the significant effects in the models. As in ANOVA without repeated measures, in repeated measures analyses with categorical factors, main effect tests comparing more than two means are usually followed by pairwise comparisons of the means or comparisons of all means to the mean of a control group, while interactions are followed by testing or estimation of simple effects (i.e., comparisons of the means of one factor at the levels of the other factors). When there are significant main or interaction effects of time in longitudinal studies, often it is of interest to assess whether the mean change over time can be described by a straight line or by a parabola and hence, testing of linear or quadratic trends is indicated.

We already illustrated post hoc testing on several of the data sets introduced in Chapter 1. In particular, we showed how to describe the significant trend over time in the augmentation depression study by comparing post-baseline time points to baseline, and by testing linear, quadratic and cubic effects (Section 3.8.1), we illustrated testing of simple effects in the serotonin levels in the mother–infant pairs study (Section 3.8.2), in the fMRI study of working memory in schizophrenia (Section 3.8.3), and in the COMBINE study of alcohol dependence (Sections 4.2.4, 4.3.4, and 5.4.1). We also showed how to perform focused mean comparisons in the meta–analysis of clinical trials in schizophrenia (Section 3.8.4) and illustrated how to estimate effect sizes in GEE and GLMM applied to self-rated health in the Health and Retirement Study (Sections 4.2.5 and 4.3.5). In almost all instances of post hoc testing so far, we used an uncorrected significance level of 0.05 for hypothesis testing and a confidence level of 0.95 for confidence interval construction. When there are multiple comparisons, this leads to inflation of the type I error rate (i.e., increased chance of finding significant effects when there are no differences) in the family of comparisons. For example, if we have three groups and compare all pairs of means (i.e., perform three comparisons: mean 1 versus 2, mean 1 versus 3, and mean 2 versus 3), each with a probability of 0.05 of finding a difference when there is no difference, the probability of finding at least one of the three differences to be statistically significant when there are no differences can be as high as 0.14. When the number of comparisons is much higher, the probability can become almost 1, or 100%. A similar issue occurs with confidence intervals. If we construct just one 95% confidence interval, then in all likelihood, the interval includes the parameter of interest (or difference of parameters, e.g., differences of population means). Only in 5% of the cases, the true parameter is not in the confidence interval. But if we construct multiple confidence intervals, then the probability that at least one of the confidence intervals does not include the parameter increases, often dramatically.

Multiple comparison procedure is any simultaneous statistical inference that allows error rates or confidence levels to be controlled in a family of tests or confidence intervals. For example, in clinical trials several treatment groups may need to be compared in terms of their mean response, by either performing multiple hypothesis tests or constructing simultaneous confidence intervals for mean differences. This is the case in the COMBINE study, where there are eight different treatment groups depending on the pharmacological and behavioral treatments that patients are randomized to. There are different sets of comparisons that can be performed, as illustrated later in this chapter, for each outcome measure.

In addition, in clinical trials there are often multiple efficacy and safety outcome measures that need to be analyzed. With multiple measures, there is increased likelihood that a new treatment will be found beneficial on at least one of the measures by chance and hence, the probability of such chance occurrence needs to be controlled. This situation is sometimes referred to as "multiple testing," rather than "multiple comparisons," in order to emphasize that different measures are compared. Also "multiple testing" often refers to hypothesis testing while "multiple comparisons" refers to simultaneous confidence intervals. In this chapter, we use "multiple comparisons" and "multiple testing" interchangeably when referring to hypothesis tests, and "multiple comparisons" when we refer to simultaneous confidence intervals.

Multiple comparison procedures must be used if there is a chance that some of the effects that are found are false positives, to claim that the observed effects from confirmatory or exploratory are real with high level of confidence, and especially when the cost of false positive results is high (e.g., a new experimental treatment with largely unexplored side effects profile is mistakenly declared to be better than a standard treatment). There are many different multiple comparison procedures that address different inferential objectives. Some methods are specific to hypothesis testing, others to confidence intervals, and some may be used in either context. Procedures also differ in terms of the errors that they control. Most commonly, procedures control the *familywise error rate* (FWER), which is the probability of at least one false positive result or the *false discovery rate* (FDR), which is the proportion of falsely rejected null hypotheses. In some cases, there are big differences in results depending on which method is used. In other cases, the results are the same.

Arguably the most important aspect of multiple comparison testing is selecting the family of inferences over which one controls the error rates. If too many separate hypotheses or confidence intervals are constructed, then the correction may be too severe and important effects may be missed. On the other hand, if the family consists of a small set of hypotheses or confidence intervals but those are selected based on extensive data dredging, then the correction may not be sufficiently strict and may result in false positive results that fail to replicate.

In this chapter, we first provide a brief historical overview of approaches for multiple comparisons. Then we describe different settings in which multiple comparison procedures may be needed and present logical choices of families of statistical inferences. In the third section, we describe classical approaches such as Bonferroni's, Tukey's and Scheffé's procedures that control the FWER. Stepwise modifications of the Bonferroni method and FDR-based approaches are considered next with a brief mention of simulation-based, bootstrap, and permutation tests. Finally, some of the data examples from Chapter 1 are used for illustration. The emphasis herein is on assumptions, interpretation of results, and applicability. For interested readers, a comprehensive reference, complete with SAS code and data examples for the use of multiple comparison procedures, is Westfall et al. (2011). Another good reference that covers most procedures is the book by Hsu (1996). Multiple comparison procedures in the context of clinical trials are described in detail by Dmitrienko et al. (2010), while Dudoit and Laan (2008) cover multiple testing in genomics experiments.

6.1 Historical Overview of Approaches to Multiple Comparisons

Some of the earliest approaches of correction for multiple comparisons are due to Tukey (Tukey, 1953) who focused on all pairwise comparisons among means, and Scheffé (1952, 1953) who focused on linear contrasts among group means. Dunnett proposed an adjustment method for multiple comparisons when multiple treatment groups are compared to a control group (Dunnett, 1955). These procedures are most commonly used in the context of post hoc testing in ANOVA, when it is of interest to understand what drives a significant overall finding of mean differences.

Another commonly used approach is the Bonferroni correction credited to Dunn (1961). This method is perhaps the most widely known and used because of its simplicity and wide applicability. It can be used not only for mean comparisons but in any situation where multiple statistical inferences are performed (e.g., when multiple efficacy endpoints are assessed in clinical trials). However, the Bonferroni correction is also the most conservative in many situations. More liberal modifications of this procedure have been proposed (Marcus et al., 1976; Holm, 1979; Hommel, 1988) and have grown in popularity in recent years.

All approaches mentioned so far are focused on controlling the *familywise error rate* (FWER), which is the probability of at least one type I error among multiple (possibly correlated) hypothesis tests. If constructing simultaneous confidence intervals is the focus, these procedures control the *familywise confidence* at pre-specified level. While Bonferroni-type and some of the classical procedures may be too conservative, simulation-based methods (Edwards and Berry, 1987) provide good control of FWER and can be used seamlessly with dependent observations in clustered and longitudinal studies.

In contrast to classical procedures that protect against a single false positive result, more recent developments are often centered on controlling the *false discovery rate* (FDR), which is the expected proportion of rejected null hypotheses that are false discoveries (i.e., incorrect rejections). The idea of FDR was first formalized by Benjamini and Hochberg (1995) and was based on previous research by Schweder and Spjøtvoll (1982), Soric (1989) and Hochberg and Benjamini (1990), as acknowledged by Benjamini (2010a). However, it was not until a few years after the seminal Benjamini and Hochberg publication that the idea received wide acceptance and use. With the explosion of technology developments in genomics and other high throughput sciences, it was necessary to test simultaneously a large number of hypotheses when data were collected on relatively few individuals. For example, in genomics or proteomics, thousands of genes or protein expressions are often evaluated simultaneously using microarrays and need to be compared between individuals with a particular disease and healthy controls. Classical familywise error rate corrections, in such situations, result in a drastic loss of power for signal detection and hence new types of multiple correction procedures are necessary. FDR procedures and related modifications have better power than FWER procedures and allow simultaneous testing of large numbers of hypotheses (in the hundreds or thousands) in relatively few individuals, without sacrificing too much power.

Nowadays, researchers can choose from a variety of FWER and FDR procedures that are incorporated in software packages. The key issue is which procedure is most appropriate in a particular situation with theoretical and empirical research still in full swing. In this chapter, we focus on post hoc comparisons to explain significant main effects and interactions in linear models, present the key concepts in multiple testing, and illustrate some of the most popular procedures on data examples. A succinct overview of multiple correction methods, multiplicity-related error rates, their interpretation, and applicability is provided in Benjamini (2010b).

6.2 The Need for Multiple Comparison Correction

6.2.1 Hypothesis Testing

When a single hypothesis test is performed at 5% significance level, there are two possible outcomes—the null hypothesis is rejected if the corresponding p-value is less than 0.05 and it is not rejected, otherwise (Table 6.1). Consider the situation when the null hypothesis is rejected. There is up to 5% probability that the null hypothesis was rejected in error (type I error). Most people would be comfortable with one in twenty probability of a type I error and would feel comfortable concluding that the null hypothesis is false.

However, suppose that k independent tests are performed and in each case there is 5% probability of falsely rejecting the null hypothesis. Then, the probability of at least one false rejection (the *familywise error rate, FWER*) is $1-0.95^k$, which is equal to 40% when $k=10$ and to 99.4% when $k=100$. Most people would probably not be comfortable having such high probability to commit a type I error. Thus multiple comparison correction for the family of hypothesis tests is necessary.

Any correction involves performing individual tests at levels lower than 5%. However, when type I error rate is decreased in a statistical test, the probability of type II error (i.e., the probability to fail to reject the null hypothesis when it is indeed false) increases and hence power (i.e., the probability to reject the null when it is false) decreases. Thus all corrections that control the FWER need to be evaluated also in terms of the loss of power when the alternative hypotheses are true. Since it is not known which of the underlying null hypotheses in the family of tests are true and which are false, a good balance needs to be maintained between the probabilities of type I and type II error over different possible scenarios.

Table 6.2 shows the possible outcomes when m hypotheses tests are performed simultaneously. Here m_0 is the (unknown) number of true null hypotheses and hence $m-m_0$ is the

TABLE 6.1

Results When Testing a Single Hypothesis Test

	Null Hypothesis Not Rejected	Rejected Null Hypothesis
True null hypothesis	Correct	Type I error
False null hypothesis	Type II error	Correct

TABLE 6.2

Results When Testing m Hypothesis Tests

	Null Hypothesis Not Rejected	Rejected Null Hypothesis	Total
True null hypothesis	T_{NR}	F_R	m_0
False null hypothesis	F_{NR}	T_R	$m-m_0$
Total	$m-R$	R	m

number of false null hypotheses. Of the m_0 true null hypotheses F_R are rejected in error and thus the FWER is the probability that F_R is 1 or more, i.e., $P(F_R \geq 1)$.

Another important measure to consider is the *per-comparison error rate* (PCER) which is the expected proportion of all hypotheses that are falsely rejected null hypotheses, i.e., $E(F_R/m)$. If all comparisons in the set are performed at a 5% significance level (i.e., no correction for multiple tests is applied), then the PCER is controlled at 5%. Depending on how many of the hypotheses in the set are true null hypotheses, this leads to a potentially substantial increase in the FWER. If all hypotheses are true null hypotheses, the increase is large even with a moderate number of hypotheses in the test, which has motivated the development of classical multiple comparison procedures that control the FWER. But if only a few of the hypotheses are true null hypotheses, then the increase may not be as large and strict FWER control may be at the expense of missing important signals, which has motivated the development of procedures that control the false discovery rate (FDR).

There are two types of FWER control with some procedures controlling only the first one but not the second one. The first type is *FWER control in the weak sense,* which means that FWER control is guaranteed to be at level α only when all null hypotheses are true (i.e., $m_0 = m$). The second type is *FWER control in the strong sense,* which means that FWER control is guaranteed to be at level α for all possible configurations of true and false null hypotheses. Procedures that control the FWER in the strong sense are, in general, preferable to procedures that control the FWER in the weak sense. However, when many of the null hypotheses are false and there is a large number of comparisons, procedures that control the false discovery rate should be considered.

The *false discovery rate* (FDR) is the expected proportion of rejected hypotheses among the set of hypothesis tests that are false discoveries (i.e., differences are found when no differences exist). Based on the notation in Table 6.2 it is defined as $E(F_R/R)$. Unlike the PCER, which has the total number of hypothesis tests in the denominator, the FDR uses only the number of rejected null hypotheses in the denominator. Thus depending on how many of the actual hypotheses are true null, it can be close to the FWER (it is equal to the FWER when all hypotheses are true null hypotheses, i.e., $m_0 = m$). When all null hypotheses are false (i.e., when $m_0 = 0$), or when there are no rejected null hypotheses (i.e., $R = 0$), the FDR is 0 by definition.

Compared to the FWER, FDR is more permissive and thus is more powerful in general. Because of this property, it is much better suited for situations when the number of simultaneous tests is large. To understand the rationale for this correction, consider the following example: if one performs 1000 simultaneous hypothesis tests, keeping the FWER (i.e., the probability of at least one false positive result) below the commonly used threshold of 5% would require a very severe correction in each individual hypothesis test and thus will lead to a significant loss of power to detect differences, even when differences exist. In comparison, controlling that no more than 5% of the rejections among the 1000 tests are false rejections (i.e., controlling the FDR within 5%) is still reasonable and would require much smaller adjustment and thus, will have better power. If among 60 rejected null hypotheses, three are false rejections this is still a good result although we have some false rejections. In contrast, if among six rejected null hypotheses, there are three false rejections, this is most likely not acceptable. If we can control the FDR at 5%, we will be assured that only a small percent of the rejections are expected to be false rejections.

When all null hypotheses are true (i.e., there are no differences in any of the hypothesis tests), the FDR is equal to the FWER since all rejections are false rejections. In general, FWER $\geq$ FDR and some of the rejections are false rejections. The more non-true null hypotheses there are, the more powerful the FDR correction is. Also, the greater the number of simultaneous tests, the greater the advantage of the FDR over the FWER if there are at least some true alternative hypotheses. That explains why FDR-type corrections are the preferred approach in genomics or proteomics experiments and other areas where high dimensional data are analyzed.

6.2.2 Confidence Intervals

When a confidence interval is constructed for a single parameter at some confidence level, say 95%, there is 95% probability that the true parameter is inside the confidence interval. That is, if the process of construction of a confidence interval is repeated many times, 95% of the time the confidence interval will be correct in that it will contain the parameter of interest. But when simultaneous intervals are constructed for multiple parameters, each at a 95% confidence level, the probability that all of them are correct can be significantly lower than 95% and hence the probability that at least one of them is incorrect (which is the familywise error in the context of confidence intervals) can be significantly higher than 5%. In many situations, there is direct correspondence between hypothesis tests and confidence intervals, and confidence intervals can be used to test the corresponding hypotheses by checking whether the parameter values under the null hypotheses are in the corresponding intervals. For example, if we are interested in all pairwise comparisons in a set of means, we can construct simultaneous confidence intervals for all pairwise differences and check which of these confidence intervals include 0. If a confidence interval includes 0, then the corresponding null hypothesis that the two means are equal is not rejected. If a confidence interval does not include 0, then the corresponding null hypothesis is rejected and the confidence interval indicates which mean is larger than the other mean. If the entire confidence interval is above 0, then the first mean is significantly larger than the second mean. If the entire confidence interval is below 0, then the second mean is significantly larger than the first mean.

While many FWER correction procedures can be applied to both confidence intervals and hypothesis tests, some are specifically designed for multiple hypothesis testing only and FDR multiple comparison procedures are mainly for hypothesis testing.

6.3 Standard Approaches to Multiple Comparisons

Standard approaches are single-stage procedures and are most commonly used for least squares mean comparisons in ANOVA designs with independent observations. These procedures have been developed for the simple linear model where the assumptions of linearity, normality, constant variance, and uncorrelated errors are satisfied. We first focus on the single-stage procedures of Bonferroni, Tukey, Scheffé, and Dunnett, and consider a scenario where k means need to be compared. Technical details about these and additional classical procedures can be found in Montgomery (2013) and Kutner et al. (2005). If the goal is to rank the means from largest to smallest value and to figure out which of the mean differences are statistically significant, then all pairwise comparisons of the means are performed. With k means, there are $k(k-1)/2$ possible comparisons of the form $\mu_i-\mu_j$. It is easy to see that the number of comparisons increases very fast. For example, with three means there are three possible comparisons. With four means there are six possible comparisons, with five means there are 10 possible comparisons. If pairwise comparisons are performed at uncorrected α level, then the probability of finding at least one false significant difference among a set of m comparisons can be much higher than α. Therefore, it is necessary to apply a correction and in the classical procedures this is done in such a way as to keep the probability of finding at least one significant difference within a certain limit, that is, to control the familywise error rate (FWER).

6.3.1 The Bonferroni Multiple Correction Procedure

The most commonly used multiplicity correction is the *Bonferroni procedure*. It consists of testing each of m comparisons at α/m significance level and thus guarantees a FWER of α for the set of comparisons. For example, if five comparisons are to be performed with the goal of limiting the probability of at least one false positive at 0.05, then each individual comparison needs to be performed at 0.01 significance level in order to guarantee that the FWER is no higher than 5%.

Equivalently, each of the raw p-values for the comparisons is multiplied by the number of comparisons to obtain *adjusted p-values*, which are then directly compared to α. The adjusted p-value approach is illustrated in Table 6.3 where raw and Bonferroni-adjusted p-values are shown in the first two columns. Since there are five comparisons in this example, each raw p-value is multiplied by 5 in order to obtain Bonferroni-adjusted p-values which are then compared to the chosen significance level (namely 0.05). While four out of five raw p-values are below 0.05, only one of the adjusted p-values is below 0.05 and thus only one of the comparisons is declared statistically significant after Bonferroni adjustment. Prior to Bonferroni adjustment four out of five comparisons are statistically significant. Note that it is possible for the adjustment to result in values larger than 1, in which case adjusted p-values are truncated at 1 and reported as 1. Adjusted p-values are interpreted as the lowest FWER for which the corresponding comparisons are statistically significant. The smallest p-value in the set of five raw p-values in Table 6.3 is 0.001, which corresponds to a Bonferroni-adjusted p-value of 0.005 and hence for any FWER that is equal or greater than 0.005 this comparison will be statistically significant. The second smallest Bonferroni-adjusted p-value is 0.06, which is not significant at 0.05 level but will be significant if we set the FWER to be 0.06 or higher. Traditionally, the desired FWER is set to 0.05. However, in specific studies it can be set to be higher or lower if one needs to be more liberal or more conservative.

Confidence intervals can also be constructed using the Bonferroni approach by using $1\text{-}\alpha/m$ confidence level for each interval rather than $1 - \alpha$ confidence level. For example, if we want to be 95% confident that five confidence intervals constructed simultaneously contain the respective parameters of interest (which means that $\alpha = 0.05$, $1 - \alpha = 0.95$), we need to construct each individual interval at $1 - 0.05/5 = 99\%$ confidence level. This leads to increased widths of the confidence intervals compared to using uncorrected 95% confidence level for each, but we are almost guaranteed that we have captured all parameters of interest. Simultaneous confidence intervals are considered in more detail in the data examples section of this chapter.

The advantages of the Bonferroni procedure are that it can be applied very easily, it can be used both for simultaneous hypothesis testing and confidence intervals construction, it is valid even when the comparisons are statistically dependent, and it can be used in a wide variety of situations when multiplicity correction is necessary, not just for comparisons of means in ANOVA. The main disadvantage is that this approach is very conservative, that is, in many situations the FWER is maintained at a level lower than α and too few

TABLE 6.3

Raw and Adjusted p-Values for a Set of Five Hypothetical Comparisons

Raw p-Values (Ordered)	Bonferroni	Bonferroni–Holm	Bonferroni–Hochberg	Hommel	Benjamini–Hochberg	Benjamini–Yekutieli
PCER Controlled	**FWER Controlled**				**FDR Controlled Under Independence**	**FDR Controlled Under any Dependence**
0.001	**0.005**	**0.005**	**0.005**	**0.005**	**0.005**	**0.0114**
0.012	0.060	**0.048**	**0.048**	**0.040**	**0.030**	0.0685
0.024	0.120	0.072	0.060	**0.048**	**0.0375**	0.0856
0.030	0.150	0.072	0.060	0.060	**0.0375**	0.0856
0.100	0.500	0.100	0.100	0.100	0.100	0.2283

Note: p-values below 0.05 are considered statistically significant and are indicated in bold.

null hypotheses are rejected. This leads to substantial loss of power to detect differences when there are more than a few comparisons and to confidence intervals that may be unnecessarily wide. There are a number of stepwise modifications of the Bonferroni procedure aimed at increasing power, as described in Section 6.4, and more appropriate procedures depending on the goal of multiple comparisons such as Tukey's, Scheffé's, and Dunnett's, as described next.

6.3.2 Tukey's Multiple Comparison Procedure

A less conservative correction than Bonferroni, in the context of multiple mean comparisons in ANOVAs and other linear models, is *Tukey's honest significance difference procedure* (also known as *Tukey's range test*). It was developed for a balanced one-way ANOVA design, that is, when the means of k groups with an equal number of independent observations per group are compared. Extensions apply to unbalanced designs with an unequal number of observations in each group (the *Tukey–Kramer method*) and dependent data (i.e., when there are correlations between the observations). Tukey's method is based on the precise distribution of the pairwise statistics and thus controls the FWER exactly (under the assumptions of the model and when the design is balanced), rather than conservatively, as in the Bonferroni method. That is, the probability of at least one false positive result is equal to the desired FWER, rather than smaller than that. This is possible because it properly takes into account the correlations between different pairs of means.

Application of Tukey's multiple comparison procedure with balanced data is easy as it involves performing multiple t-tests or setting up multiple confidence intervals just as one would do for a single test or a single confidence interval but with critical values that come from the *studentized range distribution* (Tukey, 1949) rather than from a t-distribution. Before the wide use of computers and proliferation of statistical software programs, tabled values were used to calculate the test statistics or to set up the confidence intervals. However, nowadays all statistical software programs have options to perform Tukey's multiple comparisons in ANOVAs and in linear models. Even with unbalanced data, all the calculations are performed behind the scenes and the end user just sees the constructed confidence intervals or the adjusted p-values for the pairwise comparisons. However, when the data are unbalanced, the overall confidence level is greater than $1 - \alpha$ and hence, the procedure is conservative. Tukey's test assumes that the observations are independent within and among the groups, that the outcome distributions in the different groups are normally distributed and that the variances in the different groups are the same. Therefore, it is quite appropriate as a multiple testing procedure in ANOVA for independent observations. When there are dependencies of the observations, as occurs with clustered or longitudinal data, appropriate error estimates need to be used (e.g., Hochberg and Tamhane, 1983). In general, Tukey's procedure is considered the best when all pairwise differences are tested, when confidence intervals are needed, or sample sizes are equal. In cases where many comparisons need to be performed, Scheffé's method may be preferred.

In Section 2.1.3, we used part of the COMBINE data to illustrate the one-way ANOVA approach for endpoint analysis. In particular we tested whether there were any differences in the average number of drinks per day during the last month of the treatment period among participants who drank on the following treatment combinations: naltrexone and CBI; naltrexone without CBI; placebo and CBI; placebo and no CBI. The overall test of the group effect resulted in a small p-value ($F(3,717) = 3.34$, $p = 0.02$) and thus we concluded that there were significant differences among the treatment groups. However, this overall test did not show which mean(s) were different. To understand the nature of the treatment effect, we visualized the least square means and their standard errors by treatment group and performed t-tests for all pairwise comparisons among the means. In Chapter 2, we reported unadjusted p-values and confidence intervals and concluded that all active treatment groups (naltrexone and CBI; naltrexone and no CBI; and placebo and CBI) had significantly better outcomes than the control group (placebo and no CBI). Here we compare several different classical methods of multiple comparisons, in order to illustrate the usefulness of the confidence intervals approach and the differences among the methods.

Table 6.4 gives all pairwise confidence intervals prior to adjustment and after various adjustments that keep the simultaneous confidence level at 95%. Thus, we are 95% confident that all constructed confidence intervals contain the target mean differences. P-values are also provided for completeness although they are not needed to make a decision about which treatment differences are significant. When it is possible to construct simultaneous confidence intervals, they are preferred to p-values because they indicate the direction of the differences (i.e., which means are larger and which are smaller) and they are directly used to test the corresponding multiple hypotheses at FWER of 5% or lower. Confidence intervals that do not contain zero and hence, correspond to statistically significant differences, are denoted in bold.

The results in Table 6.4 confirm the theoretical expectations that Tukey's adjustment results in the narrowest confidence intervals when the family of tests is all pairwise comparisons.

The Bonferroni method in this example leads to only slightly wider confidence intervals and to the same substantive conclusions as Tukey's adjustment. Mainly, CBI is associated with lower drinks per drinking day compared to subjects not receiving active treatment. The combined naltrexone and CBI treatment, and the naltrexone only treatment, are significantly better than the control before adjustment for all pairwise comparisons.

The results from the analysis of all pairwise comparisons can be graphically illustrated using a *mean-mean scatterplot* (Hsu, 1996), also known as a *diffogram* in SAS. Figure 6.1 shows such a plot based on the Tukey-adjusted comparisons generated for the COMBINE data. The mean values for each treatment group can be read off from the vertical and/or from the horizontal axis. Not all groups are shown on each axis because only non-redundant group pairs are displayed. Mean differences are represented as intersections of the horizontal and vertical lines corresponding to each pair of groups. The confidence intervals for the mean differences are shown as straight lines centered at these intersections and spreading out in a symmetrical fashion from them. The lines are scaled in such a way that if they cross the 45° dashed line, the corresponding confidence interval contains 0 and hence the two means are not significantly different, while if the confidence interval line does not cross the 45° dashed line, the corresponding confidence interval does not contain 0 and the two means are significantly different. Note that because the means for the naltrexone and no CBI, and the naltrexone and CBI groups are almost the same (within precision of up to two digits after the decimal point), the lines for these two groups are overlapping and appear as one thicker line.

In Figure 6.1, the line representing the confidence intervals for the mean comparison of the CBI only versus neither does not cross the 45° dashed line and hence indicates a significant difference, while the rest of the lines do cross it and hence indicate non-significant differences. This graphic display allows us to spot significant and non-significant differences easily, and the ordering of the means of the different groups. However, it becomes very busy when many treatment groups are compared.

TABLE 6.4

Unadjusted and Adjusted Confidence Limits for Pairwise Comparisons in the Analyses of Drinks per Drinking Day at Month 4 in the COMBINE Study

Treatment Group	Comparison Treatment Group	No Adjustment Mean Difference (95% CI) Adjusted p	Bonferroni Adjustment Mean Difference (95% CI) Adjusted p	Tukey Adjustment Mean Difference (95% CI) Adjusted p	Scheffé Adjustment Mean Difference (95% CI) Adjusted p	Dunnett Adjustment Mean Difference (95% CI) Adjusted p
Naltrexone and CBI	Naltrexone only	0.001 (−0.16, 0.17) p=0.99	0.001 (−0.22, 0.22) p=1.00	0.001 (−0.22, 0.22) p=1.00	0.001 (−0.24, 0.24) p=1.00	N/A
Naltrexone and CBI	CBI only	0.03 (−0.13, 0.19) p=0.69	0.03 (−0.19, 0.25) p=1.00	0.03 (−0.18, 0.25) p=0.98	0.03 (−0.20, 0.26) p=0.98	N/A
Naltrexone and CBI	**Neither**	**−0.19** **(−0.35, −0.03)** **p=0.02**	−0.19 (−0.40, 0.02) p=0.11	−0.19 (−0.40, 0.02) p=0.09	−0.19 (−0.42, 0.04) p=0.14	**−0.19** **(−0.38, 0.00)** **p=0.05**
Naltrexone only	CBI only	0.03 (−0.13, 0.19) p=0.70	0.03 (−0.19, 0.25) p=1.00	0.03 (−0.18, 0.25) p=0.98	0.03 (−0.20, 0.26) p=0.99	N/A
Naltrexone only	**Neither**	**−0.19** **(−0.35, −0.03)** **p=0.02**	−0.19 (−0.41, 0.02) p=0.11	−0.19 (−0.40, 0.02) p=0.09	−0.19 (−0.42, 0.04) p=0.14	**−0.19** **(−0.38, 0.00)** **p=0.05**
CBI only	**Neither**	−0.22 (−0.38, −0.07) p=0.005	**−0.22** **(−0.43, −0.01)** **p=0.03**	**−0.22** **(−0.43, −0.02)** **p=0.03**	**−0.22** **(−0.44, −0.00)** **p=0.05**	−0.22 (−0.41, −0.04) p=0.01

Note: Comparisons indicated in bold are statistically signficant at 0.05 level.

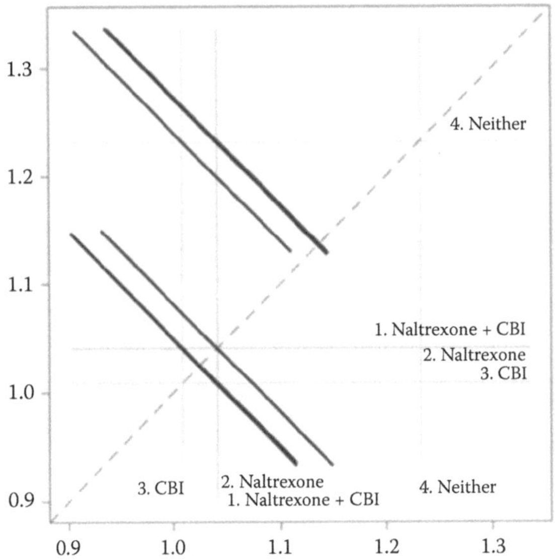

FIGURE 6.1
Diffogram for Tukey-adjusted pairwise differences in drinks per day at month four in the COMBINE study.

6.3.3 Scheffé's Multiple Comparison Procedure

Scheffé's multiple comparison method (Scheffé, 1953, 1999) is also a single-step procedure for mean comparisons developed in the context of ANOVA designs, but it can be used for any possible contrasts among the factor level means, not just pairwise differences. For example, one may be interested in testing whether each mean is equal from the average of the remaining means, whether the means are different from a control, or in linear or quadratic trends in the means when the factor levels are ordered. All these comparisons can be represented by linear contrasts, which are linear combinations of the means defined as $C = \sum c_i\mu_i$, where the c_is are constants such that $\sum c_i = 0$. Some examples are as follows:

- When two means μ_i and μ_j are compared: $c_i=1$, $c_j=-1$ while all other constants are 0 and hence the contrast C is $\mu_i-\mu_j$.
- A contrast where the fourth mean is tested to be equal to the average of the remaining three means is coded as $(\mu_1+\mu_2+\mu_3)-3\mu_4$ (i.e., $c_1=1$, $c_2=1$, $c_3=1$, $c_4=-3$).
- A linear contrast among four ordered means can be coded as $(-3\mu_1-\mu_2+\mu_3+3\mu_4)$ (i.e., $c_1=-3$, $c_2=-1$, $c_3=1$, $c_4=3$).

One can see that there are many possible contrasts that can be formulated, but only some of them are of substantive interest. Scheffé's procedure keeps the FWER at the selected alpha level for all possible contrasts when it follows an overall significant F-test for the factor of interest. Because of this, it is guaranteed to find a significant contrast when the overall F-test of the effect is statistically significant. However, this contrast may not be one of the few of interest. Like Tukey's and Bonferroni's procedures, Scheffé's procedure can be used for both simultaneous hypothesis testing and confidence interval construction. When only a few contrasts are of interest, it may be too conservative, as is the case with the pairwise comparison of the COMBINE data, shown in Table 6.4, where confidence intervals adjusted with Scheffé's method are the widest.

6.3.4 Dunnett's Multiple Comparison Procedure

In contrast to Tukey's and Scheffé's procedures, *Dunnett's multiple comparison test* (Dunnett, 1955) is specific to the situation when each of the means of several experimental treatments ($\mu_1, \mu_2, \ldots \mu_{c-1}$) is compared to the mean of a control treatment (μ_c). If only such comparisons are of interest, Tukey's and Scheffé's procedures lead to confidence intervals that are wider than necessary and to hypothesis tests that are too conservative (familywise error rate is below the target level). Similar to the other multiple comparison procedures considered so far, the only difference between this test and performing unadjusted t-tests (or equivalently between single confidence intervals and multiplicity-adjusted confidence intervals) are the critical values that are used. Those are based on the multivariate analogue of the t-distribution and are tabulated by Dunnett in the original publication introducing this method.

In the context of the COMBINE example, Dunnett's test is appropriate if we may be interested in testing only whether the combination of naltrexone and CBI, naltrexone alone, or CBI alone, are better than not getting treatment but not in the comparisons among the active treatments. Table 6.4 shows the three simultaneous confidence intervals with the control after Dunnett's adjustment. All three confidence intervals do not contain 0 and the intervals are narrower than those based on the other adjustment methods. Unlike Tukey's method, which adjusts for all pairwise comparisons, and Scheffé's method, which adjusts for all contrasts among the means, Dunnett's method adjusts only for the comparisons with the control, and thus retains more power and allows us to estimate the effects comparing the different treatments to the control more precisely. However, it does not provide estimates for the other comparisons, which may also be of interest. Note that the family of comparisons must be pre-specified rather than chosen after seeing the data, in order to avoid increasing the chance to overstate the significance of the findings.

Dunnett's approach can also be used to construct one-sided confidence intervals and hypothesis tests. In the COMBINE example, this will be appropriate if one is interested only in whether the mean drinks per day are lower in the active treatment groups than in the control group and doesn't care about differences in the other direction. This increases power but can miss differences in the other direction, so the one-sided approach should be used with care.

6.3.5 Other Classical Multiple Comparison Procedures

Another popular procedure for multiple comparisons is *Šidák's correction* (Šidák, 1967). It is similar to Bonferroni, but is slightly less conservative for independent tests or confidence intervals and hence, is recommended in such situations. However, for dependent tests or confidence intervals, it may fail to protect the FWER.

There are also procedures aimed at comparing all other treatments to the best/worst treatment in the set (e.g., Hsu, 1981). This procedure is similar to Dunnett's method but the control group is not known beforehand.

Simulation-based methods (Edwards and Berry, 1987) are very useful, especially with unbalanced data since, in these cases, the approximations of the critical values by classical methods may not be precise (e.g., as in the Tukey–Kramer procedure). These methods approximate the appropriate critical values in hypothesis tests or confidence intervals by simulation, which can be made as precise as needed. However, there is a degree of randomness in these methods and results from analyses of the same data may be slightly different.

A number of classical procedures for multiplicity correction do not control the FWER and nowadays are less frequently used (e.g., *Fisher's least significant difference approach, Duncan's multiple range procedure* [Duncan, 1955], *(Student-)Newman-Keuls procedure* [Newman, 1939]). In particular, Fisher's LSD approach attempts to protect the FWER by performing unadjusted comparisons among treatment means only if the overall F-test for the treatment effect is statistically significant. However, it is possible that the overall F-test is significant while all pairwise comparisons are not, and for the overall F-test for the treatment effect to be non-significant while one or more pairwise comparisons are statistically significant. Thus, Fisher's LSD approach does not sufficiently control the FWER.

Hochberg and Tamhane (1987) describe classical single-step and stepwise multiple correction procedures and modifications in detail. Note that results from all multiple comparisons procedures are valid only when assumptions of the underlying models are reasonably well satisfied. When the assumptions are not satisfied (e.g., a model for normal data is used when the data are not normally distributed), the FWER may not be adequately controlled.

6.3.6 Classical Multiple Comparison Procedures for Repeated Measures Data

The classical multiple comparison procedures can be used for data that are dependent and have heterogeneous variances, with a few caveats. The variance–covariance structure needs to be properly estimated (see Chapter 3) and when the data are not balanced, the appropriate approximations to the degrees of freedom need to be used (see Westfall et al., 2011). Even then, the methods are approximate and may be too conservative or too liberal depending on how unbalanced the data are and how well the chosen variance–covariance structure matches the data. Simulation-based procedures may be preferred for dependent data in that they can closely approximate the critical values for the mean comparisons. Alternatively, stepwise modifications of the Bonferroni procedure can be used for p-value adjustment, as described in Section 6.4.

6.3.7 Families of Comparisons and Robustness to Assumption Violations

As mentioned in the context of the COMBINE data example, the choice of the family of multiple comparisons is very important. If the family includes too many comparisons, some of which are not of particular interest, power may be adversely affected. But if the family is selected after a number of exploratory analyses and data peeks, then the FWER correction may be too small and the significance of results may be overstated.

In general, a family of simultaneous hypothesis tests or confidence intervals should correspond to a set of questions of interest that are related, and the overall conclusion or decision depends on the answers to all the questions. The most common scenarios are: comparisons of treatments with the goal of identifying the best one; ranking the treatments from best to worst; comparing treatments to a control, or comparing treatments or groups in terms of multiple outcome measures (e.g., multiple efficacy and safety measures in clinical trials, multiple gene, or protein expression levels). A study can have multiple sets of questions of interest and the results will be dependent on how the sets are defined. Note that the control over the familywise error rate is for the entire family of interferences and only for that family. Since our focus in this book is on models for repeated measures data, we primarily discuss and illustrate methods for post hoc testing in linear models, in which case FWER correction methods are often preferable. We also briefly mention correction for multiple outcome measures later in this chapter.

6.3.8 Post Hoc Analyses in Models for Repeated Measures

For post hoc analysis in models for repeated measures on a single outcome variable, the most common approach is to perform all tests of main effects and interactions at unadjusted significance level (e.g., 0.05). If the analysis is exploratory and/or if there are no *a priori* comparisons of interest, significant interactions and main effects are identified and multiplicity adjustments are performed only for the post hoc analyses to explain these significant effects. Separate adjustments are used to explain the different significant effects or interactions.

For example, in a study with two between-subject factors (A and B) and repeated measures on individuals over time, a linear mixed model with all possible interactions is fit. Suppose that the interactions A × time and B × time are significant. If this approach is adopted, two families of post hoc tests can be formulated: one to explain the significant interaction A × time and the other to explain the significant interaction B × time. For each set, separate FWER adjustment should be used. While this approach will not necessarily protect the FWER for all comparisons that are performed, it will maintain power better than a stricter approach that corrects for all comparisons in both sets of post hoc analyses.

Note that in clinical trials, there are usually *a priori* hypotheses about comparisons that are expected to be statistically significant. In this case, one should directly test these comparisons with a multiplicity adjustment as necessary regardless of the overall significance of effects. More information about different multiplicity situations in clinical trials and various adjustments can be found in Dmitrienko et al. (2010). Herein, we continue considering the situations of post hoc analyses with multiplicity adjustments.

Post hoc analyses in linear models should start with the highest order interaction and proceed with lower order interactions and main effects, as indicated. In general, if the highest order interaction is qualitative (i.e., the effect of one factor changes dramatically depending on the level[s] of the other factor[s]), only the highest order interaction is interpreted. If the interaction is quantitative (i.e., the effect of one factor varies in magnitude but not in direction depending on the levels of the other factors), then interpretation of lower order interactions and/or main effects may be indicated.

The following general guidelines show what post hoc analyses are indicated to explain significant effects in linear models (listed from simple to more complicated effects):

- When the levels of a categorical factor with a significant main effect are of equal interest and unordered, all pairwise comparisons should be performed. Tukey–Kramer adjustment, simulation-based adjustment, or Bonferroni-type adjustments (including those described in the next section) can be used. If there are other factors in the model, the means that are compared are averaged over the levels of the other factors.
- When the levels of a categorical factor with a significant main effect are ordered, focused comparisons should be performed. For example, if dose-response is of interest, one can construct contrasts for linear, quadratic, etc. dose effects. One can also compare each of the doses with the control. Bonferroni-type adjustments (including those described in the next section) may work best, especially if the

number of post hoc tests is small. If the number of post hoc contrasts is large, Scheffé's method may work better. Simulation-based methods can be used in both cases.

- When there is a significant main effect of a categorical factor, and it is of interest to compare all factor levels with a control, the methods of Dunnett, Bonferroni, or simulation can be used.
- When there is a significant two-way interaction between two categorical factors, post hoc testing should consist of tests of simple effects, i.e., comparisons of the means of one of the factors within each level of the other factor. Note that depending on how many levels each factor has, this can become complicated. The simplest case is when each factor has two levels. Then, we just need to compare the levels of the first factor at each level of the second factor and/or vice versa. For example, in the COMBINE study, the significant interaction between naltrexone and CBI in Chapter 2, for drinks per day during the last month, should be followed by testing the simple effect of naltrexone for those on CBI (i.e., comparison of naltrexone versus placebo on CBI) and the simple effect of naltrexone for those not on CBI (i.e., comparison of naltrexone versus placebo not on CBI). We can also test the simple effect of CBI at each level of naltrexone, which will add two comparisons to the family. If we are not interested in all four and we would like to focus on naltrexone (which should be decided *a priori*) we can adjust for only two tests.
- A slightly more complicated example is if one of the factors has three levels and the other—two levels. Then we can perform all pairwise comparisons of the levels of the first factor within each level of the second factor. This involves performing six post hoc comparisons. If the three levels of the first factor are ordered, we can test for linear and quadratic effects.
- With more levels, post hoc testing becomes quite complicated. The logic of specific post hoc testing for interactions should be decided *a priori* but should be focused on simple effects. Bonferroni-based procedures (including the ones in the next section) may be most flexible in these situations.
- When there are interactions involving categorical and continuous predictors, post hoc analysis involves comparisons of slopes for the relationship between the continuous predictor and the response at different levels of the categorical predictor. One can also select particular meaningful levels of the continuous predictor and test the simple effects of the categorical predictor at these levels. For example, if time is treated as a continuous predictor with a linear effect, and time interacts with treatment (active versus control), one can estimate slopes for change over time within each treatment group. On the other hand, one might be interested in the difference between the active and the control group at the beginning of the study, at the mid-point, and at the end.
- Significant interactions of higher order are also interpreted by testing or estimating simple effects but this may be within combinations of levels of the other factors. For example, if there is a three-way interaction $A \times B \times time$, one can look at the effect of A within each level of B at each time point. Slope comparisons may also result from interactions involving categorical and continuous predictors.

Specific examples of logical families of post hoc tests are provided in the context of the examples given further in this chapter. We also consider a situation of multiple testing when there are multiple outcome measures. With different outcome measures analyzed simultaneously (e.g., several drinking measures in COMBINE), the most logical assumptions are Bonferroni-type adjustments that are less conservative. These stepwise procedures are considered next.

6.4 Stepwise Modifications of the Bonferroni Approach

When the focus is on simultaneous testing of multiple hypotheses, rather than on confidence intervals, *stepwise procedures* are more powerful than single-step procedures, while still maintaining the FWER. Using these methods, p-values in a set of hypothesis tests are sequentially compared to different cutoffs (or adjusted in different ways) depending on the other p-values in the set. Stepwise procedures are examples of *closed testing procedures,* which involve testing extra intersection hypotheses (i.e., testing whether several hypotheses in the set are simultaneously true) in an order that allows us to effectively ignore multiplicity (Marcus et al., 1976). Westfall et al. (2011) described how these procedures work at a non-technical level. Closed testing procedures can be applied to any set of hypothesis tests (pairwise differences, sets of contrasts, or independent hypotheses).

6.4.1 The Bonferroni–Holm Multiple Comparison Procedure

The *Bonferroni–Holm method* (Holm, 1979) is one of the first stepwise modifications of the Bonferroni procedure that improve power while still controlling the FWER. It involves ordering the p-values of m hypothesis tests from lowest to highest. We denote the ordered p-values as $p_{(1)} \leq p_{(2)} \leq \ldots p_{(m)}$ and the corresponding hypotheses as $H_{(1)}, H_{(2)}, \ldots H_{(m)}$. For a given significance level α, one first tests whether $p_{(1)} < \alpha/m$. If it is, one checks whether $p_{(2)} < \alpha/(m-1)$. If this is also the case, then one continues checking whether $p_{(k)} < \alpha/(m-k+1)$ until one reaches the first k for which this condition is not satisfied. At this point, one reaches the conclusion to reject all hypotheses $H_{(1)}, H_{(2)}, \ldots H_{(k-1)}$ and to not reject the hypotheses $H_{(k)}, H_{(k+1)}, \ldots H_{(m)}$. If even the first inequality is not satisfied (i.e., if $p_{(1)} \geq \alpha/m$) then none of the hypotheses are rejected and no significant differences are found. If $p_{(m)} < \alpha$ then all null hypotheses are rejected. This procedure ensures that the FWER is smaller or equal to α. A simple example how to apply it is as follows:

Suppose that we are performing four simultaneous tests that result in p-values $p_1 = 0.10$, $p_2 = 0.03$, $p_3 = 0.001$, $p_4 = 0.015$. Uncorrected tests at 0.05 significance level would result in rejection of H_2, H_3, and H_4. The classical Bonferroni correction would require comparing all p-values to $0.05/4 = 0.0125$ and hence, would lead to rejection of only H_3. The Bonferroni–Holm procedure would involve ordering the four p-values so that $p_{(1)} = p_3 = 0.001$, $p_{(2)} = p_4 = 0.015$, $p_{(3)} = p_2 = 0.03$, $p_{(4)} = p_1 = 0.010$, comparing the smallest p-value $p_{(1)} = 0.001$ to $\alpha/m = 0.05/4 = 0.0125$, the second smallest p-value $p_{(2)} = 0.015$ to $\alpha/(m-1) = 0.05/3 = 0.0167$, since the smallest p-value is smaller than the corresponding cut off, and comparing $p_{(3)} = 0.03$ to $\alpha/(m-2) = 0.05/2 = 0.02$. Since the last inequality is not satisfied, the Bonferroni–Holm procedure results in a rejection of H_3 and H_4, which is an intermediate result between not correcting and using the conservative Bonferroni correction.

Table 6.3 also shows the results from the Bonferroni–Holm procedure applied to the hypothetical set of five hypotheses we considered earlier in this chapter. Column 3 shows the adjusted p-values from the test, which can be compared directly to the chosen FWER (0.05 in this case), in order to decide which hypotheses are rejected and which are not. An elegant explanation of how adjusted p-values are calculated can be found in Westfall et al. (2011). Two of the five hypotheses in this example are rejected, compared to four out of five when no adjustment is applied, and only one out of five when the conservative Bonferroni approach is applied.

Indeed, the main advantage of the Bonferroni-Holm procedure over the classical Bonferroni procedure is that it is less conservative and more powerful. However, there are other methods for controlling the FWER that are even more powerful, such as *Hochberg's procedure* (Hochberg, 1988) and *Hommel's procedure* (Hommel, 1988). They both rely on some of the theoretical framework developed by Simes (1986).

6.4.2 Hochberg's Multiple Comparison Procedure

Hochberg's procedure is similar to the Bonferroni–Holm approach in that it uses the same cutoff values for the ordered p-values but it is a *step-up* (starts with testing less significant test statistics and moves toward testing more significant test statistics) rather than a *step-down* approach (starts with testing more significant test statistics and moves toward testing less significant test statistics). The p-values and the corresponding hypotheses are again ordered so that $p_{(1)} \le p_{(2)} \le \ldots \le p_{(m)}$, but then we start by comparing the largest p-value (corresponding to the least significant test statistic) to the significance level α. If $p_{(m)} \le \alpha$ then all hypotheses are rejected and we stop. If $p_{(m)} > \alpha$ then we do not reject $H_{(m)}$ and evaluate how the next p-value (corresponding to the second most non-significant test statistic) compares to its cutoff (n) i.e., whether $p_{(m-1)} \le \alpha/2$. If it is, then all remaining hypotheses (i.e., $H_{(1)}, H_{(2)}, \ldots H_{(m-1)}$) are rejected and we stop. If not, we continue checking. The kth p-value is compared to $\alpha/(m-k+1)$ but we allow the p-value to be equal to the cutoff in order to reject, i.e., we check whether $p_{(k)} \le \alpha/(m-k+1)$. If it is, then we reject all remaining hypotheses (i.e., $H_{(1)}, H_{(2)}, \ldots H_{(k)}$). If none of the p-values are less or equal to their corresponding cutoffs then none of the null hypotheses are rejected.

Note that because the inequalities are strict in Holm's procedure while the p-values are allowed to be equal to the cut off in Hochberg's approach, Hochberg's approach is more powerful. However, Hochberg's procedure is guaranteed to protect the FWER in case of independent or positively dependent hypotheses, while Bonferroni–Holm can be applied in any situation.

Similar to Bonferroni–Holm's procedure, adjusted p-values can be calculated for Hochberg's procedure and directly compared to the selected overall alpha level. Adjusted p-values from Hochberg's procedure are always smaller or equal to the adjusted p-values from Bonferroni–Holm's procedure.

The fourth column of Table 6.3 includes the adjusted p-values from Hochberg's step-up procedure applied to the hypothetical set of five hypotheses. As expected those are equal or smaller to the adjusted p-values from Bonferroni–Holm's procedure, which in turn are smaller than the Bonferroni-adjusted p-values. The same two hypotheses are rejected using Hochberg's and Bonferroni–Holm's approaches.

Hochberg's approach protects the FWER when the p-values are independent or positively dependent. If the p-values are negatively dependent then the FWER may be inflated.

6.4.3 Hommel's Multiple Comparison Procedure

Hommel's approach is even more powerful than Hochberg's approach but it is more difficult to understand and takes more computational time. Like the other two modifications of the Bonferroni procedure considered here, the method also orders the p-values from smallest to largest. Then it seeks to identify the largest integer k (less than or equal to the number of comparisons m), such that $p_{(m-k+j)} > j\alpha/k$ for all $j=1,\ldots k$. If there is no such k then all hypotheses are rejected. If there is, then all hypotheses for which $p_{(i)} \le \alpha/k$ are rejected and the remaining are not rejected. Like Hochberg's approach, Hommel's method requires that the p-values be either independent or positively dependent in order to control the FWER at the desired level. If the p-values are negatively dependent, it can result in a FWE level greater than the desired level.

In the hypothetical data example from Table 6.3, the adjusted p-values based on Hommel's approach are in the fifth column. Three of those p-values are less than 0.05 and hence three of the hypotheses are rejected. This is one more than the number of hypotheses rejected using the Bonferroni–Holm and Hochberg procedures.

6.5 Procedures Controlling the False Discovery Rate (FDR)

While FWER has been the preferred approach to multiple corrections for a long time, it is too conservative in many situations, which has led to some researchers not using the control at all and just keeping the per-comparison error rate at a pre-specified alpha level. FWER does protect against inflation of type I error but such strict control may not be always needed. In general, if the overall result from the simultaneous testing can be considered invalid even if there is just one mistake, then FWER may be essential. This is the case when out of several treatments, one wants to select the best one. But, when an experimental treatment is compared to a control treatment on a number of outcome measures, and some of the rejections are false rejections, the overall conclusion of superiority of the experimental treatment may not be invalidated by these false rejections. We now turn our attention to more appropriate corrections in cases when strict control of FWER may not be needed and/or when the number of comparisons is so high that FWER correction leads to significant loss of power to detect any differences.

As described previously, the false discovery rate (FDR) is the expected proportion of false rejections. When it is likely that there are going to be many rejections (as is the case in large scale genomics, proteomics, and other high throughput studies), then this interpretation is quite intuitive. However, if it is likely that there are no or very few rejections and/or the number of hypotheses is small, then the interpretation of the FDR is not clear. In such cases it is better to use methods that control the FWER.

Note that the FDR correction assures that the proportion of false rejections is less than the desired FDR level only on average. Therefore, it is quite possible that in some samples the ratio of false versus all rejections can be higher than intended.

The FDR can be controlled at any level but it is typically controlled at the same level as the FWER, namely 5%. Procedures that control the FDR also control the FWER at the same level, but typically the FDR is much lower than the FWER, and when the goal is to control the FDR, a number of less conservative procedures than the FWER-controlling procedures are available.

6.5.1 Benjamini–Hochberg's Multiple Comparison Procedure

The first and most frequently used procedure that controls the FDR, is *Benjamini–Hochberg's procedure* (Benjamini and Hochberg, 1995). It is simple to implement and is very similar to the modifications of the Bonferroni procedure considered in the previous section, in particular the step-up procedures. For a given level α, one needs to find the largest number k, such that $p_{(k)} \leq k\alpha/m$ and then reject the null hypotheses $H_{(1)}, H_{(2)}, \ldots H_{(k)}$. As before, k needs to be between 1 and m inclusive. If no such k exists then none of the null hypotheses are rejected. Note that the thresholds to which the p-values are compared are larger than the thresholds in Hochberg's test and thus more hypotheses can be rejected. The Benjamini–Hochberg procedure is valid when the tests are independent or positively dependent.

As with the other multiplicity control methods, this procedure is usually implemented by comparing adjusted p-values to the chosen FDR threshold. Table 6.3 shows the adjusted p-values based on Benjamini–Hochberg's method for the simple data example. It is indeed less conservative than the other methods in that it rejects four out of the five hypotheses. Note, though, that in this situation the interpretation of the FDR is not clear since there are only five hypotheses in total and the expected number of rejections is small. Typically, the Benjamini–Hochberg correction is used when the number of tested hypotheses is large.

6.5.2 Benjamini–Yekutieli's Multiple Comparison Procedure

A modification of Benjamini–Hochberg's procedure, when there is dependence between the hypothesis tests, as often encountered with multiple outcome tests on the same individuals, is due to Benjamini and Yekutieli (2001). This procedure modifies the threshold so that the dependence is taken into account. The inequalities that are evaluated are

$$p_{(k)} \leq \frac{k}{m \times c(m)} \alpha,$$

where $c(m) = \sum_{i=1}^{m} 1/i$ under arbitrary dependence while $c(m) = 1$ under independence and positive dependence. Note that in the latter scenario, Benjamini—Yekutieli's procedure reduces to Benjamini–Hochberg's procedure.

The adjusted p-values based on Benjamini–Yekutieli's correction for the example in Table 6.3 show that this correction can be quite conservative when we are unsure about the dependence of the structure of the hypotheses. Only one out of five hypotheses is rejected in this case. However, this is hardly an appropriate example to illustrate the advantages of FDR correction procedures since the family set is small.

Both Benjamini–Hochberg's and Benjamini–Yekutieli's procedures control the FDR, so that $FDR \leq m_0\alpha/m$ and therefore, they can be conservative if the number of true null hypotheses is smaller than the total number of hypotheses in the set. If one knew the number of true null hypotheses m_0, then one could formulate a more powerful FDR-controlling procedure. There are indeed adaptive FDR adjustments that use an estimate of the number of true null hypotheses.

Many other procedures that control the FDR and related error rates (e.g., the *positive false discovery rate* (pFDR), or the *false discover proportion* (FDP)) have been considered in recent years (see Benjamini (2010b) for a review). Most of them improve on the Benjamini–Hochberg procedure in order to make it more powerful (e.g., Storey, 2003; Genovese and Wasserman, 2004; Benjamini et al., 2006).

6.5.3 Simultaneous Confidence Intervals Controlling the False Coverage Rate

The FDR equivalent for confidence intervals is the *false coverage rate* (FCR) (Benjamini and Yekutieli, 2005). It is a measure of interval coverage following the selection of a number of parameters from a larger set of potential parameters, based on statistical significance. The procedure constructs individual CIs for each selected parameter with the confidence level adjusted for the number of selected parameters. The FCR indicates the average rate of false coverage, namely, the expected proportion of parameters not covered by the CIs among the selected parameters. The proportion is 0 if no parameter is selected. There are different FCR procedures depending on how the parameters are selected and what adjustment is applied to the construction of confidence intervals for the selected parameters (e.g., Bonferroni-Selected-Bonferroni-Adjusted, Adjusted Benjamini–Hochberg-Selected-CIs). In the Adjusted Benjamini–Hochberg-Selected CIs, first the Benjamini–Hochberg FDR procedure is applied, and the parameters for which the null hypotheses are rejected at level α are selected. Then $1 - R\alpha/m$ level confidence intervals are constructed for each of these R parameters.

6.6 Procedures Based on Resampling and Bootstrap

Another class of procedures for multiple comparisons is based on resampling of the data with replacement (bootstrap) and without replacement (permutation). This results in multiple simulated data sets based on the original data. The basic idea is to use these simulated data sets to approximate the distributions of the minimum p-value (which is a key to most multiplicity corrections) and to use these approximations to adjust the individual p-values. Resampling methods are computationally intensive but have advantages over the other methods in seamlessly taking into account correlations and distributional characteristics. They can be used in situations when the distributional assumptions of other models are not satisfied. See Westfall and Young (1993) for a detailed description of these approaches and Dudoit and Laan (2008) for a more up-to-date but very technical description. More recent research is focused on improving the computational performance of the procedures (e.g., Zhang et al., 2012).

6.7 Data Examples

6.7.1 Post Hoc Testing in the COMBINE Study

Earlier in this chapter, we focused on the log-transformed number of drinks per day during the last month of treatment in the COMBINE Study and illustrated classical multiplicity corrections for all pairwise tests among four treatments (naltrexone and CBI, naltrexone only, CBI only, and neither naltrexone nor CBI). However, in this analysis we ignored the third active treatment (namely acamprosate), the factorial nature of the study design, and the fact that there is more than one outcome measure of interest. Herein, we present additional analyses of these data in order to compare the FWER and FDR correction procedures, to discuss the challenges in specifying the family of inferences and the sensitivity of conclusions to the choice of family and methods. Note that in the first subsection we consider a rather artificial family of comparisons (i.e., one would not normally perform so many unfocused comparisons for such data) but it demonstrates how the FDR methods allow us to retain power better than FWER methods.

6.7.1.1 *Correction for Simultaneous Pairwise Comparisons on Different Outcome Measures*

We can consider a family of inferences that focuses on all possible pairwise comparisons among the eight treatments (all possible combinations of levels of naltrexone, acamprosate, and CBI) for two outcomes measured during the last month of treatment that we considered previously in separate analyses: average number of drinks per day and number of drinking days. This unfocused set of tests consists of 56 comparisons ($7\times8/2$ pairwise comparisons for each of the two outcome measures). To assess whether there is an indication of some non-null hypotheses, one can graphically view the results using the *Schweder-Spjøtvoll p-value plot* (see Figure 6.2). This plot depicts the relationship between the ordered p-values and their rank order. On the horizontal axis is the rank (going from 1 for the largest p-value to 56, in this example, for the smallest p-value). On the vertical axis each p-value is shown after being subtracted from 1. If there are no differences among the means (i.e., all null hypotheses are true), then the p-values should fall approximately on a straight diagonal line going from the lower left corner to the upper right corner. When there are some actual differences, then the corresponding p-values for these differences are smaller than expected under the null hypotheses and hence the circles in the graph corresponding to these comparisons will be in the upper right corner above the straight

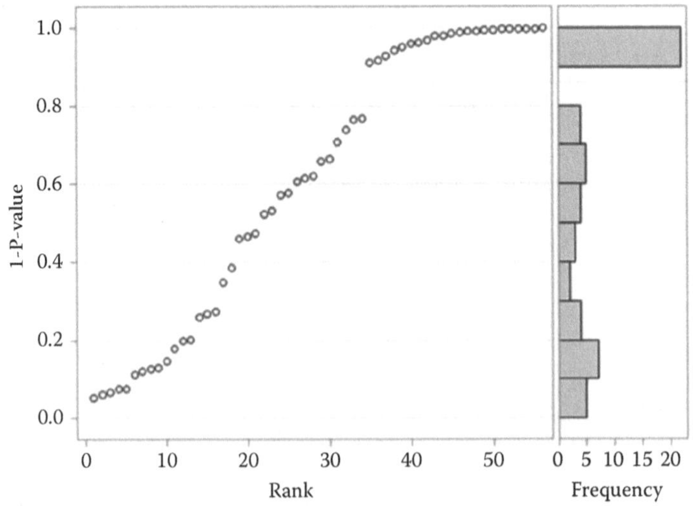

FIGURE 6.2
Schweder-Spjøtvoll p-value plot for all pairwise comparisons on two outcome measures during month four in the COMBINE study.

diagonal line. In this particular example, we see that a number of the comparisons are indeed above the straight line so they might correspond to genuine differences. The plot as created by PROC MULTTEST in SAS also includes a histogram of the 1 − p-values which should be uniform if all null hypotheses are true. If there are genuine differences then there should be more values at the top, which is what we see in Figure 6.2.

Although the graphic display indicates that some differences are likely true differences, we need to apply formal multiple comparison correction in order to figure out which differences are statistically significant when multiplicity is taken into account. Since the family consists of a mix of pairwise mean comparisons on the same variable and tests on different variables, we can't directly use corrections such as Tukey's and Scheffé's. However, Bonferroni-type FWER corrections and FDR corrections are appropriate. We can also apply Tukey–Kramer's method for all pairwise comparisons on each outcome variable at a Bonferroni corrected level of $\alpha/2$ per variable. We considered the Bonferroni, Bonferroni-Holm, Hochberg, and Hommel methods. We also applied the Benjamini–Hochberg and Benjamini–Yekutieli corrections. The results of the stepwise Bonferroni procedures were very similar and led to the same substantive conclusions that there are no significant differences after adjustment hence we show the p-values from the Hommel method only. The Benjamini–Yekutieli correction and the Tukey–Bonferroni combination also made all results non-significant and are not shown here. All results are available in the online materials. Eighteen of the 56 comparisons are significant prior to correction for multiplicity. Ten out of the 18 comparisons remain significant at 0.05 level with the Benjamini–Hochberg method and none are significant at familywise 0.05 level with the other corrections we considered. Table 6.5 shows the raw and adjusted p-values for the comparisons that were significant before adjustment for the different methods.

This example illustrates that with such a comparatively large family of tests, controlling the FWER results in a severe correction and probably misses the identification of genuine differences. FDR corrections maintain power but the corresponding FWER is likely (much) higher than 5%. In such a situation, a more focused testing or estimation strategy, which takes into account the factorial nature of the design, followed by procedures that control the FWER, is preferable, as illustrated in the next subsection.

6.7.1.2 Post Hoc Testing of Significant Main Effects and Interactions

Due to the factorial design of this study, it is more appropriate to assess main effects and interactions, and to perform follow-up tests for the significant effects in the model following the guidelines presented in Section 6.3.7. In Section 2.1.3, we performed all tests of main effects and interactions for the outcome measure of drinks per day at the end of treatment for subjects who drank in COMBINE, using 0.05 significance level. We also considered these data earlier in this chapter to illustrate differences among the classical multiple comparison procedures.

The results from the three-factor ANOVA analysis showed that the interaction between naltrexone and CBI ($F(1,713) = 3.77$, $p = 0.05$) (see Table 2.3) was statistically significant at 0.05 significance level. The general strategy in such a situation is to test all main effects and interactions at uncorrected alpha level of 0.05, then to interpret any significant interactions first by assessing simple effects and to perform post hoc analysis for main effects as needed.

In this particular example, the simple effects of naltrexone to explain the naltrexone by CBI interaction are simply comparisons between the least square means on active naltrexone and on placebo naltrexone at each level of therapy (CBI and no CBI). Similarly, the simple

TABLE 6.5

Raw and Adjusted p-Values for the Pairwise Comparisons Significant at 0.05 Level Prior to Adjustment in the Analysis of Endpoint Drinks per Day and Number of Drinking Days in the COMBINE Study

Outcome	Treatment	Versus Treatment	Unadjusted	Hommel	Benjamini–Hochberg
Number of drinking days	Naltrexone, acamprosate, and CBI	Placebo naltrexone, acamprosate, and no CBI	**0.0414**	0.9465	0.1363
	Naltrexone, acamprosate, and CBI	Placebo pills and no CBI	**0.0036**	0.1678	**0.0400**
	Naltrexone, placebo acamprosate, and CBI	Placebo pills and no CBI	**0.0383**	0.9465	0.1342
	Naltrexone, acamprosate, and no CBI	Placebo pills and no CBI	**0.0075**	0.3292	**0.0465**
	Naltrexone, placebo acamprosate, and no CBI	Placebo pills and no CBI	**0.0056**	0.2505	**0.0401**
	Placebo naltrexone, placebo acamprosate, and CBI	Placebo naltrexone, acamprosate, and no CBI	**0.0487**	0.9465	0.1516
	Placebo naltrexone, placebo acamprosate, and CBI	Placebo pills and no CBI	**0.0044**	0.2021	**0.0401**
Drinks per day	Naltrexone, acamprosate, and CBI	Placebo naltrexone, acamprosate, and no CBI	**0.0208**	0.7922	0.0834
	Naltrexone, acamprosate, and CBI	Placebo pills and no CBI	**0.0035**	0.1656	**0.0400**
	Naltrexone, placebo acamprosate, and CBI	Placebo naltrexone, acamprosate, and no CBI	**0.0156**	0.6067	0.0726
	Naltrexone, placebo acamprosate, and CBI	Placebo pills and no CBI	**0.0024**	0.1172	**0.0400**
	Naltrexone, acamprosate, and no CBI	Placebo naltrexone, acamprosate, and no CBI	**0.0083**	0.3584	**0.0467**
	Naltrexone, acamprosate, and no CBI	Placebo pills and no CBI	**0.0012**	0.0607	**0.0400**
	Naltrexone, placebo acamprosate, and no CBI	Placebo naltrexone, acamprosate, and no CBI	**0.0317**	0.9465	0.1182
	Naltrexone, placebo acamprosate, and no CBI	Placebo pills and no CBI	**0.0057**	0.2577	**0.0401**
	Placebo naltrexone, acamprosate, and CBI	Placebo pills and no CBI	**0.0203**	0.7723	0.0834
	Placebo naltrexone, placebo acamprosate, and CBI	Placebo naltrexone, acamprosate, and no CBI	**0.0123**	0.5046	0.0627
	Placebo naltrexone, placebo acamprosate, and CBI	Placebo pills and no CBI	**0.0018**	0.0909	**0.0400**

Note: Values in bold are statistically significant at 0.05 level.

TABLE 6.6

Raw and Adjusted p-Values for the Simple Effects of Naltrexone and CBI in the Analysis of Endpoint Drinks per Day in the COMBINE Study

Effect	At Level of the Other Factor	Unadjusted	Bonferroni	Bonferroni–Holm	Hochberg	Benjamini–Hochberg
Active versus placebo naltrexone	CBI	0.6851	1.0000	1.0000	0.9825	0.9135
	No CBI	**0.0189**	0.0756	0.0567	0.0567	**0.0378**
CBI versus no CBI	Naltrexone	0.9825	1.0000	1.0000	0.9825	0.9825
	Placebo	**0.0050**	**0.0200**	**0.0200**	**0.0200**	**0.0200**

Note: Values indicated in bold are statistically significant at 0.05 level.

effects of CBI are comparisons between the least square means on CBI and without CBI at each level of naltrexone (active and placebo). Figure 2.1 visualizes these simple effects in a convenient way. The p-values for these simple effects, together with various adjustments for multiple testing, are provided in Table 6.6. Note that we are testing a subset of the possible comparisons among the levels of all factors after pre-specifying that we will interpret significant interactions with simple effects and thus we do not need to adjust for all possible pairwise comparisons. In this situation, all the Bonferroni adjustments lead to the same substantive conclusions, namely that all tests of simple effects are non-significant except the comparison of CBI versus the control. The Benjamini–Hochberg correction retains the significance of both the simple effect of naltrexone when CBI is not provided and the simple effect of CBI when naltrexone is not given. Note that since the Benjamini–Hochberg and the step-down Bonferroni procedures can't be used for confidence intervals, a better approach that also provides effect size estimates is to focus on confidence intervals. Confidence intervals can be Bonferroni corrected. Although such an analysis will not alter the substantive conclusions regarding statistical significance, it provides meaningful effect size estimates. In the next section, we focus on constructing confidence intervals for focused post hoc comparisons in a linear model.

6.7.1.3 Multiple Comparison Adjustments for Post Hoc Analysis in Models for Repeated Measures Data

In Chapter 4, we used GEE and GLMM to assess treatment effects on the number of drinking days per month during treatment in the COMBINE study. We constructed 95% confidence intervals to explain the significant effects in the models but did not apply correction for multiple testing. Herein, we show how confidence intervals and p-values can be adjusted to take into account that multiple inferences are being made simultaneously. We focus on the negative binomial GEE for the number of drinking days. The overall tests of main and interactive effects showed that there was a significant interaction between CBI and time, a significant main effect of time, and a significant naltrexone by CBI interaction at 0.05 significance level (see Section 4.2.4). To explain the significant interactions, a simple effects estimation is performed. Note that many statistical programs automatically perform all possible pairwise comparisons of different time points between groups (e.g., baseline of one group versus endpoint of another group) and adjust for all of these comparisons. This rarely makes sense. Usually, only the pairwise comparisons within group or the between-group comparisons at each time point are interpretable.

TABLE 6.7

Raw and Adjusted Confidence Intervals for Mean Ratios for the Significant Effects in the Negative Binomial GEE with Log Link Fitted to Number of Drinking Days per Month in the COMBINE Study

Effect	Level	Comparison Level	Unadjusted Rate Ratio (95% CI)	Adjusted Rate Ratio (Bonferroni-Corrected CI)
Naltrexone × CBI interaction	Naltrexone + CBI	Naltrexone	1.10 (0.91, 1.33)	1.10 (0.85, 1.43)
	Naltrexone + CBI	CBI	1.04 (0.86, 1.25)	1.04 (0.81, 1.34)
	Naltrexone + CBI	Neither	0.85 (0.71, 1.02)	0.85 (0.67, 1.08)
	Naltrexone	CBI	0.95 (0.78, 1.15)	0.95 (0.73, 1.23)
	Naltrexone	Neither	0.77 (0.64, 0.93)	0.77 (0.60, 0.99)
	CBI	Neither	0.82 (0.68, 0.98)	0.82 (0.64, 1.04)
CBI × time	CBI in period 1	No CBI in period 1	1.06 (0.91, 1.22)	1.06 (0.88, 1.27)
	CBI in period 2	No CBI in period 2	0.96 (0.83, 1.11)	0.96 (0.80, 1.15)
	CBI in period 3	No CBI in period 3	0.90 (0.78, 1.04)	0.90 (0.75, 1.08)
	CBI in period 4	No CBI in period 4	0.88 (0.76, 1.03)	0.88 (0.73, 1.06)
Main effect of time	Period 1	Period 2	0.85 (0.82, 0.89)	0.85 (0.80, 0.90)
	Period 1	Period 3	0.85 (0.80, 0.90)	0.85 (0.79, 0.92)
	Period 1	Period 4	0.83 (0.79, 0.89)	0.83 (0.77, 0.91)
	Period 2	Period 3	1.00 (0.96, 1.04)	1.00 (0.95, 1.05)
	Period 2	Period 4	0.98 (0.93, 1.03)	0.98 (0.92, 1.04)
	Period 3	Period 4	0.98 (0.95, 1.02)	0.98 (0.94, 1.03)

Table 6.7 shows the confidence intervals for the pairwise time comparisons prior to and after Bonferroni correction. Correction is applied only within the post hoc tests of each hypothesis. Tukey is not appropriate here since we do not consider all possible pairwise comparisons. Stepwise and FDR procedures work with p-values rather than confidence intervals and the number of comparisons is relatively small, so FWER control is better than FDR control in this situation. The familywise confidence level in the simultaneous intervals is 95% or higher.

As expected, the adjusted confidence intervals for the post hoc comparisons of the treatment groups are wider than the non-adjusted and one of the comparisons is not significant after adjustment (the comparison of CBI versus the control). The adjusted confidence intervals for the CBI by time interaction, and the main effect of time, are also wider but the statistical significance of the results does not change remarkably.

6.7.2 Post Hoc Testing in the fMRI Study of Working Memory in Schizophrenia

In Section 3.8.3, we used a LMM to determine whether there were differences between schizophrenia patients and healthy controls on activation measures during a working memory task. The overall analysis revealed a significant group by phase interaction which was followed by post hoc assessment of simple effects within each phase of the task (encoding, maintenance, and response). We did not adjust these multiple analyses (see Table 3.8). In Table 6.8, we show the results after several adjustments for multiple testing. Since we are focusing on p-values here, rather than confidence intervals, we use some of the stepwise closed testing procedures. Hommel is the only procedure that shows the comparison between schizophrenic patients and controls during maintenance to be statistically significant at the familywise significance level of 0.05. The comparison during response is significant before but not after correction for multiple testing.

TABLE 6.8

Raw and Adjusted p-Values for the Tests of the Simple Effect of Group within Each Phase of the Working Memory Task in the fMRI Study in Schizophrenia

Comparison	Phase	Unadjusted p-Value	Bonferroni-Adjusted p-Value	Bonferroni-Holm Adjusted p-Value	Hommel Adjusted p-Value
Schizophrenic versus control	Encoding	0.8631	1.0000	0.8631	0.8631
	Maintenance	**0.0248**	0.0745	0.0745	**0.0497**
	Response	**0.0288**	0.0865	0.0745	0.0577

6.8 Guidelines to Multiple Comparison Procedures

Since there are so many options for multiple comparison corrections, it is a challenge to choose the most appropriate method in different situations. Westfall et al. (2011) propose some general guidelines:

- For graphical summary, use the Schweder-Spjøtvoll p-value plot. Graphic displays should also be used to supplement formal analyses, especially when there is a large number of comparisons.
- Bonferroni and Šidák corrections are easy to apply both for hypothesis testing and for confidence intervals. Bonferroni can be used in any situation and Šidák is preferred for independent tests.
- When confidence intervals are not required, the stepwise modifications of the Bonferroni procedure are preferable in order to control the FWER.
- Tukey's procedure is most powerful for all pairwise comparisons of a set of means. However, with repeated measures data, this procedure is only approximately correct. Simulation-based methods can be used in order to properly account for the correlation structure and potential deviations from distributional assumptions.
- Dunnett's procedure is preferable for comparisons of multiple groups with a control group.
- FDR procedures are preferable in large scale studies where some percentage of false positive results can be tolerated.

Note that multiple comparison corrections are necessary both for independent and for correlated tests. Westfall et al. (2011) recommend resampling methods because they readily adjust only for the comparisons of interest, properly address the correlated comparisons, and can be used in virtually all situations.

6.9 Summary

In this chapter, we reviewed different methods for multiplicity corrections and provided some general guidelines for when to use them. Although the choice of the best procedure for each scenario is challenging, the biggest issue is the definition of a proper family of comparisons over which to apply the corrections. Our focus was mainly on post hoc testing in the context of linear models for correlated data, in which case, classical one-step and stepwise FWER control procedures of pairwise comparisons, comparisons to a control, or assessment of simple effects are usually most appropriate. The issues of controlling for multiple outcome measures and controlling the FDR in the simultaneous analysis of a large number of hypotheses, as occurring in high throughput experiments, were only briefly mentioned. Further reading on these topics is offered in the books by Dmitrienko et al. (2010), who describe issues and methods for multiple comparisons in the context of clinical trials, and by Dudoit and Laan (2008), who focus on multiple testing in genomics experiments.

A particular problem with the specification of the family of inferences, is that sometimes the selection is based on multiple peeks at the data. This leads to inflation of the reported FWER and FDRs. Therefore, an appropriate strategy of multiple testing needs to be developed at the design stage of the study and results need to be reported accurately.

One must also always keep in mind that the results from multiple comparison procedures are only as valid as the assumptions of the underlying model. For example, if a model for normal data is selected when data clearly deviate from the model assumptions, or correlations are not taken into account, the results from both the overall tests of main and interactive effects, and post hoc multiple comparison tests, can't be trusted. Simulation-based methods are preferred in situations when data assumptions are suspect.

Missing data can also severely affect the results from statistical modeling and multiplicity adjustment. We now turn to this very important topic, especially in the context of longitudinal studies where missing data are paramount.

7

Handling of Missing Data and Dropout in Longitudinal Studies

The term *missing data* refers to data that were intended to be collected but for whatever reason were not. Missing data are of paramount importance in clinical trials and observational studies. Subjects drop out or do not show up for some scheduled study visits, refuse to answer specific questions, data are incorrectly recorded or lost. There are two types of missing data in longitudinal studies: *intermittent missing data* (also referred to as *in-study non-response*) and *dropout*. Intermittent missing data occur when there is a gap in data collection followed by further measurements. For example, a participant might have been traveling and missed a scheduled visit. Dropout occurs when a participant stops providing any data in the study. There might be varying reasons for dropout (e.g., death, withdrawal of consent to participate, relocation) that may or may not be related to the outcome being analyzed. Thus, the presence of missing data may or may not be informative about the outcome of interest and care must be taken when interpreting summary statistics and results from statistical analyses.

Traditional methods for repeated measures analysis such as repeated measures ANOVA (rANOVA), repeated measures MANOVA (rMANOVA), and endpoint analysis can be severely affected by missing data. Usually, statistical software programs implementing these methods automatically drop individuals with missing data from the analyses. This leads to a loss of power because part of the information is lost and, even more importantly, to potential bias since dropouts and subjects with missing data may be systematically different from subjects with complete data. Alternatively, simple substitution methods such as last observation carried forward or mean substitution are used to fill in the missing values, and then classical analyses are performed as if all values in the data set were observed. This almost always results in bias, since it is usually unreasonable to assume that a subject's response would remain the same after dropout or that the mean value (whether within the individual or across individuals within a specific time point) corresponds to the unobserved value well. It also underestimates the variability associated with substituting missing values since a constant value is substituted for all missing values for the individual.

Recent developments in the theory of missing data, such as multiple imputation, full information maximum likelihood estimation, and weighting methods, allow missing data to be handled properly so that bias in statistical inference is minimized and the variability in the data is properly accounted for. These methods deal with both intermittent missing data and dropouts and provide valid results when data are randomly missing (i.e., missing data do not provide information about the unobserved outcome). However, even these methods can provide biased results when data are not randomly missing (i.e., dropout is related to the unobserved outcome). Many methods for sensitivity analyses are available in such situations. The complexity in dealing with missing data and the continuing ignorance of applied researchers of approaches for handling missing data have hindered progress in the transition from naive to modern methods for missing data. This chapter is intended to clarify concepts, illustrate the available methods with examples, point out useful references, and present guidelines for handling missing data.

In Section 7.1, we describe the basic terminology introduced by Rubin (1976) and explained in detail in Little and Rubin (2014) regarding types of missing data. We illustrate different scenarios of dropout and intermittent missing observations and provide an overview of the potential effects of the different types of missing data. In Section 7.2, we briefly mention simple substitution methods and point out their shortcomings in handling missing data. The subsequent three sections focus on the state-of-the-art methods for missing data; namely, multiple imputation (MI) (Section 7.3), full information maximum likelihood (FIML) (Section 7.4), and inverse probability weighting methods (Section 7.5). Methods for analysis when data are informatively missing are described briefly in Section 7.6 and references are provided for interested readers. The chapter concludes with illustration of the methods on data examples (Section 7.7) and general guidelines for handling missing data in studies with longitudinal and clustered data (Section 7.8).

Detailed technical information about missing data and approaches to handle them can be found in the books of Little and Rubin (2014) and Molenberghs et al. (2014). More non-technical presentations are available in the books of Allison (2002) and C. K. Enders (2010). A special chapter in Widaman (2006) and the manuscripts by Graham (2009) and Schlomer et al. (2010) provide brief, non-technical, and fairly comprehensive reviews of the issues and methods. Specific publications that focus on missing data in longitudinal studies are Ibrahim and Molenberghs (2009), Spratt et al. (2010), and Enders (2011). The tutorial of Hogan et al. (2004) is a very useful introduction for applied statisticians and quantitatively oriented researchers. Since our focus in this book is on missing data in longitudinal studies, we make a distinction between missing data on predictor and repeatedly measured outcome variables and emphasize available methods for dealing with both situations.

7.1 Types of Missing Data

Missing data can lead to a variety of issues with analysis and interpretation of results in longitudinal studies: in particular, bias in estimation and hypothesis testing, and loss of power to detect effects of interest. However, the extent to which this presents a problem depends on the amount of missing data, the mechanism by which the data became missing, and the robustness of statistical analysis methods to the effects of missing data.

There is no clear-cut rule about what amount of missing data presents problems for analysis. The effect is dependent on the sample, the question of interest, and the analysis method. As expected, the larger the proportion of missing data, the larger the potential bias and efficiency loss. Therefore, in longitudinal studies there is usually a concentrated and intensive effort to prevent or minimize missing data. Nevertheless, it is unrealistic to expect that missing data can be entirely avoided. Mallinckrodt et al. (2013) have presented different strategies for minimizing missing data in clinical trials.

In this section, we focus on the hierarchy of three different types of missing data, as defined in Little and Rubin (2014), based on whether the missingness gives us information about the outcomes that are missing. If a participant misses a visit because they moved, then missingness is likely unrelated to the unobserved outcome and is non-informative or ignorable. On the other hand, if sicker individuals are more likely to miss visits, then missingness does contain some information about the unobserved outcome and may be informative or non-ignorable. Intermittent missingness is usually considered ignorable, while dropout may be ignorable or non-ignorable.

The three different types of missing data are *missing completely at random* (MCAR), *missing at random* (MAR), and *missing not at random* (MNAR) (also referred to as *not missing at random* or NMAR). MCAR and MAR are considered non-informative or ignorable, while MNAR is considered informative or non-ignorable. MCAR is a special case of MAR. There are also some related missing data types such as covariate-dependent missingness and sequentially missing at random that are mentioned later in this section. Different analysis methods make different assumptions about the types of missing data. For more information see Hogan et al. (2004).

The MCAR, MAR, and MNAR are also referred to as three different *missing data mechanisms.* Note that investigators do not control the mechanisms. Rather, the mechanisms reflect different assumptions that are made regarding the missing data and these assumptions may or may not hold for the data at hand. The results are valid if the assumptions hold and an appropriate analysis is chosen that corresponds to the missing data mechanism. Modern methods for the analysis of repeated measures data, such as mixed models, deal well with non-informative (ignorable) missing data, but special methods are necessary to handle informative (non-ignorable) missing data.

To explain the three different mechanisms in longitudinal studies from a practical perspective we consider the augmentation depression study from Chapter 1. This is a double-blind randomized clinical trial of augmentation versus control treatment in major depression, with subjects receiving treatment for six weeks and depression severity measured weekly by the Hamilton Depression Rating Scale (HDRS). About 30% of the subjects in this trial dropped out or missed visits (i.e., had intermittent missing data). Subjects who missed visits do not have HDRS data from these visits. We consider a statistical model with treatment, time, and their interaction, with HDRS as the dependent variable. Presume also that some subject characteristics (e.g., gender) are included in the model as additional predictors.

In this context, missing data on the HDRS would be MCAR if the missingness does not depend on any observed or unobserved outcomes. That is, whether a particular HDRS score is missing does not depend on any previous, current, or future HDRS values. MCAR may or may not depend on covariates, with some authors preferring the definition of MCAR that allows for dependent missingness (in which case it is commonly referred to as *covariate-dependent MCAR*) and some preferring the definition of MCAR as a completely chance mechanism not dependent on either outcome or covariates. We focus on the simpler situation, when MCAR does not depend on covariates. In this case, a consequence of the MCAR assumption about missing data is that subjects who drop out or have intermittent missing data are a random sample from all participants. For such data, all methods of analysis provide valid results but there might be loss in efficiency in estimates (i.e., standard errors of estimates may be larger, which may lead to decreased power) if subjects with missing data are dropped from the analysis. Note that if MCAR is covariate-dependent, then the subjects with missing data are a random sample of the participants with the same characteristics receiving the same treatment, and analyses need to include such characteristics as predictors. In general, it is often difficult to justify the MCAR assumption since whether subjects drop out often depends on their treatment response or longitudinal trajectory. In particular, some subjects are expected to drop out of the augmentation depression study because of lack of improvement.

A more realistic assumption in the context of the augmentation depression study is that missing HDRS scores are MAR, which means that missingness depends on observed outcomes (and potentially on covariates) but not on unobserved outcomes (i.e., on responses that should have been obtained but were not). That is, whether a subject is missing some data points may depend on previous depression severity but not on the current and unobserved depression severity scores. For example, if a subject drops out due to inefficacy and the lack of improvement is measured by the investigator, their past responses can be used to predict dropout. In such situations, the MAR assumption is reasonable but the data are not MCAR. Under MAR, participants with missing data are not a random sample of the population of interest but their future trajectories can be predicted based on the data from other individuals with the same set of observed values prior to dropout.

The name MAR is a bit of a misnomer as the data are not strictly missing at random. Some alternative terminology has been proposed, such as *conditionally missing at random* (CMAR) (Graham, 2009), but has not gained much popularity due to the possible confusion of this term with MCAR. Mixed-effects models provide valid results when data are MAR and the model (fixed effects and variance–covariance structure) is specified correctly.

A concept related to MAR is *sequentially missing at random* (S-MAR) dropout. Data are S-MAR if missingness depends on observed covariates and outcomes prior to dropout. While GEE models do not in general provide valid inference under MAR assumptions, modifications are available that provide valid results under S-MAR dropout and with additional assumptions as explained in Section 7.5.

When missingness is related to the specific values that should have been obtained but were not, in addition to the ones already obtained, the data are said to be *missing not at random* (MNAR) or *not missing at random* (NMAR). In the context of the depression example, if subjects miss visits because their depression suddenly becomes worse and the investigator is not able to observe the deterioration, then data are MNAR. Individuals' responses up to the point of dropout fail to predict their dropout because dropout is related to the unobserved depression severity. Such data are *informatively missing* because dropout tells us something about the missing values. They are also *non-ignorable,* because to analyze such data properly one needs to specify a model for the missing data mechanism and fit this model jointly with the model for the primary outcome. Results depend on the choice of the missing data model. On top of that, the assumptions about the missing data are unverifiable from the observed data. Hence, analyses of MNAR data are usually considered only as sensitivity, and not as primary, analyses.

In summary, in longitudinal studies, missing data on the dependent variable are MCAR when the probability of dropout or missing data is not related to observed outcomes. When the probability of dropout or missing data is related to observed but not to unobserved outcomes, data are MAR, and when it is related to unobserved outcomes, data are MNAR. There is a test of the MCAR assumption (R. J. A. Little, 1988) that distinguishes between MCAR and MAR scenarios, but the MAR and MNAR assumptions cannot be distinguished based on the observed data. MNAR is used mainly in a sensitivity framework.

Less frequently, data on predictor variables may be missing. Data on predictor variables are considered MCAR when the missingness does not depend on any observed or unobserved values of the predictors or response, that is, the subjects with missing data on the predictors are a random sample of all individuals. Data are MAR when missingness depends on observed but not unobserved values, and data are MNAR when missingness depends on unobserved values of the predictors. In the augmentation depression study, no data are missing on predictor variables, so we will consider a hypothetical example. Suppose that individuals are asked whether they use a prohibited substance at baseline and the researcher is interested in using this as a predictor of an outcome in the statistical model. The data on this variable are MCAR if whether a subject replied to this question is not related to their substance use or any other observed data. The data are MAR if whether a subject replied to this question is related to other subject characteristics (e.g., gender, race, age) but not to the substance use itself, and data are MNAR if subjects who used the prohibited substance are more likely to refuse to reply to this question. Since predictors are usually measured at baseline (although it is possible to have time-dependent covariates) we do not specifically consider the scenario when missing data on predictors may depend on the response.

We now focus on different statistical approaches for missing data and their ability to handle data of the three different types. Keep in mind that if only a small portion of the data are missing (e.g., less than 5%–10%), the resulting bias and efficiency loss even when using a suboptimal analysis method will likely be small and unlikely to jeopardize interpretation.

7.2 Deletion and Substitution Methods for Handling Missing Data

Due to the inability of traditional approaches to handle missing data, the earliest approaches have been to delete individuals/cases with any missing data and perform complete case analysis, or to substitute missing values with "reasonable" guesses and then analyze the augmented data set with the substituted values as if these were the observed data. The most popular simple substitution method for missing values on the dependent variable in longitudinal studies has been last observation carried forward (LOCF), while mean or regression substitution has been used for imputing values on predictor variables. These approaches have major drawbacks, as detailed below.

Complete case analysis means that only subjects with complete data on the dependent and independent variables are included in the statistical analysis. In Chapter 2, we demonstrated endpoint, rANOVA, and rMANOVA analyses on subjects with complete data in the augmentation depression study. These analyses were performed on only about 70% of the available sample. Losing a high percentage of the sample before analysis can lead to major issues with results and interpretation. In particular, the sample of individuals with complete data may not be representative of the entire population of subjects, and thus the estimates obtained from these individuals may be systematically biased. For example, if individuals who fail to improve selectively drop out, then we might overestimate the magnitude of treatment-induced change over time. Or if subjects in the treatment group selectively drop out due to side effects and subjects in the control group selectively drop out due to inefficacy, the treatment versus control comparison based on the subjects with complete data will be biased.

Furthermore, there is a loss of power in statistical tests and increased uncertainty in the estimates due to the decreased sample size. The loss of power may be quite severe if a large proportion of the subjects are excluded from the analysis. Thus, complete case analysis may be used only when a very small proportion of the data are missing. However, there is no general agreement about what constitutes a small proportion. Some thresholds that have been proposed are less than 1% or less than 5% since in these cases loss of power is indeed small. But even with a small proportion of missing data, if the individuals with missing data are very different from the rest of the sample, some bias may occur. Nowadays, with readily available methods for analysis of incomplete data across time, there really is no good reason for using methods that require complete data.

Note that complete case analysis is often referred to as *listwise deletion*. A less extreme deletion of missing data is *pairwise deletion*, which means that, in each analysis assessing the relationship between a pair of variables, only those observations that have missing values on these two variables are deleted. Pairwise deletion is not often used with longitudinal data as separate analyses are rarely done for pairs of variables. In contrast, in cross-sectional data, pairwise correlations and regression analyses may be performed on a subset of the variables. If we are interested in assessing the pairwise correlations among ten variables, with listwise deletion we first delete all observations with missing values on any of the ten variables, while with pairwise deletion for each pair of variables, we drop only observations that are missing values on these two variables. The latter approach loses less power, but a different sample is used for each pairwise correlation and, hence, it is difficult to generalize and interpret the results for the entire sample.

Last observation carried forward substitution for longitudinal data involves replacing missing observations on the dependent variable with the last available observation prior to dropout or intermittent missing data. This results in a "complete" data set that can then be analyzed using any method. Figure 7.1 shows how the missing data for a couple of individuals in the augmentation depression study are substituted (one subject in the augmentation and one in the control group) using different approaches. The black dotted line with circles shows what LOCF substitution does to the profile of repeated observations over time for these individuals. The individual on the left is from the augmentation group and drops out after the second post-randomization visit. We observe some improvement over the first two weeks of the study, but we do not know what happens to the participant after dropout. Nevertheless, it seems unlikely that the slope of the change in depression scores over time suddenly levels out and depression severity remains the same. The individual on the right is from the control group and drops out after the first post-randomization visit without showing any improvement. While the LOCF substitution continues the trend of no improvement prior to dropout, it is unlikely that it describes the missing response well since depression treatment takes time to work and this individual did get the standard treatment. LOCF also implies a perfect correlation between the last observed

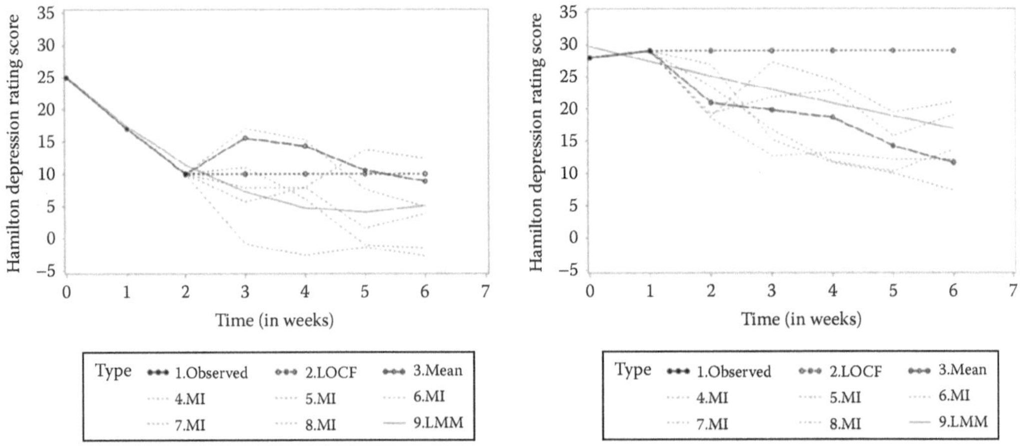

FIGURE 7.1
Observed, substituted, imputed, and predicted values for missing Hamilton Depression Rating Scale scores on two individuals who dropped out: one in the augmentation group (on the left) and one in the control group (on the right). LOCF = last observation carried forward substitution, Mean = mean substitution, MI = multiple imputation, LMM = linear model prediction.

measurement and all unobserved measurements, whereas in longitudinal studies correlations in the range of 0.4 to 0.6 are much more likely (rather than a correlation of 1). Thus, the flat line of projected response is probably unreasonable.

LOCF substitution is valid only if the response of an individual does not change after dropout. This is in most cases an unreasonable assumption but, nevertheless, this approach has been used for a long time because of its simplicity and since it was believed to be conservative. That is, it was believed to underestimate the treatment effect in simple parallel group clinical trials with an active and control group. However, in some situations, LOCF may actually overestimate the treatment effect and in all scenarios it is virtually guaranteed to give biased results. Thus, this approach should not be used for the analysis of longitudinal data.

A number of other *substitution approaches* have been used for longitudinal data. In particular, missing values on the dependent variable can be replaced with the mean value of all individuals in the group to which the subject belongs at the particular time point. This does not change the marginal means at the particular time point, but affects the estimated variances and covariances of the repeated measures so that both are underestimated. Also, it is not reasonable to assume that, regardless of the previous responses of an individual, the missing response is equal to the sample mean. Figure 7.1 illustrates this type of substitution for the two individuals in the augmentation depression study with the dashed gray lines. For the individual in the augmentation group, mean substitution after dropout results in an apparent abrupt deterioration, while for the individual in the control group, mean substitution leads to apparent significant improvement over time. While it is likely that the individuals will regress to the group means, assuming that their unobserved responses are equal to the group means is not reasonable. As described in Section 7.4, a reasonable estimate of the missing data for an individual is a weighted average of the trend of the subject's response estimated from the available data up to the point of dropout and the group average over time. However, this simple substitution method does not allow this.

A more appropriate approach than mean substitution is *regression substitution*, whereby a regression model is formulated for repeated observations with previous responses and other covariates as fixed predictors. The predicted values from the regression model corresponding to missing observations then replace the missing observations. This is better than mean substitution, because it maintains the relationship among the observations, not just the mean values. However, it still underestimates the variability of the data since it does not take into account the uncertainty in predicting the missing value.

Also, regression and mean substitution may not work well for binary or categorical outcomes. For binary and ordinal data, extreme case substitution is often performed. For example, in alcohol clinical trials where outcome is often a binary indicator of heavy or any drinking, missing data are coded as heavy (any) drinking. Whereas this may be a reasonable assumption for the majority of subjects, it certainly is not true in general, and leads to the same problems as other oversimplified methods such as last observation carried forward (D. Hedeker et al., 2007; Nelson et al., 2009; Blankers et al., 2016). However, extreme case substitution for binary or ordinal data has its place in the context of sensitivity analysis. In particular, if missing values are coded first at one of the extremes (e.g., 1 for binary data, the highest category for ordinal data) and the data analyzed, and then all missing values are coded at the other extreme (0 for binary data, the lowest category for ordinal data) and the data analyzed, and the results are substantively the same, then one can be confident in the conclusions. Since the rates of missing data may be different across groups, the process may need to be performed differentially by group (e.g., coding all missing binary data as 1 in one of the groups and 0 in the other group, and then the reverse). If we obtain consistent results in all these scenarios, then the findings are robust to the treatment of missing data. An extension of this approach has been considered by Delucchi (1994). On the other hand, if the results are not all consistent a more appropriate analysis method or additional sensitivity analyses are needed.

Another class of substitution methods is based on matching the individuals with missing data to other individuals on different baseline characteristics or using external information and then substituting the values from these individuals for the missing values. These are called *pattern-matching imputation* methods (Schlomer et al., 2010) and include *hot-deck* and *cold-deck* imputation methods. In hot-deck imputation, data from similar individuals in the sample are used to replace the missing values, while in cold-deck imputation data from similar individuals in other samples are used to replace the missing values. Pattern-matching imputation methods have the same disadvantages as the other simple substitution methods as they underestimate the variability in the data. In order to represent the variability in the data properly with a substitution approach, one needs to introduce a stochastic component and repeat the substitution multiple times (i.e., do multiple imputation). In the next section, we provide an overview and discuss the benefits of multiple imputation.

Before proceeding with multiple imputation, we also focus on the most important and appropriate *single imputation approach based on the EM algorithm.* The EM algorithm is a statistical method for maximum likelihood estimation that allows us to obtain maximum likelihood estimates when there are missing data. Technical details about the method are available in Little and Rubin (2014) while a more non-technical description can be found in Graham (2009). As an imputation method, it is commonly used to obtain the mean and variance–covariance matrix of a set of variables that are assumed to have a multivariate normal distribution and which are then used as an input to different statistical procedures (e.g., regression). Alternatively, a single set of imputed values is generated based on the observed mean and covariance matrices by adding random variability according to the assumptions of the statistical model.

The advantage of this approach is that it guarantees that the estimates are true maximum likelihood estimates and hence are unbiased when data are missing at random. The disadvantage is that it does not provide valid standard errors. In order to obtain standard errors, one can use the method of *bootstrapping* (Efron, 1994). That is, one can draw many samples with replacement from the original sample, produce EM estimates for each sample, and calculate the standard errors of all regression coefficients across samples. This allows one to properly account for the uncertainty due to missing data and produces accurate standard errors. However, this may require some programming, as software packages usually provide just single EM imputation. An alternative method for obtaining both estimates and correct standard errors is multiple imputation.

7.3 Multiple Imputation

Multiple imputation (Schafer, 1999; Rubin, 1996) as an approach for analyzing data sets with missing data consists of three steps:

1. Several "complete" (also referred to as *imputed*) data sets are created using stochastic imputation based on a selected imputation model.

2. Each "complete" data set is analyzed separately.
3. The results from the separate analyses are combined to obtain a single set of estimates, test statistics, and inferences.

To illustrate, consider the regression substitution approach. Single substitution underestimates the variability in the data, attenuates the relationship among variables, and may produce bias in some parameter estimates and, hence, randomness needs to be introduced in the imputation process. Rather than replacing missing values with the predicted values from the regression model, random perturbations can be added to these values according to the estimated distribution of the errors. Thus, each missing value is replaced with slightly different imputed value in different "complete" data sets. Figure 7.1 shows five sets of values generated using multiple imputation for the two individuals from the augmentation depression study. We see that the values are all different and their spread indicates the uncertainty in imputing missing values for these individuals. Multiple imputation uses information both about the observed response of the individual up to the point of dropout and from the responses of other individuals in order to generate reasonable values for the missing data points.

Analysis of the "complete" data sets is then performed according to the chosen statistical model. The final parameter estimates are simply the averages of the parameter estimates from the different "complete" data sets and as such have minimal bias and are efficient. The variances of the parameters are obtained as weighted averages of the "between" and "within" data set variances. The "between" variance estimates the sampling variability produced by the imputation process, while the "within" variance is the mean of the squared standard errors from the separate analysis of the different data sets. Exact formulae can be found in Carpenter and Kenward (2013), among others.

Multiple imputation has optimal statistical properties but it is sometimes challenging to implement, mainly because the results depend on the chosen imputation method and variables included in this model, and also on the amount and type of missing data. Note that multiple imputation produces unbiased results only if data are MCAR or MAR. If data are informatively missing, some amount of bias remains. Also, imputation of values on categorical variables is more challenging than imputation of values on continuous variables.

In general, the imputation model is different from the analysis model and includes observed variables and interactions of variables that are related to the missing data. Variables that are included in the imputation but not in the analysis model are often referred to as *auxiliary variables*. Usually, all variables in the analysis model are included in the imputation model in the particular form (after transformation, with interactions) which they take in the analysis model. This makes the imputation model consistent with the analysis model and is done because omitting variables from the imputation model assumes that they are uncorrelated with the variable with missing data, which is rarely the case. In particular, when there are missing values on a predictor variable and it is related to the dependent variable, one needs to include the dependent variable in the imputation model for the predictor variable, otherwise bias may occur (see e.g., Allison, 2000). The imputation model can have many more variables than the analysis models, for example additional baseline and time-dependent covariates. Auxiliary variables that are correlated with the variables with missing data or are predictive of missingness can dramatically improve the quality of the imputation from the imputation model by reducing uncertainly and variability in imputed values.

With longitudinal data, missing data can form different patterns. When subjects drop out of the study, the patterns are usually *monotone*. That is, if the observation at the kth time

TABLE 7.1

Pattern of Missing HDRS Scores in the Augmentation Depression Study. Plus (+) Indicates Data Are Present. Minus (–) Indicates Data Are Missing

Pattern	Week 1	Week 2	Week 3	Week 4	Week 5	Week 6	Week 7	Number of Individuals(%)
CompleteData	+	+	+	+	+	+	+	35 (70)
Pattern 1	+	+	+	+	+	+	–	2 (4)
Pattern 2	+	+	+	+	+	–	+	1 (2)
Pattern 3	+	+	+	+	+	–	–	4 (8)
Pattern 4	+	+	+	+	–	+	+	1 (2)
Pattern 5	+	+	+	–	–	–	–	2 (4)
Pattern 6	+	+	–	–	+	+	+	1 (2)
Pattern 7	+	+	–	–	–	–	–	4 (8)

point is missing, then all subsequent observations on that individual are also missing. In contrast, if a subject misses a scheduled visit or does not provide information on a variable of interest at a particular visit but then returns for subsequent visits, we have *intermittent* missing data. Table 7.1 shows the different missing patterns in the augmentation depression study. Patterns 1, 3, 5, and 7 are monotone and patterns 2, 4, and 6 are intermittent.

Whether patterns are monotone or intermittent, subjects often have missing values on more than one variable or on more than one repeated occasion. This adds additional complexity to the imputation of missing values for longitudinal data as a series of models may need to be iteratively fit to impute all missing data. The two most flexible approaches are the *Markov chain Monte Carlo (MCMC) imputation approach* (Schafer, 1997) and the *full conditional specification (FCS) imputation approach* (e.g., White et al., 2011; Van Buuren et al., 2006). The MCMC approach is computationally efficient, and can be used with any pattern of missing data, but as implemented in software packages it may not be appropriate for some types of categorical data. The FCS approach can also be used with any pattern of missing data, is appropriate for imputation of categorical data, but is computationally more demanding. Other commonly used imputation algorithms available in PROC MI in SAS are *regression imputation* and *propensity score imputation*, but they require that data have a monotone missing pattern, so are not in general appropriate for non-monotone missing data. More information about multiple imputation algorithms can be found in Carpenter and Kenward (2013), Van Buuren (2012), White et al. (2011), and Little and Rubin (2014).

Another decision that one needs to make with multiple imputation is how many "complete" data sets to generate. The general recommendations are that five to ten data sets are sufficient, but some say that 20 data sets are needed. Nevertheless, the sensitivity of conclusions to the number of data sets can always be assessed by generating a larger number and comparing the estimates. Note that since there is a degree of randomness in multiple imputation the results will vary slightly when the procedure is repeatedly implemented. In order to be able to replicate the results, it is important to fix the random seed to allow for exact replication of the results. If the program automatically selects the random seed, then full replication is not possible.

While multiple imputation is one of the preferred approaches for dealing with missing data in longitudinal studies, it may be daunting to apply, due to the different decisions that one needs to make. In particular, one needs to decide what imputation model and what analysis model to use, what algorithm is appropriate, whether to change default settings of the algorithm, and how many imputation data sets to generate. Each of these decisions is non-trivial and needs to be justified. We illustrate how to go through these steps on a data example in Section 7.7, but before that we turn our attention to another method of analysis in the presence of missing data that gives asymptotically unbiased and efficient results when data are missing at random, namely *full information maximum likelihood* (FIML).

7.4 Full Information Maximum Likelihood

In FIML, the parameter estimates are obtained by maximizing the likelihood based on all observed data. The likelihood function is summed or integrated over the missing data, which means that the missing data are allowed to vary over all possible values according to the model assumptions, and the observed data likelihood is like a weighted average over the possible values for the missing data. The "weights" are determined based on the distributional and model assumptions. In the case of continuous variables, the averaging is actually integration. This approach allows one to seamlessly incorporate the uncertainty due to the missing values, to use all available data on individuals, and to produce the same result every time the algorithm is run. The latter is not the case with multiple imputation, which can produce different results as the algorithm is repeated. This is one of the reasons FIML is preferable to multiple imputation. Others are that it is more efficient, it is easier to implement, and since everything is done under the same model, there is no potential discrepancy between the imputation and the analysis model. The main factor limiting the use of FIML is that it is not always available in software packages, especially when there are missing data on predictor variables in longitudinal data. Also, FIML provides valid results when the model is correctly specified. If important covariates are omitted then bias may occur.

In the context of longitudinal data, the mixed-effects models presented in Chapters 3 and 4 are fit according to the FIML approach when data are missing on the dependent variable only. Subjects who drop out provide information in the likelihood based on their observed responses prior to dropout. When there are intermittent missing data, all remaining observations on the individual are again used to derive the likelihood. Mixed-effects models provide asymptotically unbiased results that are also maximally efficient as long as the data are missing at random, all variables that predict dropout or intermittent missing data are included in the model, and the variance–covariance structure is correctly specified. For example, if the probability of dropout is related to treatment and possibly previous responses, mixed models that include treatment as a predictor and model all repeated responses provide unbiased results. However, if the probability of dropout is also related to the unobserved response or some other predictors that are not measured or not included in the model, results may be biased. Since it is not possible to distinguish whether data are MAR or MNAR, the mixed model is often the best analysis that one can do. Sensitivity analyses under MNAR assumptions can help ascertain the robustness of the results to the effects of missing data. Such models are considered further in this chapter.

Note that mixed models, as implemented in most software programs, automatically drop subjects with missing values on the predictor variables (as opposed to the outcome variable) from the analyses. MPlus and PROC CALIS in SAS with the FIML option are exceptions, with PROC CALIS applicable only for multivariate normal data. When there are missing values on predictor variables and the software does not have a FIML option, there are two approaches that can be taken. One is to use the EM algorithm with bootstrap standard errors as described in Section 7.2. The other approach is to use multiple imputation for the predictor variables. Note that the imputation and the analysis models in multiple imputation can be any statistical models. Therefore, it is completely acceptable to impute missing values on predictor variables using multiple imputation, to use mixed-effects models as the analysis models for each imputed data set, and to combine the results of the different analyses to obtain the final results. This is a combination of multiple imputation and FIML analysis since FIML is used for the missing data on the dependent variable and multiple imputation is used to handle missing values on the predictor variables. Note that in longitudinal data, some values of the dependent variable are almost guaranteed to be missing, while missing data on predictor variables are encountered much less frequently.

7.5 Weighted GEE

Unlike likelihood-based mixed models that provide unbiased results when data on the dependent variable are MAR, classical GEE models provide unbiased results only when data on the dependent variable are MCAR. However, modifications are available for MAR data, such as *inverse probability weighting* methods (see Li et al. (2013) or Rotnitzky (2009) for a technical review) and combined imputation (mean or multiple) and GEE methods (e.g., Paik, 1997; Chapter 11 in Molenberghs and Kenward, 2007).

Inverse probability weighting attempts to correct the underrepresentation of certain response profiles in the sample. For example, if a large proportion of subjects with increasing depression severity drop out from the study, there will be fewer fully observed trajectories of deterioration in the sample. Average depression scores will be biased toward better scores because some of the "bad" scores are missing from the data set due to dropout, and this phenomenon is more pronounced as more participants drop out. Inverse probability weighting allows one to put more weight on the trajectories of the subjects who remain in the sample but show similar deterioration to those subjects who drop out, and thus corrects the bias. This allows one to base estimation on the observed responses but weigh them according to the probability of dropout. The probability of dropout can be estimated using statistical models (e.g., logistic regression) with covariates, observed responses, and auxiliary variables, and then the weights are calculated from these estimated probabilities. The weights can be interpreted as the number of observations that a particular observed value represents. The more individuals there are who have dropped out with a similar response pattern and covariates to the individual with the observed value, the higher the weight on this observation, since it represents many missing data points. The GEE approach then takes into account the weights and produces valid estimates as long as the model that is used to estimate the weights (i.e., the model used to predict the dropout probabilities) is correctly specified. We illustrate the inverse probability-weighted GEE approach in Section 7.7.

7.6 Methods for Informatively Missing Data

We first focus on extensions of the FIML approach to deal with informatively missing data and then proceed with description of weighting and imputation approaches. There are three types of likelihood-based models for MNAR analyses: *shared parameter models, selection models*, and *pattern-mixture models*. Detailed descriptions of these methods are available in Molenberghs and Kenward (2007) and Molenberghs et al. (2014). All of these approaches involve treating missingness as an additional outcome and relating the missingness and the response processes. To be a little bit more specific, we consider the outcome Y_{ij} at time j for individual i and define the missing data binary indicator R_{ij} to be equal to 1 if Y_{ij} is observed, and to 0 if Y_{ij} is unobserved. In Chapters 3 and 4, we showed different types of models for Y_{ij}, but so far we have ignored R_{ij}. When data are MCAR and MAR, it is not in general necessary to specify a model for R_{ij} (except in the weighted GEE approach). However, when data are MNAR, one needs to define a model for R_{ij} and relate the substantive and the missingness models. The three approaches differ in how this is done.

Shared parameter models consist of two sub-models—one for the primary outcome and one for the dropout/missingness. The two are linked by shared random effects, latent variables, or latent classes. For example, we can have a linear mixed model for the Y_{ij} with a random intercept, b_{i0}, and a random slope, b_{i1}. We considered such a model for the augmentation depression study in Chapter 3. It may be reasonable to assume that the probability of missing outcome also depends on the intercept and slope. For example, subjects with higher intercepts (i.e., more severe depression at baseline) and/or with narrower slopes (i.e., little improvement over time) may be more likely to drop out. To take this potentially informative dropout process into account, we can specify a generalized linear mixed model for R_{ij} with binary response, logit link, and the random intercept b_{i0} and the random slope b_{i1} as predictors. Fitting the two related models together allows us to account for potentially nonignorable dropout or intermittent missing data. Note that there is no way to test whether this particular joint model fits the data best and, hence, such modeling is usually done as sensitivity analysis rather than primary analysis. It is also possible for random effects to interact with treatment in predicting dropout (i.e., controls who are not improving drop out, whereas treated subjects who improve quickly drop out). The model needs to be modified by considering these interactions in order to provide a good fit to the data.

The shared parameters between the substantive and the missingness processes are not necessarily random effects. A special case of shared parameter models is when a latent class variable links the two processes. Thus, one can assume that there are different types of individuals in the population (represented by different latent classes that are not known *a priori*) and that conditional on the type of individual, the dropout and the outcome are independent. As before, there is no way to verify the form of the model from the data at hand. One needs to rely on substantive considerations.

Selection models also consist of two sub-models, but the dependent variable from the substantive model is included as a predictor in the model for the dropout or missing value. As an example, we can again have a linear mixed model for the outcome, Y_{ij}, and a generalized linear mixed model for the missingness indicators, R_{ij}. We can then include the corresponding values of Y_{ij} (some of which are unobserved), and, potentially, interactions of those with treatment in the linear predictor of the elements of R_{ij}. Note that the linear predictor may (and often should) include previous observed outcomes and covariates. The model should be defined based on substantive considerations as it relies on unverifiable assumptions. Since some of the outcomes, Y_{ij}, are unobserved, numerical integration is necessary to obtain estimates. Thus, selection models are in general difficult to fit with existing software which limits their use in practice.

Pattern-mixture models reverse the order in which the substantive model and the missingness model are related. That is, a model for R_{ij} is considered, and then R_{ij} is included as a predictor in the model for Y_{ij}. We can relate R_{ij} to concurrent and future response values. This approach essentially leads to different substantive models corresponding to each dropout pattern, and then the overall estimates of the effects are obtained by averaging over patterns weighted by their estimated probabilities. Patterns are most often defined by the time of dropout, but other definitions are possible (e.g., reason for dropout). Pattern-mixture models are not fully identifiable since some of the data in different patterns are entirely missing, and thus some parameter constraints are necessary to estimate all parameters. As do the other two approaches, this one relies on unverifiable assumptions and is mostly used as sensitivity analysis. Pattern-mixture models are especially useful when the number of dropout times is small and when subjects drop out due to death (i.e., their unobserved outcomes cannot be observed). We consider pattern-mixture models on an example in Section 7.7.

As already described, each class of model relies on unverifiable assumptions. Even more importantly, it has been shown (Molenberghs et al., 2009a) that for every MAR model there is an equally well-fitting MNAR model to the observed data but with different predictions for the unobserved data. Hence, the primary analysis model is usually an MAR model (such as a linear or generalized linear mixed model) and then different types of MNAR models are used for sensitivity analysis. Sensitivity analysis involves simultaneous consideration of several plausible statistical models and/or evaluation of different estimates of quantities of interest with confidence intervals under different possible deviations from the primary model. If conclusions and effect size estimates are consistent, then one can have more confidence in the results. We show an example of primary and sensitivity analyses based on MAR and MNAR models in the context of the data examples in Section 7.7. Detailed explanations of different approaches including diagnostic type measures of local and global influence, and intervals of ignorance and uncertainty, are available in Molenberghs et al. (2009b).

Another approach to dealing with informatively missing data is to perform multiple imputation under MNAR rather than under MAR assumptions. One such technique is *reference-based imputation*, where the imputation model is derived from the control group only, and is applied to both the control and the treatment groups. (The usual way to apply multiple imputation is to develop separate models for the active and the control groups). For example, subjects who discontinue in the active group may be assumed to follow the trajectory of outcomes in the control group immediately after dropout. This would mean that whatever benefit might have been accrued with treatment disappears right after treatment discontinuation. Performing such sensitivity analysis and comparing the results to the results from the primary analysis shows how sensitive the conclusions are under the fairly drastic assumptions of an abrupt loss of benefit from treatment.

Weighted GEE models can also be used for sensitivity analysis based on different models for the probability of non-response that are used to calculate the weights. While under MAR the probability of non-response is usually estimated as a function of covariates and observed responses, dependence on unobserved responses can also be incorporated in these methods (e.g., Rotnitzky and Robins, 1997; Scharfstein et al., 1999). *Doubly robust estimates* (Rotnitzky et al., 2012) of the effects of interest can then be obtained under MNAR assumptions. Doubly robust means that they provide valid results if either the substantive model or the missing data model is correct. This method is also considered in the next section.

7.7 Data Examples

We will now illustrate different MCAR, MAR, and MNAR approaches on data from the augmentation depression study and from the Health and Retirement Study. The first example focuses on the continuous and approximately normally distributed depression score, while the second focuses on the ordinal measure of self-rated health. We compare the performance of mixed models, GEE methods, multiple imputation, and pattern-mixture models in the presence of missing data. Since there are many possible models (especially MNAR models) that can be considered this is not intended to be a comprehensive set of examples. Rather, we illustrate some of the techniques, mainly the ones that can be fairly easily implemented with existing software. SAS code and output for all results are available in the online materials. Detailed examples of different methods can be found in Molenberghs and Kenward (2007), Molenberghs et al. (2014), Hedeker and Gibbons (2006), and Mallinckrodt et al. (2014), among others.

7.7.1 Missing Data Models in the Augmentation Depression Study

As mentioned earlier in this chapter, 30% of the subjects in the augmentation depression study had missing data and 24% dropped out before the end of the double-blind treatment phase. As a first step toward assessing the potential impact of missing data on inferences, the data on the response variable are plotted by time of dropout. This allows one to assess whether participants who drop out have similar or different trajectories to individuals who stay in the study. Figure 7.2a and b visualize the raw HDRS means of different sets of subjects. The left panel of Figure 7.2a shows the means (by treatment group) based on all available observations at each time point while the right panel of Figure 7.2a shows the means based on data only for completers. The two graphs are fairly similar, with the lines for the two treatment groups a little bit closer together for completers. Both figures suggest that there are substantial improvements in both treatment groups but no obvious differences between groups.

The left panel of Figure 7.2b shows the mean depression scores of subjects who dropped out before the mid-point of the study (three weeks), while the right panel shows the mean scores of subjects who dropped out after the mid-point of the study. A divergence of mean scores by treatment group is evident in both graphs. In particular, it appears that subjects who drop out in the control group do not improve much, if anything it seems they deteriorate prior to dropout. At the same time, subjects in the active group drop out after their depression scores have

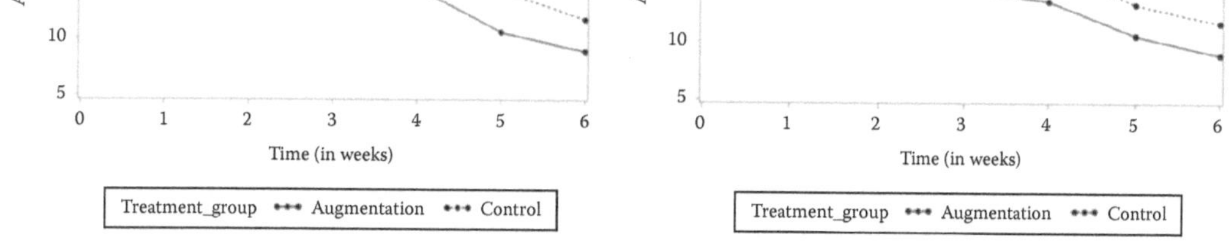

FIGURE 7.2A
Mean Hamilton Depression Rating Scale scores based on all available data (on the left) and only on data of completers (on the right).

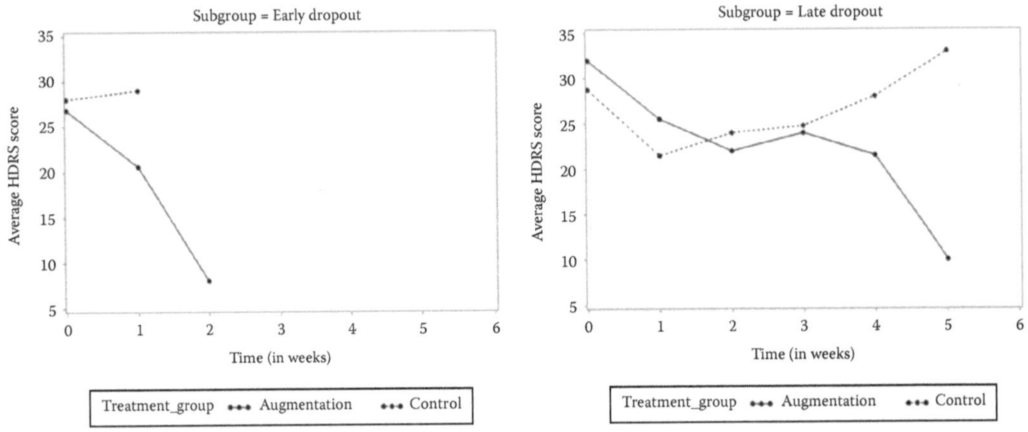

FIGURE 7.2B
Mean Hamilton Depression Rating Scale scores based on the data from subjects who dropped out early during treatment (on the left) and subjects who dropped out late during treatment (on the right).

gone down. Thus, it does not appear that dropout is MCAR, although we cannot decide based on these graphs if dropout is more likely to be MAR or MNAR. Thus, we follow the general recommendation in such a case and select a linear mixed model as our primary analytic method with secondary analysis based on pattern-mixture models as sensitivity analysis. We also compare the GEE approach under MCAR with two imputation approaches (under MAR and MNAR) with GEE on the imputed data sets. Since the outcome is normally distributed, linear mixed-effects models and the corresponding GEE specification with the same linear predictor estimate the same mean effects. Remember that, in general, GEE models provide valid results even if the correlation structure of the repeated measures is incorrectly specified, but this nice property is guaranteed when data are complete or MCAR. When data are MAR or MNAR, we need to use either weighted GEE methods or use multiple imputation to fill in the missing data. We chose to illustrate the second approach on this study based on a GEE with a normal response and an identity link function. The weighted GEE is illustrated in the second data example (i.e., the Health and Retirement Study).

For simplicity of presentation and to facilitate comparisons among models, we consider linear effects in terms of log time; thus, our main focus is on estimating and comparing the slopes of the two treatment groups. As shown in Chapter 3, this parsimonious mean pattern matched the raw data fairly well. The linear mixed-effects model (LMM) under a MAR assumption has fixed effects of treatment group, time (log-transformed), the interaction between group and time, and random intercept and slope. Both random effects and random errors are assumed to be normally distributed as usual and the random intercept and slope are correlated.

The corresponding pattern-mixture model (PMM) under the MNAR assumption includes a binary dropout indicator (equal to 1 for subjects who drop out and equal to 0 for subjects who complete the study) and all its interactions with treatment group and time, and has different random intercept and slope distributions for completers and for subjects who drop out. Thus, in this model there are twice as many parameters as in the LMM. We chose a simple dropout indicator since the sample size was small and would not allow us to estimate separate coefficients for subjects who dropped out early and late. In general, pattern-mixture models consider different coefficients for different dropout patterns as long as the sample size can support it. Table 7.2 shows the estimates from the two models

TABLE 7.2

Estimates and 95% Confidence Intervals from a LMM with Random Intercept and Slope (MAR model) and a Pattern-Mixture Model (PMM) with Dropout Indicator (MNAR model) Fit to the HDRS Scores in the Augmentation Depression Study

	Intercept in Augmentation Group	Slope in Augmentation Group	Intercept in Control Group	Slope in Control Group	Difference in Intercepts	Difference in Slopes
LMM (MAR)	29.8 (27.2, 32.4)	−10.4 (−12.6, −8.3)	31.5 (28.8, 34.1)	−8.7 (−10.9, −6.5)	−1.7 (−5.4, 2.0)	−1.7 (−4.8, 1.3)
PMM (MNAR) completers	30.4 (27.3, 33.5)	−10.9 (−13.1, −8.7)	32.7 (29.5, 35.8)	−10.5 (−12.7, −8.2)	−2.3 (−6.7, 2.2)	−0.5 (−3.6, 2.7)
PMM (MNAR) dropouts	28.4 (25.6, 31.1)	-9.4 (−13.0, −5.8)	26.0 (22.8, 29.3)	0.5 (−3.4, 4.6)	2.3 (−1.9, 6.6)	-9.9 (−15.2, −4.6)

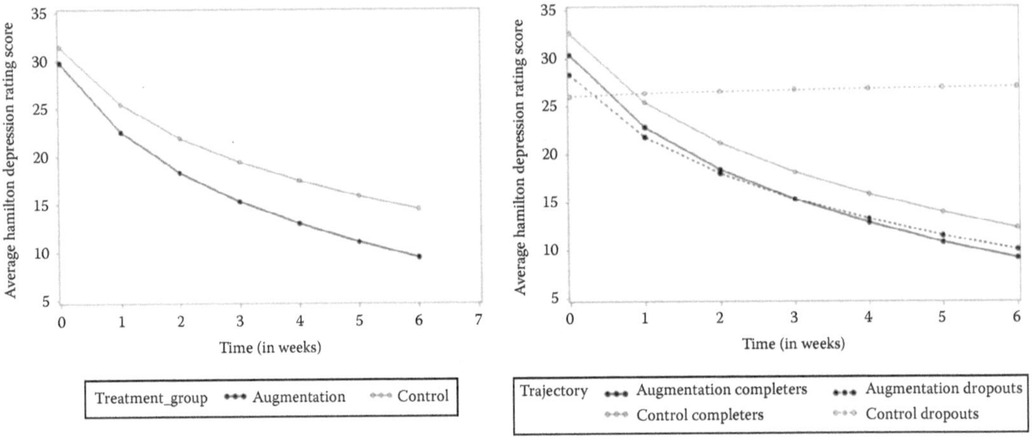

FIGURE 7.3
Predicted Mean Hamilton Depression Rating Scale scores based on the Linear Mixed Model (on the left) and on the Pattern Mixture Model (on the right).

while Figure 7.3 shows the corresponding predictions for the mean HDRS scores based on the LMM (in the left panel) and based on the PMM for completers and dropouts (in the right panel).

The estimates from the LMM (which provides valid results under MAR assumptions) show that the slopes for both groups are significantly negative, and the difference in slopes is not statistically significant as the confidence interval in the last column of Table 7.2 includes zero. The estimates from the PMM show that, for completers, the slopes in both groups are almost identical (–10.9 and –10.5). However, for subjects who drop out, the slope in the control group is slightly positive rather than negative, and the difference in slopes between the augmentation and control group is statistically significant. Figure 7.3 illustrates this more dramatically, as it shows a very different estimated trajectory for subjects in the control group who drop out. Since there are only 12 subjects who dropped out (seven in the augmentation group and five in the control group) caution should be applied when interpreting these results. Also, since no information is available after drop-out, the trajectories for dropouts toward the end of the period are extrapolations. Although the right panel of Figure 7.3 suggests that dropout might be informative (non-ignorable), there is no way to check this. Note that if we calculate weighted averages of the slopes of completers and dropouts from the PMM, they are going to result in similar trajectories to the ones shown in the left panel of Figure 7.3. Thus, although dropout may be informative in this data set, due to the relatively small percentage of subjects who drop out, the impact on the results is limited.

We also considered GEE models and combinations of MI and GEE, since they allow us to explore differences in estimates under different missing data assumptions. The simple GEE model (MCAR model) is based on all available data on individuals, has the same linear predictor as the mixed model, and uses an AR(1) working correlation structure. Results from this model are shown in the first row of Table 7.3. The code to perform MI and GEE analysis in SAS is included in the online materials.

In order to make valid inferences under MAR assumptions, we performed MI of missing HDRS scores separately for each treatment group using the FCS method and then fit a GEE model to each of the complete data sets. We generated ten imputed data sets, fitted

TABLE 7.3

Estimates and 95% Confidence Intervals from a GEE Model with Normal Distribution, Identity Link, and AR(1) Correlation Structure (MCAR model), MI under MAR + GEE model, and MI under MNAR + GEE Model Fit to the HDRS Scores in the Augmentation Depression Study

	Intercept in Augmentation Group	Slope in Augmentation Group	Intercept in Control Group	Slope in Control Group	Difference in Intercepts	Difference in Slopes
GEE (MCAR)	29.1 (26.8, 31.4)	−9.9 (−11.9, −8.0)	31.0 (28.5, 33.4)	−8.5 (−10.6, −6.5)	−1.8 (−5.2, 1.5)	−1.4 (−4.2, 1.4)
MI + GEE (MAR)	30.7 (26.8, 34.5)	−10.6 (−14.4, −6.8)	33.5 (29.4, 37.6)	−10.5 (−13.4, −7.7)	−2.8 (−8.4, 2.7)	−0.1 (−4.5, 4.3)
MI + GEE (MNAR)	31.5 (28.0, 34.9)	−11.8 (−14.7, −8.9)	31.8 (27.0, 36.5)	−8.1 (−12.3, −3.8)	−0.3 (−6.1, 5.5)	−3.7(−8.6, 1.2)

the same GEE model on the imputed data sets, and combined the results. These results are shown in the second row of Table 7.3.

Finally, we performed sensitivity analysis with MI using the FCS method with adjustment to the imputed HDRS values (shown in the third row of Table 7.3). Generated HDRS values in the control group were artificially increased by two points, while generated HDRS values in the augmentation group were decreased by 0.2 points to account for potentially different reasons for dropout in the two groups. This was intended to allow assessment of the sensitivity of the results when subjects who dropped out in the control group were worse off, while subjects who dropped out in the augmentation group were slightly better off, than indicated by the extension of their respective observed trajectories.

Note that in such sensitivity analysis, one would normally fit a series of models under potentially different assumptions. That is, one changes the perturbations and investigates how far from MAR they need to be to influence the results. We did consider different perturbations (+1, +2, +3, and +4 in the control group; −0.1, −0.2, −0.4, and −1 in the augmentation group), but larger perturbations than the ones shown in Table 7.3 corresponded to unreasonable values for the HDRS scores. For example, for one subject in the augmentation group, most imputed values were negative when the scores were decreased by 0.4 and 1, and for one subject in the control group, most imputed values were larger than the possible maximum on the HDRS (53 points) when the scores were increased by +3 and +4. Thus, such large perturbations are not reasonable. Also, perturbations in the other direction (e.g., smaller than anticipated values in the control group, larger than anticipated values in the augmentation group) are not likely, since the observed trajectories suggest otherwise. If unobserved values are in these unexpected directions, this will make the null hypothesis of no differences between the two treatment groups even more likely. The results for the slope comparison can theoretically change only if dropouts pull the group trajectories in different directions. Many other MNAR models are possible, as indicated previously in this chapter, but are not considered here.

Note that when using multiple imputation we can get individual imputed values outside of the range of the data (in this case values less than 0 or larger than the maximum possible HDRS score). It is not recommended in such situations to truncate the values, since this artificially decreases the estimate of the variability in the data. Nevertheless, it is good to keep the average imputed values for each missing data point inside the range of possible values, as otherwise the considered perturbations are unrealistic.

Table 7.3 shows the estimates from the three different models we considered. As expected based on the results from the LMM shown above, the slopes of both groups are significantly negative under MCAR and MAR and there are no statistically significant differences in slopes. Under the specific MNAR multiple imputation, the slope estimate for the augmentation group is larger in magnitude, and since it is negative there is a faster decrease in scores than under MCAR and MAR assumptions. At the same time, the slope estimate in the control group is smaller in magnitude, and hence there is slower decrease in scores than under MCAR and MAR assumptions. The difference in slopes, while still not statistically significant, is larger in absolute value (−3.7, 95% CI: (−8.6, 1.2)), indicating a larger degree of separation between groups. Because all three models suggest that there are no statistically significant differences between groups in slopes of change in log time, we can conclude that the results are fairly robust to the effects of missing data. This does not preclude the speculation that a larger study could find a significant influence of missing data.

We selected a parsimonious model to describe the time trend in order to illustrate the methods more easily. However, in the presence of missing data, the "correctness" of the mean model is even more important than with complete data, especially in the context of the GEE approach. While model diagnostics can help assess different aspects of the model, they can also be influenced by missing data. Assessing the robustness of results should involve not only sensitivity analysis with respect to different models and assumptions for the missing data but also different plausible model specifications.

7.7.2 Missing Data Models in the Health and Retirement Study

In Chapter 4, we presented GLMM and GEE analyses of the ordinal measure of self-rated health assessed biennially over a period of 14 years in individuals transitioning into retirement. We focused on assessment of gender differences and effects of smoking at baseline on the time trends in self-rated health. In the previous analyses, we ignored the issue of missing data. This is reasonable in the GLMM model, which provides valid results under MAR assumptions when full maximum likelihood estimation is used. However, the GEE model produces valid results only under MCAR assumptions. In this section, we explore different types of missing data in the study, present several GEE models under varying assumptions, and assess the potential impact of missing data on the substantive conclusions. As in any large longitudinal survey, there are all kinds of missing data in the HRS. In particular, there are missing data on predictor variables, intermittent missing data on the response variable, and dropouts. Dropouts are further separated in individuals who died and who dropped out for other reasons. Our focus here is on missing data on the dependent variable (self-rated health) and on dropouts. Since data are complete on the primary predictors (gender and smoking status) at baseline, we do not consider the issue of missing data on predictors. Figure 7.4 shows the patterns of mean self-rated health scores in subjects who completed the study or dropped out for a different reason than death (in the left panel, separate lines shown for different dropout times) and in subjects who died during the study period (in the right panel, separate lines shown for different dropout times). Separate plots of patterns of change among completers and dropouts for other reasons, and subjects with intermittent missing data did not reveal any obvious changes, so the left panel lumps all these individuals together. We further omitted subjects with intermittent missing data from the analyses in order to simplify interpretation and be able to apply the inverse probability weighting method in a GEE context that is targeted toward dropout.

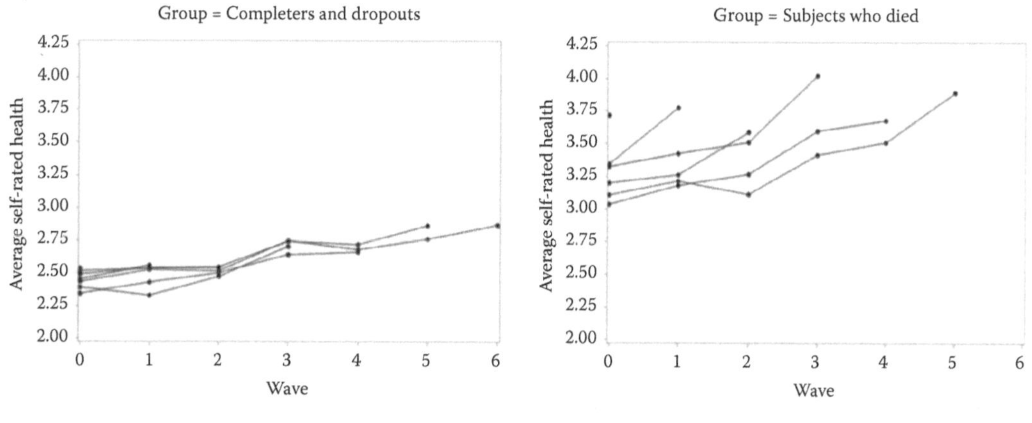

FIGURE 7.4
Mean self-rated health scores by dropout status in the Health and Retirement study.

Figure 7.4 shows that subjects who died had significantly worse self-rated health and showed faster deterioration prior to dropout compared with subjects who provided data at all time points or dropped out for other reasons. Thus, it appears that dropout can be predicted from the available data and therefore can be considered MAR, or if it also depends on unobserved data then it can be considered MNAR. Among subjects without intermittent missing data (8365), 1244 (14.9%) died during the study, while 1267 (15.2%) dropped out. Although not overwhelming in terms of percentage of the entire sample, dropout and death could have an effect on inferences, so considering different models and assessing sensitivity of results is desirable.

Unlike the analysis of the augmentation depression study, the outcome here is not normally distributed, and hence, estimates from GLMM and GEE are not expected to be the same. We first fit the same GLMM and GEE models as in Chapter 4. The results are substantively very similar, as the only difference in these basic analyses is that, in this chapter, individuals with intermittent missing data are dropped. In both the GLMM and GEE models there are significant smoking by time effects that we focus on in order to illustrate and compare different missing data models. The fixed slope estimate for non-smokers and smokers from the GLMM are 0.20 (95% CI: (0.19, 0.22)) and 0.26 (95% CI: (0.23, 0.28)), respectively. Thus, the cumulative log odds of worse health increase for both non-smokers and smokers with time, but at a lower rate for non-smokers. Subtracting the two slopes and exponentiating gives a cumulative odds ratio for the comparison of rate of change over time in non-smokers relative to smokers of 0.95 (95% CI: (0.92, 0.98)), indicating that not smoking is protective in terms of slowing deterioration in self-rated health. Since the GLMM provides valid estimates under MAR missingness and the focus is on individual change over time, this would be the preferred approach for this example.

Nevertheless, we consider GEE models for these data in more detail in order to compare the results under the three possible mechanisms and to present and illustrate the inverse probability weighting approach. The usual GEE model with multinomial response, cumulative logit link, and independent working correlation matrix (the only such structure available for ordinal data in SAS) provides valid results only when data are MCAR. Next, we also fit a weighted GEE model with the same assumptions about the response, link, and working correlation structure but weigh the contribution of individual observations to the results using the inverse probability approach as described below. This type of model provides valid results under S-MAR assumptions (i.e., when data are MAR, depending only on the previous observed responses). Finally, we tweak the weights in order to simulate a MNAR process and compare the results for the overall tests of the treatment effects and the individual slope estimates and comparisons in order to assess the sensitivity of the results to missing data assumptions.

In the models, we consider gender and smoking status as categorical predictors, and wave as a continuous predictor. We model a linear effect of time.

We first report the significant results from the tests of main and interactive effects of the fixed factor. In the GEE model without weights, which provides valid results under MCAR mechanism, there is a statistically significant interaction between smoking status and time ($\chi^2(1) = 3.79$, $p = 0.05$) and significant main effects of smoking ($\chi^2(1) = 166.0$, $p < 0.0001$) and time ($\chi^2(1) = 374.3$, $p < 0.0001$). Interestingly, in contrast to our analysis in Chapter 4, there are no significant gender effects. This might reflect a loss of power due to dropping subjects with intermittent missing data. Since our main interest here is in comparing the results of models under different assumptions of missing data, we focus on the effects of smoking and, in particular, on changes over time by smoking status. Additional estimates for the main effects can be obtained as discussed in Chapter 4.

TABLE 7.4

Estimates and 95% Confidence Intervals from GEE (under MCAR) and Weighted GEE (under S-MAR and MNAR) for Self-Rated Health in the Health and Retirement Study

	Slope for Non-Smokers	Slope for Smokers	Cumulative Odds Ratio for the Difference in Slopes
GEE (MCAR)	0.08 (0.07, 0.09)	0.10 (0.08, 0.11)	0.98 (0.97, 1.00)
Weighted GEE (S-MAR)	0.10 (0.10, 0.11)	0.14 (0.12, 0.15)	0.97 (0.95, 0.99)
Weighted GEE (MNAR) Model 1	0.15 (0.14, 0.16)	0.17 (0.15, 0.19)	0.98 (0.96, 1.00)
Weighted GEE (MNAR) Model 2	0.14 (0.13, 0.15)	0.17 (0.15, 0.18)	0.98 (0.96, 0.99)

Table 7.4 shows the estimated slopes for change in self-rated health over time by smoking status and based on these, the estimated cumulative odds ratios when comparing the increase in odds of worse self-rated health per wave for smokers and non-smokers. Intercepts are not shown, since there are four different intercept parameters for all cumulative odds of the five-level ordinal response. All these estimates are available in the online materials. Positive slopes show that self-rated health deteriorates over time, and the cumulative odds ratios show the estimated decrease in odds of worse self-rated health assessment per wave for non-smokers compared with smokers. The first row of Table 7.4 shows the results from the GEE under MCAR, that is, GEE based on all available data without weighting. The results show significantly positive slopes for both smokers and non-smokers, indicating that self-rated health assessment worsens with time. The deterioration is statistically significantly, but slightly less so for non-smokers compared with smokers (about $1-0.98=0.02$, or 2% lower per wave for non-smokers compared with smokers). Next, we assess how these results change when we weigh the observations under MAR assumptions.

The weights used in the weighted GEE, calculated under S-MAR assumptions, are based on the estimated probabilities of individual self-rated health measures being observed. We estimate the probabilities by fitting a logistic regression model with a missing data indicator ($R_{ij}=1$ if self-rated health was observed and $R_{ij}=0$ if self-rated health was missing for individual i at wave j) as the response variable and the following predictors, updated at the previous wave: self-rated health at the previous visit, gender, smoking status, wave, age at study entry, indicator variables for ever having cancer, heart attack, stroke, high blood pressure, diabetes, or lung disease. Note that we include additional variables here that are not part of our main model but which may be related to death and dropout from the study. This helps us improve the prediction of dropout or death. We denote these estimated probabilities as p_{ij}, with i for subject and j for wave. These probabilities are obtained for all post-baseline measurement occasions on which self-rated health is observed, and for the first occasion after dropout for individuals who drop out. Since at baseline there is no information about previous self-rated health but complete information about current self-rated health, $p_{i1}=1$ for all individuals at baseline. A subject who drops out at wave 2 contributes $R_{i1}=1$ and $R_{i2}=0$ to the logistic regression, while a subject who drops out at wave 4 contributes $R_{i1}=R_{i2}=R_{i3}=1$ and $R_{i4}=0$. We estimate p_{i1} and p_{i2} for the first individual, and p_{i1}, p_{i2}, p_{i3}, and p_{i4} for the second individual.

The inverse probability weights are then calculated as follows:

$$w_{ij}=\frac{1}{p_{i1}\times p_{i2}\times\ldots p_{i,j-1}}$$

Obviously, the weight at the first time point is equal to one (i.e., $w_{i1} = 1$), and it increases (perhaps substantially) over time for subjects who are likely to drop out, as we keep multiplying by numbers less than one in the denominator. The idea behind this weighting is that data on individuals who are likely to drop out based on their previous response measure and covariates need to be more heavily weighted in order to account in the analysis for individuals with similar characteristics and covariates who actually drop out. Figure 7.5 shows the estimated weights according to the logistic model above.

As expected, the weights increase over time, with some weights as large as ten at the last wave. Note that if weights are very high, undue emphasis is based on some observations and another approach for dealing with missing data, such as multiple imputation, may be more appropriate. See Hogan et al. (2004) for more discussion. In this data example, there are only a few weights that are relatively high, which do not affect the results considerably.

The second row of Table 7.4 shows the estimated slopes and the contrast of interest under the weighted GEE model under MAR assumptions. Note that the same overall tests as in the unweighted GEE are statistically significant, with the interaction between wave and smoking much more strongly significant than before ($\chi^2(1) = 11.5$, $p = 0.0007$ for the interaction, $\chi^2(1) = 160.7$, $p < 0.0001$ for the main effect of smoking, and $\chi^2(1) = 524.5$, $p < 0.0001$ for the main effect of time). The slope estimates for both non-smokers and smokers in the weighted GEE are steeper than in the unweighted GEE, reflecting that under MCAR assumptions the deterioration in self-rated health over time is underestimated. The difference in slopes between smokers and non-smokers is more pronounced in the weighted GEE than in the unweighted GEE (cumulative odds ratio = 0.97 compared with 0.98, see last column of Table 7.4).

The third and fourth rows of Table 7.4 show the estimated slopes and the contrasts of interest under the considered MNAR-weighted GEE models. In both models, we estimate the probabilities of missingness with a logistic regression model as specified above except that we use the current (potentially unobserved) self-rated health in the linear predictor rather than self-rated health at the previous visit. Since self-rated health is not observed for

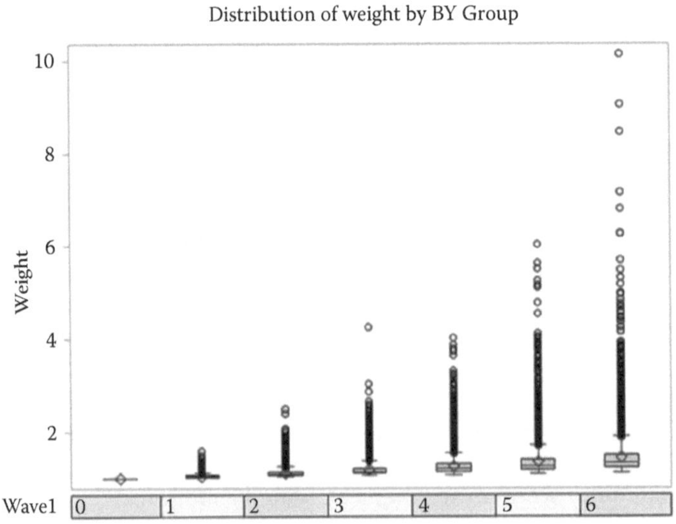

FIGURE 7.5
Distribution of estimated individual weights based on the inverse propensity score approach in the Health and Retirement Study.

subjects and dropouts at the last time point that is used in the logistic regression model, we add 0.5 to the previous self-rated health for dropouts and use this as the current unobserved self-rated health value. For subjects who died, we assign values of 5.5 for self-rated health for the first assessment after dropout. This is 0.5 higher than the code for "poor" self-rated health in the first model. In the second weighted GEE under MNAR assumptions, we do the same "imputation" of values for subjects who died regardless of smoking status, but for dropouts we add 0.5 to previous self-rated health for smokers and 0.2 for non-smokers.

These decisions are fairly arbitrary, and one can argue that for subjects who died we should not even be considering any values post-dropout. Note though that subjects might have died at any point in the two-year period between visits, including right before the missed assessment, and we are imputing a value only for the first visit past dropout. Thus, to a certain extent, the "imputation" we make is reasonable, since "health" of subjects who died in the last interval should have been worse than for those alive. For dropouts from causes other than death, it is reasonable to assume that they have a further deterioration in self-rated health that is not observed, and this deterioration might depend on smoking status. We can perform multiple sensitivity analyses using different values or by modeling the informative dropout in different ways. Herein, we just illustrate the point that the weights in the GEE model can be manipulated to reflect different MNAR mechanisms.

The slope estimates for both non-smokers and smokers are further increased under both considered MNAR mechanisms, and the estimate for the cumulative odds ratio reflecting the rate of deterioration in self-rated health between smokers and non-smokers is between the estimates from the MCAR and S-MAR models. The estimate from the first MNAR scenario, when our assumptions about dropout and death do not differ by smoking status, is closer to the MCAR estimate, while that from the second MNAR scenario, when we allowed self-rated health to vary for dropouts by smoking status, is closer to the S-MAR estimate. Thus, the conclusions do not change substantively under these particular MNAR mechanisms.

As expected, the slope estimates from the GLMM are larger than those from the GEE model; this is consistent with the expected relationship between subject-specific and population-averaged estimates, as explained in Chapter 4. Furthermore, the estimated slopes for smokers are steeper than for non-smokers, with cumulative odds ratio estimates that are more highly statistically significant than in the GEE models. Although there are substantial differences between subjects who die during the study and subjects who complete or drop out for other reasons, the substantive results under MAR are not much different compared with the MNAR models we considered. Thus, we can conclude that the results are robust to deviations from the MAR assumption.

7.8 Guidelines for Handling Missing Data

Many publications have appeared in recent years that give guidelines for handling missing data (e.g., Graham, 2009; Schlomer et al., 2010; Little et al., 2012; Mallinckrodt et al., 2013; https://www.ncbi.nlm.nih.gov/books/NBK209904). Perhaps the most active area is missing data in clinical research (Molenberghs and Kenward, 2007) due to the important implications in interpreting results from clinical trials. Mallinckrodt et al. (2014) identified three pillars for dealing with missing data: "(1) providing clearly stated objectives and causal estimands; (2) preventing as much missing data as possible, and (3) combining a sensible primary analysis with sensitivity analyses to assess robustness of inferences to missing data assumptions."

In clinical trials, an important distinction in objectives is made between *efficacy* and *effectiveness* analyses. Efficacy is the effect of treatment if applied as directed (i.e., drug taken as directed, behavioral therapy delivered and received as directed) and the corresponding analysis is done *per protocol*. Effectiveness is the effect of treatment as actually applied (i.e., subjects may stop receiving treatment, change doses, switch to another medication) and the corresponding analysis is *intention-to-treat*.

Missing data are handled differently in these two situations. The per-protocol analysis is performed only on completers and the results are generalizable only to individuals who are able to receive treatment as intended. Intention-to-treat analysis is performed on all randomized subjects; results are generalizable to the entire population, but the estimated effect is not of the treatment itself, but rather of how treatment is intended to be applied. Effectiveness analysis can also be performed to assess the effectiveness of the initially randomized treatment, but data on subjects who drop out, change dose, or switch to another treatment after the change are not used in the analysis. Instead, their data may be imputed.

This illustrates the importance of clear objectives in making a decision of how to handle missing data in the analysis. Of course, it is even more important to prevent or at least minimize missing data. While prevention of all missing data is unrealistic, missing data can be minimized using different strategies (Mallinckrodt et al., 2013). Regarding the primary analysis plan, most often this is a MAR approach since it is both reasonable and fairly straightforward to implement. The three MAR approaches most often used are likelihood-based analyses (in this category are all mixed models we considered in Chapters 3 and 4), multiple imputation, and weighted generalized estimating equations. Methods for informatively missing data under different MNAR assumptions are most often used as sensitivity analyses, since they can never be definite because they rely on unverifiable assumptions about the missing data. If the primary MAR analysis and a reasonable set of secondary MNAR analyses lead to the same conclusions, we have confidence in the conclusions from the study. If there are discrepancies, then the secondary analyses provide a measure of how much the results depend on the MAR assumption.

7.9 Summary

In this chapter, we reviewed the basic terminology and explained at a non-technical level the modern approaches to analysis of longitudinal data with missing data. The methods were illustrated on a fairly simple data example and general guidelines were presented.

The most important take-home message is that the primary analysis of longitudinal data sets with missing data needs to be performed under MAR assumptions, and it is recommended that sensitivity analyses under reasonable MNAR mechanisms are used to assess how robust the results are to deviations from MAR. When data are missing only on the dependent measure, the preferred approach is LMM or GLMM analysis, since it is simple to perform and interpret and provides valid and efficient results under MAR assumptions. PMM can be used as sensitivity analyses with selection and shared parameter approaches as other good choices that are somewhat more complicated to perform with existing statistical software.

Although mixed models are the preferred approach for longitudinal data, the inferences from LMM or GLMM are valid if all aspects of the model reflect the data well (e.g., both mean and variance–covariance structure are reasonably well modeled). When this is difficult to ensure, an alternative is to use doubly robust weighted GEE models, which provide valid estimates when either the missing data mechanism or the main model are correctly specified. These methods also require just a working correlation structure. The inverse probability-weighted GEE is fairly easy to apply in existing statistical software and allows manipulation of the weights under different MNAR assumptions in order to address the sensitivity of the results.

When data are missing on both predictor and outcome variables, a preferred approach is multiple imputation together with an appropriate model for the longitudinal data. Multiple imputation is efficient even with a small number of imputations and allows multiply imputed data sets to be created separately from the modeling. That is, data can be multiply imputed and then different models can be fit to the same data sets. However, multiple imputation requires the investigator to make multiple decisions and it is not always clear what effect these have on the results. The preferred MI approaches are MCMC for missing continuous data and FCS (also known as *multiple chain equations*) for missing data of different types. Multiple imputation can also be done under MNAR assumptions to assess the sensitivity of results.

Finally, causal inference with counterfactual outcomes is considered a special case of missing data analysis, with many recent developments in the statistical literature. Since missing data is an area of continuing and very intensive research, the current chapter touches only on the tip of iceberg. The interested reader is referred to Molenberghs et al. (2014) for details and the most up-to-date methods.

8

Controlling for Covariates in Studies with Repeated Measures

In Chapters 3–7, we presented different models for the analysis of longitudinal and clustered data from experimental and observational studies. Our main focus was on the assessment of the effects of treatments and in evaluating group differences. For example, in the depression clinical trials and in the COMBINE trial of alcohol dependence, the main question of interest was whether depression severity and drinking outcomes, respectively, improved with treatment. In the Health and Retirement Study, we investigated differences and changes in health self-assessment by smoking status, and in the schizophrenia working memory data, the focus was on testing for differences between schizophrenia patients and healthy controls in brain activation. In all these examples, we would ideally like to assess the causal effect of treatment or the independent (unconfounded) effect of group. In the case of randomized studies, the treatment groups are expected to be balanced on observed and unobserved characteristics that might change the relationship between treatment and outcome, and hence treatment effects have a causal interpretation. In observational studies, non-randomized groups of subjects are compared and these groups may differ from one another on a variety of covariates. Estimating the independent effect of group in this case is difficult since it is likely to be confounded with the effects of other predictors of outcome.

Analysis of covariance (ANCOVA) is a statistical technique that allows one to adjust inferences so that individuals from different groups are compared at the same levels of the covariates (also known as *confounding variables, concomitant variables*, or *independent variables*). The classical ANCOVA approach involves adding the covariate that we want to control to the statistical model before the main predictor (treatment, group, or exposure) is added. This allows us to reduce the noise in the data and may increase power in the statistical analysis. However, when the covariate is influenced by treatment or differs by group, controlling for it may still result in bias and can lead to erroneous conclusions.

In general, for ANCOVA to be valid, it is necessary for the main predictor of interest (i.e., treatment in randomized studies and exposure or group in observational studies) to be unrelated to the potential covariates. This is common in randomized studies where any differences at baseline among groups can be attributed to chance. For example, baseline severity is likely to be associated with the outcome and thus may be important to include in the model. Since groups are expected to be balanced in terms of initial severity because of the randomization, treatment is unrelated to baseline illness severity. In this situation, ANCOVA is quite appropriate and may improve power and efficiency for the estimation of treatment effects on the outcome. However, inclusion of covariates in the model should not depend on whether there are significant differences between groups on the covariates but rather should be based on *a priori* substantive considerations in order to ensure generalizable conclusions.

In contrast, in observational studies, the main predictor of interest is often statistically associated with potential covariates. For example, smoking may be related to drinking, and hence smokers and non-smokers may differ in terms of their drinking distributions.

In this case, controlling for drinking in a statistical model can actually remove some of the effect of smoking and lead to biased and not readily interpretable results. In general, if the covariates that are controlled in the statistical model are affected by treatment or exposure, controlling for these covariates can remove some of the treatment effect and can bias the estimates. It is a common misconception that including the potentially confounding predictors in observational studies "corrects" the estimates of the main predictor effect of interest. This is true only in special situations and when appropriate statistical techniques are used.

In this chapter, we explain how to control for potentially important covariates by including them in the statistical model with the goal of improving power and precision of estimates. In Section 8.1, we focus on the classic ANCOVA in cross-sectional studies or longitudinal studies with two repeated measures (pre-treatment versus post-treatment), describe how ANCOVA is properly used in randomized studies, and discuss challenges and limitations of this approach in observational studies. In Section 8.2, we proceed to consider ANCOVA in the context of more complicated studies with repeated measures, and distinguish between situations when covariates vary between or within individuals. Attention is devoted to time-independent and time-dependent covariates in longitudinal studies. Section 8.3 presents the propensity scoring approach for reduction of bias in observational studies and discusses regression adjustments, weighting methods, and matching. With this approach, observational studies can be considered as "pseudo-experiments" in which balance on measured covariates can be achieved. The issue of controlling for unmeasured confounders is briefly discussed. Data examples are presented in Section 8.4 with the appropriate code and output included in the online materials. The chapter concludes with a summary and includes references for alternative approaches better suited for causal inference (Section 8.5).

As always, the emphasis of the chapter is on conceptual issues. A detailed and comprehensive reference on the technical details of analysis of covariance models, including models for repeated measures data, is presented in Milliken and Johnson (2008). Other useful recent references are Huitema (2011) and Rutherford (2012). A non-technical description of the caveats and inappropriate uses of ANCOVA can be found in Miller and Chapman (2001). References on the propensity scoring approach are given in Section 8.3.

8.1 Controlling for Covariates in Cross-Sectional and Simple Longitudinal Designs

In Chapter 2, we considered controlling for covariates in the context of endpoint analysis by using traditional analysis of covariance (ANCOVA) methods for cross-sectional data. Herein, we detail and expand this discussion. We start by considering randomized experiments and, in particular, the simple situation when individuals are randomized to one of t different treatments. A quantitative outcome variable and potential covariate are measured on each individual. The usual strategy in such a design is to test whether there are differences in response among the treatment groups followed by pairwise or other mean comparisons if the overall treatment effect is significant. The most simple ANOVA model is

$$Y_i = \beta_1 I_{i1} + \ldots \beta_t I_{it} + \varepsilon_{ij} \tag{8.1}$$

where:

i denotes individual

I_{i1} indicates whether individual i is assigned to the first treatment (i.e., $I_{i1} = 1$ if subject i is assigned to the first treatment and 0 otherwise)

I_{i2} indicates whether individual i is assigned to the second treatment, and so on

The usual assumptions about normality, independence, and equal variances of the errors, ε_{ij}, are made. Using this notation, we see that the β parameters correspond to the unknown means for the t different treatments and the usual null hypothesis of equality of means is H_0: $\beta_1 = \beta_2 = \ldots \beta_t$. When there are significant differences between the means, pairwise or other focused mean comparisons are performed to identify differing means or patterns of means. The ANOVA model ignores the systematic effects of other potentially important variables on the outcome and considers them random noise. This is reasonable in randomized studies where such effects are likely to be balanced across the different treatment groups and hence the estimates of the treatment effect are unbiased.

However, treatment effects could potentially vary for individuals depending on other variables. Taking those into account may improve power for the treatment comparisons. For example, in the COMBINE study, intensity of drinking at baseline is likely related to intensity of drinking during treatment and may account for some of the residual variability in the ANOVA model described. Other predictors such as gender and age can also be related to the outcome. Including such predictors in the model can decrease the residual variability and thus increase precision for the treatment comparisons. The traditional ANCOVA model with one covariate is

$$Y_i = \beta_1 I_{i1} + \ldots \beta_t I_{it} + \beta_{t+1} x_i + \varepsilon_{ij} \tag{8.2}$$

where:

x_i is the value of the covariate for the ith individual

β_{t+1} describes the effect of this covariate

This model, known as the *common slope model*, is intended to adjust the treatment effects for the covariate. That is, we estimate the effect of treatment at the same level of the covariate. Thus, even if there is chance imbalance on this covariate, as long as the covariate is not statistically dependent on the treatment, unbiased treatment effects are obtained. However, there are several implicit assumptions that are made in the common slope model that might invalidate it, if not satisfied. For example, the relationship between the covariate and the outcome is assumed to be linear and the same for all treatments. Since it is usually not known *a priori* whether this is the case in a particular situation, we need to go through several steps in order to perform a proper analysis of covariance.

8.1.1 Steps in Classical ANCOVA

Step 1: Assess the type of the relationship between the outcome and the covariate within each treatment group. Is it indeed linear? Is a transformation needed? To answer these questions, we can fit separate simple linear regressions within the treatment group, examine residuals, and assess whether remedial measures such as transformations or including higher order terms (such as x_i^2) are needed. When it is determined that remedial measures are necessary, they are performed before proceeding to the next step.

Note that when there are many treatment groups, evaluations of the relationship between the covariate and the outcome may not be straightforward. For example, a linear relationship may seem to hold in one treatment group but a log-linear relationship in another. Since we need to treat a covariate consistently (e.g., as a linear effect without transformation, or a linear effect after transformation), we may need to go through all the steps repeatedly using different forms of the covariate–outcome relationship or transformations of the covariate or outcome before deciding what best describes the relationship with the outcome. Residual plots of the entire model can help with this decision.

Step 2: Assess whether the outcome is significantly associated with the covariate. Since this relationship can vary by treatment, to perform this step we need to fit the following model:

$$Y_i = \beta_1 I_{i1} + \ldots + \beta_t I_{it} + \beta_{t+1} x_i I_{i1} + \ldots + \beta_{2t} x_i I_{it} + \varepsilon_{ij} \quad (8.3)$$

This is a full rank model with an interaction between treatment and the covariate. In this model, testing whether the coefficients β_{t+1} through β_{2t} are equal to zero tells us whether there is a statistically significant linear relationship between the covariate and the outcome for any of the treatment groups. Note that if transformations are applied to the covariate values, the x values in Equation 8.3 are the transformed covariate values. If there is a curvilinear relationship between the covariate and the treatments, then x_i^2 values are also included, and both the slopes and the coefficients of the quadratic terms are simultaneously assessed for equality to zero.

If there is no statistical relationship between the covariate and the outcome, the covariate adjustment is likely not necessary and there will be no gain in power. Thus, analysis can be done based on an ANOVA model without adjusting for the covariate and we do not need to continue following steps 3 and 4. Otherwise, if there is an indication of an association for at least some of the treatment groups we proceed to step 3.

Step 3: Assess whether the relationship between the covariate and the outcome varies by treatment group. This is accomplished by testing whether the coefficients β_{t+1} through β_{2t} in the more general, third ANCOVA model are equal to one another (but not necessarily to zero). This is actually a test of the interaction between the treatment and the covariate.

If the relationship is the same, then the simpler common slope ANCOVA model (i.e., the model in Equation 8.2) can be used for statistical inference. On the other hand, if there is an indication that the relationship between the covariate and the outcome varies by treatment (i.e., the coefficients are not all equal to one another) then we need to base inferences on the more general model with the interaction of the covariate and treatment (i.e., the model in Equation 8.3). We consider inferences under this scenario right after the description of inferences under the common slope model in step 4.

Step 4: When there is no evidence that the relationship between the predictor and the outcome varies by treatment group, the fourth step of the approach is to perform inferences based on the common slope model in Equation 8.2. This model is often described as the basic ANCOVA model, and models with interactions are not even considered in many cases. We urge caution with direct application of this model, since if there are in fact interactions between treatment and the covariate, incorrect inferences may result. Note that in the common slope model the treatment comparisons are still the focus of the inferences but they are interpreted as the differences between the treatments *adjusted for the covariate*, i.e., the treatment differences are evaluated at the same value of the covariate. It does not matter what value of the covariate we consider, since the relationship between the covariate and the outcome is described by parallel lines for the different treatment groups and hence the distances are the same for each value of the covariate.

In the case when the covariate by treatment interaction is statistically significant and we use the model in Eq. 8.3 for statistical inferences, the magnitude of the treatment comparisons depends on the value of the covariate. Thus, we get a different estimate for the mean differences between treatments at different values of the covariate. In this case, the follow-up approach is to perform treatment comparisons at several (usually three) different values of the covariate. These should be meaningful from a subject-matter perspective, and by all means not outside of the range of values for the available covariates. Often, the mean value of the covariate is used together with values one or two standard deviations above and below the mean. Alternatively, we can also estimate different slopes for the relationship between the covariate and the outcome in each treatment group and perform pairwise comparisons of these slopes.

More complex post hoc analyses involve constructing confidence bands on the regression predictions within each treatment group and establishing a range of the predictor values within which the mean outcome is different between two or more treatments. The interested reader is referred to Milliken and Johnson (2008) for examples and details.

We will mention several additional issues with analysis of covariance: controlling for multiple covariates, effects of transformations, dealing with categorical covariates and/or outcomes, effects of missing data, and advantages of ANCOVA over change score analyses in simple pre- versus post-treatment longitudinal studies.

Controlling for multiple covariates: When multiple covariates are of interest, a model selection procedure based on evaluation of residuals may need to be performed to select which covariates to use. For the equal slope scenario, this approach involves calculating residuals from the ANOVA model of the outcome on treatment and residuals from separate linear regression models of each covariate on treatment, and using stepwise model selection procedures (e.g., forward selection, backward elimination, stepwise selection) to identify important covariates. The procedure is similar, but more unwieldy, when the slopes are not equal (see Chapter 7 in Milliken and Johnson [2008]).

Effects of transformations: Note that the transformations can affect the relationship between covariates and the outcome. A linear association between the mean of a transformed response and a covariate often corresponds to a non-linear association between the mean of the original response and a covariate. Thus, the equality of slopes hypothesis and the shape of the relationship between the covariate and the response can vary depending on whether a transformation is used.

Categorical covariates: In the steps above for ANCOVA, we focused on quantitative covariates but it is possible that covariates are categorical (e.g., binary, ordinal, nominal). In this case, the same approach is used but the results are interpreted as mean differences rather than slope differences.

Categorical outcome: When the outcomes are categorical, analysis of covariance can also be used by replacing the linear model with a generalized linear model. However, since a non-linear function relates the predictors to the outcome, interpretation can become complicated and it is more challenging to identify the proper relationship between the predictors and the outcome.

Missing data: Traditional ANCOVA requires complete data on the outcome and the covariate. When there are missing data, a common approach is to impute data on the covariate and/or on the outcome and then use ANCOVA. This needs to be done with multiple rather than single imputation in order to appropriately account for the loss of information due to missing data. Thus, the appropriate algorithm is to impute missing data using multiple imputation, fit ANCOVA to each imputed data set, and combine the estimates and standard errors taking into account the variances within and between imputed data sets as outlined in Chapter 7.

ANCOVA in longitudinal studies: In simple longitudinal designs with only two repeated measurements (baseline and endpoint), ANCOVA is frequently used to control for baseline imbalance or to improve power. A number of authors have compared the performance of ANCOVA at endpoint controlling for baseline to an ANOVA analysis of change scores (endpoint minus baseline), with the unequivocal conclusion that ANCOVA is preferred to change score analysis in randomized studies. However, there are somewhat differing views as to how useful it is in observational studies where group differences in other covariates may be present (Van Breukelen, 2006; Egbewale et al., 2014; Senn, 2006). We now turn our attention to the discussion of the properties of this method in experimental versus observational studies.

8.1.2 Analysis of Covariance in Randomized Studies

In randomized studies, estimates of treatment effects from ANCOVA have causal interpretation. Since controlling for confounding variables may improve power and precision in statistical inference, many researchers look for baseline differences in any potentially important covariates and include all covariates for which there are statistically significant differences between treatments in the analysis. However, this leads to several serious issues. First, whether there are statistically significant differences at baseline depends largely on sample size. In small studies, even sizeable imbalances may not be statistically significant, while in large studies even trivial covariate differences are statistically significant. Second, adjusting for covariates that differ by group but are not prognostic of treatment outcome does not improve efficiency and in small samples may lead to bias. Third, differences in covariates are typically evaluated one at a time, thus ignoring potential statistical relationships among the covariates themselves. Since covariates may work together or against each other in unpredictable ways, including them in the statistical model jointly can have unforeseen effects on inferences. Fourth, covariates are often included as main effects without consideration of possible interactions with treatment. While the four-step approach described earlier deals with this issue, it is often not used, and covariates are directly controlled using the common slope model.

In view of these potential problems, the CONSORT guidelines developed to ensure consistency in the implementation and interpretation of clinical trials (Moher et al., 2012) recommend that covariates are selected based on *a priori* substantive considerations rather than in a post hoc fashion based on the presence of significant differences between treatment groups. This allows for seamless integration of results of different studies in meta-analyses, as the covariates that are controlled in each study are not likely to be idiosyncratic to the particular study.

8.1.3 Analysis of Covariance in Observational Studies

In observational studies, controlling for covariates is much more complex since it is possible that the main predictor of interest (treatment or exposure) is majorly or completely confounded with other predictors of outcome. Confounding with quantitative covariates manifests in no, or little, overlap of the distributions of the covariates in the different treatment\exposure groups. In this case, including the potential covariate as a main or interactive effect in the model could remove or exaggerate the treatment\exposure effect. Thus, the need for, and method of, covarying should be carefully considered and the relationship between the covariate and treatment\exposure should be examined from a substantive perspective. In general, for analysis of covariance to be valid in observational studies, the covariate should not be affected directly or indirectly by treatment or exposure and there needs to be substantial overlap between the distributions of the covariate for each level of treatment or exposure. If there is no or very little overlap, results of ANCOVA are not interpretable. If there is substantial overlap then ANCOVA could be performed, but interpretation depends on the relationship between the covariate and exposure/treatment, and the potential for bias remains.

ANCOVA can be used to control multiple covariates, but a better method is the *propensity scoring* approach (see D'Agostino (1998) and Williamson and Forbes (2014) for a tutorial and introduction, respectively). This method is considered in more detail in Section 8.3 and later illustrated on a data example (Section 8.4) but the basic idea is as follows: When comparing a non-randomized group to a control group, the propensity score is defined as the probability of being in the treatment/exposure group given the covariates. It can be used to balance the covariates in the two groups by matching or stratification, regression adjustment, or inverse probability weighting. When balance on the covariates is achieved, bias due to confounding with these covariates can be reduced or eliminated.

While ANCOVA with multiple covariates or the propensity scoring approach allows us to adjust for a set of observed variables, groups may differ not only on observed, but also on unobserved, covariates. In this case, it is very difficult to obtain unbiased estimates of the group effects. ANCOVA and propensity scoring cannot deal with variability due to unmeasured confounders. One approach that is designed with the goal of controlling for unobserved confounding is the *instrumental variable approach* (see, e.g., Hogan and Lancaster, 2004; Baiocchi et al., 2014). Instrumental variables are variables that are independent of other measured or unmeasured covariates, are associated with treatment/exposure, and have no direct effect on the outcome. That is, whatever effect they might have on the outcome is via the treatment/exposure variable. A two-stage estimation approach is usually used in order to remove bias via the use of instrumental variables. The success of this approach depends on the ability to find a good instrumental variable that is specific to the subject-matter area, and this is often a very challenging task. Perhaps for this reason, this method is still not very popular in the medical and behavioral sciences literature. However, it has been used extensively in econometrics. Describing this approach is beyond the scope of this book, but we refer the interested reader to Bowden and Turkington (1984), Angrist et al. (1996), and Imbens (2014).

8.2 Controlling for Covariates in Clustered and Longitudinal Studies

Controlling for covariates in studies with repeated measures has similar advantages as in studies with cross-sectional data. In particular, precision and efficiency may be increased and chance imbalances can be corrected in randomized experiments. However, similar cautions apply in observational studies where estimates are likely to be biased. Furthermore, there are added challenges, as there are different types of covariates in longitudinal and clustered designs that can be related in different ways to the main predictor of interest and the outcome. Covariates can vary within individual (*within-subject covariates*) or between individuals (*between-subject covariates*). For example, variables such as sex or different genotypes vary between individuals. Measures of environmental exposures or people's behaviors can vary within individuals. In longitudinal studies, covariates are classified as either *time-independent* (i.e., their values do not vary during the entire study period) or *time-dependent* (i.e., their values potentially change during the study period). For example, in COMBINE, baseline drinking intensity is an example of a time-independent covariate while medication compliance or concurrent medications are examples of time-dependent covariates. In the cross-over study of menthol's effects on nicotine reinforcement, type of cigarettes smoked (mentholated versus non-mentholated) is an example of a time-independent covariate, while baseline on each test day is an example of a time-dependent covariate. In clustered data with different levels of clustering, covariates can be measured at each level of clustering (e.g., individual characteristics at the student level, homeroom characteristics at the homeroom level, and school level characteristics at the school level).

Different covariate types are seamlessly incorporated in GEE and mixed models, but one needs to be careful not to specify effects or interactions that are not readily interpretable. For example, interaction of time-independent covariates with time can be easily interpreted, but that is not always the case for interactions of time-dependent covariates and time. Time-dependent covariates are usually included as main effects. If treatment changes over time (as in cross-over trials, for example), interactions between time-dependent covariates and treatment might be difficult to interpret.

The general strategy of handling covariates in models for repeated measures data is as follows:

Step 1: Determine the adequate form of the covariate part of the model. That is, determine whether the covariates and the outcome (or appropriate function of the outcome such as odds or log means in the case of non-normality) are related linearly and whether transformations are needed. Ideally, this needs to be done within each treatment group and by time (in balanced designs), but in unbalanced designs this is not possible. In addition, the relationship can change with time or be different by treatment group. In such cases, several different complete models might need to be considered, their residuals examined, and the decision between competing models based on interpretability and goodness of fit. Note that substantive considerations should guide the model selection, as otherwise there may be too many possibilities to consider and type I errors can be committed more easily.

Step 2: Determine the variance–covariance part of the model. That is, determine the random effects and the residual error variance–covariance structure by comparing different models as outlined in Chapters 3 and 4.

Step 3: Simplify the fixed part of the model as described in steps 2 and 3 in Section 8.1.1 for cross-sectional studies. That is, test whether the covariates are needed. Then, if they are needed, test the equal slope assumption. Note that with longitudinal data you may need to evaluate not only whether the slopes are the same across treatments, but also whether they are the same over time. Thus, one needs to carefully consider potential interactions among covariates and treatment and to evaluate whether there is evidence that they are important. Often, substantive considerations trump statistical significance as significance is frequently dependent on sample size.

Step 4: Compare treatments/exposures based on the final model identified in step 3. If an equal slope model is selected, evaluate the differences at an arbitrary value of the covariate. If the unequal slope model is selected, compare the treatments at three or more different values of the covariate, or compare intercepts and slopes between the different treatment groups. Since the results may also vary by time, additional comparisons may need to be made.

Similar to the situation with cross-sectional data, controlling for multiple covariates is challenging, transformations can change the nature and the significance of covariate effects, categorical covariates and outcomes are seamlessly handled, and missing data (especially on the covariate) can affect inferences.

An additional issue with analysis of covariance in the context of longitudinal data is that it can be performed on the repeated observations as they are (whether including baseline as part of the repeated measures or not) or on change from baseline (absolute or percent change). Absolute change is, in general, preferable to percent change because it is always well-defined and has been empirically shown to be more efficient in a variety of scenarios (Vickers, 2001). In contrast, percent change is sometimes not well-defined. For example, one cannot calculate a percent change of zero, and percent change may not be meaningful when there is a mix of positive and negative numbers. Still, in some cases when the repeated measures are all positive, an analysis on the logarithmic scale with results presented as percentages may be appropriate.

When change from baseline is the outcome, it is imperative to include the baseline values as covariates. If baseline values are not included, estimates may be biased because the analysis essentially assumes that the relationship between post and baseline values is described by a simple linear regression with a slope of 1. As with other covariates, one needs to assess whether there are equal or unequal slopes (i.e., whether baseline interacts with treatment).

Although analysis of covariance is appropriate when the goal is to improve power in randomized studies and to control for chance imbalances between treatment groups, it requires complete data on the outcome and the covariate. This is rarely the case in prospective clinical trials as subjects drop out. One solution to this problem is to use full information likelihood inference based on all repeated measures data on an individual controlling for baseline covariates. This approach can be applied seamlessly when data are missing only on the outcome. Another approach is to impute missing data using multiple imputation, fit an analysis of covariance model to each imputed data set, and combine the estimates and standard errors, taking into account the variances within and between imputed data sets as outlined in Chapter 7. This method can be applied when there are missing data on both the covariate and outcome variable.

8.3 Propensity Scoring

Propensity scoring allows one to adjust the estimates of treatment/exposure effects on an outcome for multiple measured confounders (Rosenbaum and Rubin, 1983; 1984; 1985). The ultimate goal is to estimate causal effects, and this approach attempts to do that when systematic differences between groups (defined by treatment or exposure) are expected. Propensity scoring is mainly used to adjust inferences in observational studies, but it can also be used in clinical trials, most often to adjust for dropout. Herein, we present the general propensity scoring idea in more detail and discuss how it can be applied to assess causal effects via *regression adjustment, matching, stratification,* or *probability weighting.* Examples are given in Section 8.4. We focus on the simple scenario of a binary treatment/exposure that has been considered by D'Agostino (1998) and Williamson and Forbes (2014) in their fairly non-technical introductions. Extensions to categorical predictors with more levels or to quantitative predictors have been considered in recent years (e.g., Imai and van Dyk, 2004). The books of Rosenbaum (2002, 2010) provide a detailed and technical guide to design and analysis of data from observational studies. In a recent review of the medical literature (Austin, 2008), different pitfalls with the application of the propensity scoring approach have been identified. Most often, propensity scoring is used for the analysis of cross-sectional data and when treatment is not time-varying. However, in recent years, extensions to time-varying treatment effects have also been proposed (e.g., Lu, 2005).

To understand propensity scoring we first need to define causal effects. The causal effect of treatment (active versus control) at the individual level is defined as the outcome on the active treatment minus the outcome on the control treatment. An individual receives only one of the possible treatments, and hence, only one of these outcomes is observed. The other is unobserved and is called a *counterfactual outcome*. Thus, individual causal effects cannot be directly measured or estimated. However, average causal effects in a population of individuals can be estimated in randomized parallel group experiments as the difference between the average response of subjects on active treatment and subjects on control treatment. Because of randomization, individuals receiving the active treatment and those receiving the control treatment are representative of the entire population of interest and thus the average outcome for each group is an unbiased estimate of the outcome of all individuals who could potentially have received active and control treatment, respectively. This makes randomized clinical trials well suited for causal inference, but it is immediately clear that observational studies where individuals are not randomly assigned to groups are ill-suited for causal inference. The propensity scoring approach attempts to balance the groups on observed covariates so that observational studies can be treated as *pseudo-experiments* and causal inference can be done under certain conditions. In particular, in order for this approach to result in causal estimates, it is necessary to assume that there are no unmeasured confounder variables and that the individuals do not influence each other's outcomes.

In observational studies, groups of individuals are often compared (e.g., smokers versus non-smokers, patients with a particular disease versus healthy controls). Thus, the groups differ on a variety of characteristics (both measured and unmeasured), some of which are prognostic of the outcome, and thus the group differences in outcome cannot strictly be attributed to group. Analysis of covariance in this situation usually gives biased results because it cannot adequately adjust for group differences in important covariates. In such situations, alternative approaches to analysis of covariance based on propensity scoring adjustments with matching, stratification, regression modeling, or inverse probability weighting are used. Since the propensity score method is more frequently used in observational studies, we will consider the two groups to be exposed and non-exposed individuals for the remainder of this section.

The *propensity score* is the probability that an individual is exposed given the measured confounding variables. We can estimate it by fitting a logistic regression with the confounding variables as predictors and the binary indicator of exposure as the outcome. Other approaches such as classification trees are possible but not as frequently used. The predicted exposure probabilities are the estimated propensity scores and they all are between 0 and 1. A crucial property of the propensity score is that all variables that are included in the propensity score model are balanced at each value of the estimated propensity score. Thus, the causal exposure effect can be obtained by comparing the outcome in the exposed and unexposed groups *at each value of the estimated propensity score*. Matching, stratification, and controlling for the propensity score are all valid techniques to do this. Weighting is another technique that can be used to obtain causal effects. We briefly explain these here.

Propensity score matching involves creating exposed and unexposed groups that are matched on propensity scores. Thus, for each individual in the exposed group, one or more individuals in the unexposed group with very similar propensity scores (within a certain level of closeness) to that individual are identified. If the matched samples are balanced on the covariates (which can be assessed by evaluating standardized differences in each covariate), statistical methods for matched data can be used to estimate exposure effects (e.g., conditional logistic regression, weighted regression methods). Note that creating matched samples is rarely an easy task. For example, some individuals in the exposed group might not have close matches, and in this case such individuals are discarded. Thus, the estimated exposure effect might not be representative of the exposure effect in the population of exposed individuals. There are a variety of techniques for propensity score matching with no clear winner. For example, matching can be done with or without replacement from the population of unexposed individuals, but if replacement is used, one needs to account for potentially using some subjects' data more than once. In general, the propensity score matching approach is preferred when the number of exposed individuals is much smaller than the number of unexposed individuals.

Propensity score stratification involves splitting the estimated propensity scores in several strata (e.g., the lower 20% of propensity scores, 20%–40%, 40%–60%, 60%–80%, 80%–100%), evaluating exposure effects within each stratum, and then calculating an overall average of the within-stratum effects. An advantage of this approach is that it is easy to implement, but it is not as precise as propensity score matching since there might still be lack of balance between propensity scores of the exposed and unexposed groups within stratum. Usually, there are only a few strata (e.g., five) and although the number can be increased, some residual imbalances may remain. Furthermore, it is possible that the distributions of the propensity scores in the exposed and non-exposed groups are shifted with respect to each other, in which case in some strata there might be too many individuals of one group and too few the other.

Covariate adjustment using propensity scores involves fitting a regression model with the exposure variable as the primary predictor and the propensity score itself as a covariate. Interactions between exposure and the propensity score can also be considered. This approach is the simplest to apply, as it is essentially an ANCOVA model with the propensity score as the covariate of interest. However, it may fail to correct for bias when the distributions of the propensity scores between the groups do not sufficiently overlap, and, even more importantly, it relies on the assumption that the model relating the propensity score and the response is correctly specified. For these reasons, this approach is usually not recommended.

The inverse probability weighting approach differs from the other three methods in that it does not compare individuals with the same value of the propensity score but rather weighs the individuals' data based on the estimated propensity score in an appropriate model for the outcome. If p_i is the estimated score for the ith individual, the weight is $1/p_i$ if the individual is in the exposed group and $1/(1 - p_i)$ if the individual is in the unexposed group. Thus, individuals in the exposed group with higher estimated propensity scores are given less weight than individuals with lower propensity scores in that same group. In contrast, individuals in the unexposed group with higher estimated propensity scores are given more weight than individuals with lower propensity scores in that group. Thus, subjects in a particular group who are more like the subjects in the other group in terms of their covariates are weighed more heavily. The outcome model can be any appropriate model, e.g., logistic or linear regression for a single outcome variable.

We have already considered such a weighting method in the previous chapter in the context of accounting for missing data. The same technique is used to control for lack of balance of covariates among exposure groups. This approach is easy to apply and performs well, except when the estimated propensity scores are close to 0 or 1. In this case, the weights are too high and the resulting exposure estimates are imprecise. Trimming procedures have been proposed to deal with this issue. This approach is preferable in the absence of large weights and when the exposed and unexposed groups are of similar size.

A few comments regarding propensity scoring are in order. First, all potential confounders should be included in the propensity score model. To reiterate, these are variables that are related to the exposure and predictive of the outcome. Adding variables that are related to exposure but not to the outcome may actually inflate the variance of the exposure effect, and thus decrease precision. Variables that are predictive of the outcome but not related to the exposure do not improve the fit of the exposure model but may increase precision; thus, it may sometimes be beneficial to include these.

Second, it should be checked whether the propensity score model achieves balance on the potential confounders. This is done by calculated standardized differences between the exposed and unexposed groups before and after applying the propensity score adjustment by any of the four methods. These are standardized mean differences for continuous confounders and standardized differences of probabilities for binary confounders (see Williamson and Forbes [2014] or Harder et al. [2010] for non-technical descriptions). Values of greater than 10% difference are indicative of some remaining bias. Such a level of bias is problematic for strongly predictive variables of the outcome.

Third, missing data in the exposure model (whether on the exposure itself or on covariates) can be handled by multiple imputation.

Fourth, a sizeable sample size is needed for propensity score analysis in order to carry out a logistic regression or other prediction model of exposure with multiple possible covariates. The most typical propensity score analyses are performed on observational data sets with thousands of observations.

Fifth, although we considered the simple situation with binary exposure variable here, methods have also been developed for categorical and continuous exposure variables (Imbens, 2000; Imai and van Dyk, 2004).

Finally, propensity score methods are quite attractive because most of the modeling for bias correction can be done without looking at the outcome. That is, the propensity score model for the exposure can be fitted without knowing the outcome. Thus, it can be considered as a quasi-randomization approach for observational studies.

In summary, the propensity score methods are flexible and appropriate when it is necessary to control for multiple measured confounding variables. However, the presence of bias on potentially predictive variables should be checked before and after adjustment. Bias may still remain due to unmeasured confounders. In this case, other methods of adjustment such as instrumental variable approaches may need to be considered.

8.4 Data Examples

8.4.1 ANCOVA of Endpoint Drinks per Day Controlling for Baseline Drinking Intensity in the COMBINE Study

ANCOVA is most often applied for the comparison of endpoint outcomes between groups when controlling for baseline measures. To illustrate this traditional ANCOVA, we consider again the COMBINE clinical trial in alcohol dependence and herein focus on the outcome drinks per day at the end of treatment for individuals who drink. An analysis involving all four months of treatment is considered in the next subsection. We ignore acamprosate treatment to simplify the presentation and perform an overall test of differences between the four groups (naltrexone and CBI, naltrexone only, CBI only, neither naltrexone nor CBI). This analysis was used to illustrate one-way ANOVA in Chapter 2 and here we consider it again in order to demonstrate the basic steps of ANCOVA.

If a simple one-way ANOVA model is fit to the log-transformed outcome, there is a statistically significant treatment effect ($F(3,717) = 3.34$, $p = 0.02$) with significantly fewer drinks per day on average for subjects who received at least one active treatment (naltrexone and/or CBI) compared with those not receiving an active treatment. Comparisons of least square means with confidence intervals are shown in Table 8.1. This analysis answers the question of whether treatments differ on average in their effects on intensity of drinking at endpoint in the clinical trial. However, the effect of the treatment could potentially vary for individuals depending on their baseline intensity of drinking. The treatment groups are balanced at baseline on drinks per day ($F(3,717) = 2.04$,

TABLE 8.1

Confidence Intervals for Pairwise Comparisons of Log Drinks per Day during the Last Month of the Study Period in the COMBINE Study

Treatment Group	Comparison Treatment Group	Least Square Mean Difference in ANOVA Model (95% CI)	Least Square Mean Difference in ANCOVA Model with Parallel Slopes (95% CI)
Naltrexone + CBI	Naltrexone only	0.001 (−0.16, 0.17)	−0.02 (−0.18, 0.14)
Naltrexone + CBI	CBI only	0.03 (−0.13, 0.19)	0.06 (−0.10, 0.21)
Naltrexone + CBI	**Neither**	**−0.19 (−0.35, −0.03)**	**−0.21 (−0.36, −0.06)**
Naltrexone only	CBI only	0.03 (−0.13, 0.19)	0.08 (−0.08, 0.24)
Naltrexone only	**Neither**	**−0.19 (−0.35, −0.03)**	**−0.19 (−0.34, −0.03)**
CBI only	**Neither**	**−0.22 (−0.38, −0.07)**	**−0.27 (−0.42, −0.12)**

Note: Estimates highlighted in bold indicate statistically significant differences at 0.05 level.

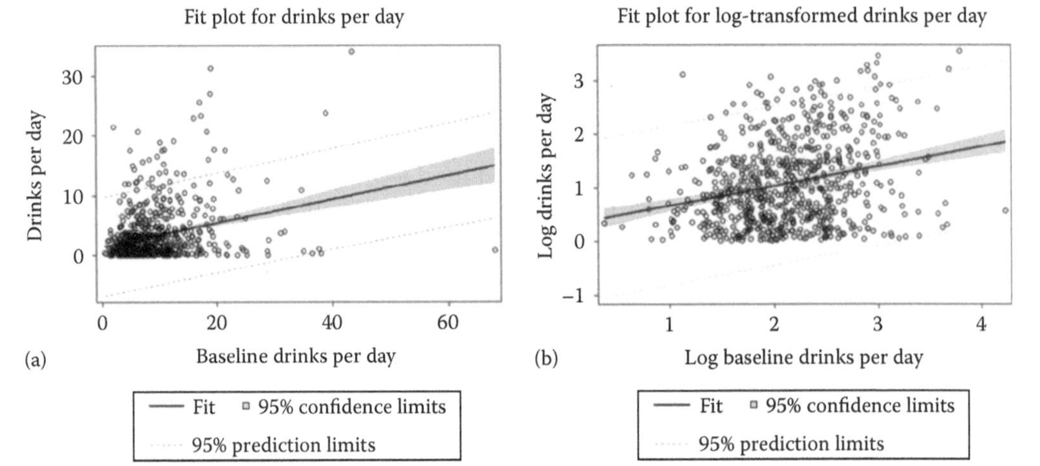

FIGURE 8.1
Simple linear regression fit of drinks per day at the end of treatment versus baseline drinks per day in the COMBINE study before (a) and after (b) log transformation.

$p = 0.11$), hence there is no reason to expect systematic bias in the estimates of the effects in ANOVA, but ANCOVA may improve power for the between-group comparisons and may increase precision in the estimates of treatment effects. The steps of ANCOVA analysis are outlined in the following.

Step 1: We assess the type of the relationship between the outcome and the covariate by fitting several different models to evaluate how intensity of drinking relates to baseline drinking by treatment group. In particular, we consider linear and quadratic regression models on raw and log-transformed measures. Figure 8.1 shows the fit of the simple linear regression models to the raw and log-transformed data. We show the results of the analysis of the entire sample together, but separate models by treatment arm look very similar. We note that there is no indication of a curvilinear relationship between intensity of drinking at baseline and during treatment. Indeed, when quadratic models are fit, the quadratic term estimates are not statistically significant for any of the treatment arms. In addition, the fit of the model is much better when both measures of intensity of drinking are log-transformed, because the transformation both stabilizes the variances and reels in potential outliers. There is still a minor issue with floor effects (since number of drinks cannot be less than zero) and there are some positive outliers outside of the prediction limits based on the regression fit, but none are too extreme. Thus, it appears that a linear relationship between the log-transformed covariate and the log-transformed outcome is justified, and we proceed to the next steps in ANCOVA using this form of the model. Residual plots (not shown) confirm that this is a good choice.

Step 2: We assess whether the outcome is significantly associated with the covariate. Figure 8.1 suggests that there is a positive association between the two variables, but the formal test of whether the slopes of the linear relationship between the covariate and the outcome are simultaneously zero is highly statistically significant ($F(4,713) = 15.63$, $p < 0.0001$), indicating that such a relationship indeed exists.

Step 3: Next, we assess whether the relationship between the covariate and the outcome varies by treatment group. The interaction test is not statistically significant ($F(3,713) = 2.03$, $p = 0.11$); hence, we conclude that the relationship between the covariate and the outcome does not vary by treatment group and we can use a common slope model.

Step 4: We perform inferences based on the common slope model. The left panel of Figure 8.2 shows the results from the application of the common slope model to the intensity of drinking outcome in the COMBINE data, while, for comparison purposes, the right panel of Figure 8.2 shows the results when different slopes are considered. Since the test of the interaction between treatment and the covariate is not statistically significant, the graph on left in Figure 8.2 is based on our final model.

Table 8.1 shows the least square mean comparisons and associated 95% confidence intervals for the contrasts between the different treatments when covarying for baseline intensity of drinking according to our final model. Note that the estimates are somewhat different from the estimates in the model without covarying since there are some differences in the covariate at baseline between groups. In ANOVA, one estimates the mean differences regardless of the values of the covariate, and in ANCOVA, the mean differences are adjusted for the covariate levels, i.e., we align the groups as if they have the same values on the covariate and then compare the means. When the covariates are well balanced across groups, the difference between ANOVA and ANCOVA estimates tend to disappear. From Table 8.1, we also notice that the confidence intervals based on ANCOVA are slightly narrower than those based on ANOVA. This is because we gain efficiency and reduce the residual variability by essentially subtracting the variability in the outcome due to the covariate. However, the gains here are minimal.

Just for illustration, we also consider the more general model with unequal slopes (i.e., with treatment by covariate interaction) that was used to produce the right panel of Figure 8.2. In this plot, the regression lines describing the relationship between the covariate and the outcome for the different treatments cross. Thus, depending on which level of the covariate we consider, we get a different estimate for the mean differences between

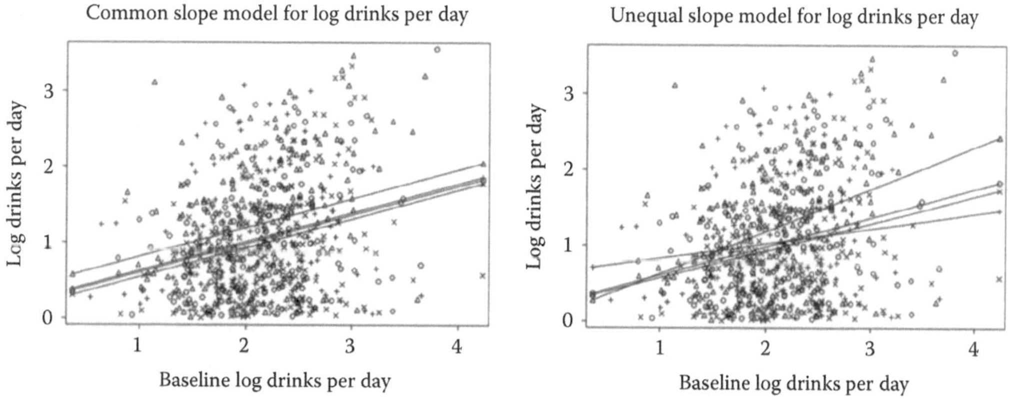

FIGURE 8.2
Analysis of covariance model for drinks per day at the end of treatment in the COMBINE study: Common slope (left) and unequal slope (right).

TABLE 8.2

Confidence Intervals for Pairwise Comparisons of Log Drinks per Day Based on the Unequal Slopes Model in the COMBINE Study

Treatment Group	Comparison Treatment Group	Least Square Mean Difference at Two Standard Deviations below the Mean Covariate Value (95% CI)	Least Square Mean Difference at Mean Covariate Value (95% CI)	Least Square Mean Difference at Two Standard Deviations above the Mean Covariate Value (95% CI)
Naltrexone + CBI	Naltrexone only	−0.22 (−0.58, 0.14)	−0.04 (−0.20, 0.13)	0.15 (−0.16, 0.45)
Naltrexone + CBI	CBI only	0.03 (−0.33, 0.39)	0.05 (−0.11, 0.22)	0.07 (−0.21, 0.35)
Naltrexone + CBI	Neither	−0.02 (−0.36, 0.32)	**−0.20 (−0.35, −0.04)**	**−0.37 (−0.66, −0.08)**
Naltrexone only	CBI only	0.25 (−0.11, 0.61)	0.09 (−0.07, 0.25)	−0.07 (−0.37, 0.22)
Naltrexone only	Neither	0.20 (−0.15, 0.54)	**−0.16 (−0.31, −0.00)**	**−0.52 (−0.82, −0.21)**
CBI only	Neither	−0.05 (−0.40, 0.30)	**−0.25 (−0.40, −0.09)**	**−0.44 (−0.72, −0.17)**

Note: Significant effects at 0.05 level are indicated in bold.

treatments. Table 8.2 shows the least square mean comparisons with 95% confidence intervals evaluated at approximately the mean value of the covariate (log number of drinks at baseline = 2), at a value that is about two standard deviations below the mean (log number of drinks at baseline = 1) and at a value that is about two standard deviations above the mean (log number of drinks at baseline = 3). These values correspond to seven, three, and 20 drinks per day (note that on the original scale the values are not equally spaced but correspond to a number of drinks at the lower end of the heavy drinking range, below the commonly used heavy drinking cutoff of 5, and very heavy drinking).

We see quite a bit of variability in the estimates and the confidence intervals depending on the value of the covariate at which we assess the effects. The confidence intervals are tighter when calculated at mean baseline intensity of drinking, and wider at baseline intensity of drinking that is either higher or lower by two standard deviations than the mean (on the log scale). There are no significant differences between the treatment groups when baseline intensity of drinking is low. In contrast, for average and high baseline drinking intensity, the active treatment is better than placebo, with more exaggerated effects at high baseline drinking intensity. Note, though, that since the overall baseline intensity by treatment interaction is not statistically significant, the equal slope model should be used to interpret treatment effects rather than this model.

8.4.2 Analysis of Monthly Drinks per Day Controlling for Baseline Drinking Intensity in the COMBINE Study

Since the outcome drinks per day for subjects who drink is assessed monthly, we perform an analysis of the repeated measures data (months one to four) using a covariance-pattern model and include baseline drinking intensity as a covariate. We follow the steps outlined in Section 8.3.

Step 1: This step is very similar in Section 8.4.1, but there are more time point by treatment combinations. The results are very similar for the longitudinal data so are not presented here. The overall conclusions are the same, so we use log-transformed drinks per day as the outcome, and log-transformed baseline drinking intensity as the covariate. The fixed portion of the model includes effects of treatment, time, log-transformed baseline drinking intensity, and all possible interactions.

Step 2: We select the best-fitting variance–covariance structure for the model with the general fixed-effects structure from step 1. We compare unstructured, autoregressive of first order, autoregressive of first order with heterogeneous variances, compound symmetry and compound symmetry heterogeneous. The unstructured has the lowest AIC, so we choose this option.

Step 3: This step aims to simplify the fixed portion of the model. However, in this case, the three-way interaction between the baseline covariate, time, and treatment is statistically significant ($F(9,946) = 2.12$, $p = 0.03$), and hence, no simplification is possible. The significant interaction means that the differences between treatments vary by time and baseline intensity level.

Step 4: Since there is a significant interaction between treatment, time and baseline intensity, we assess the treatment effects at three different levels of the covariate and at all time points. We again select the mean covariate value and values approximately two standard deviations above and below the mean. Table 8.3 shows the tests of effect slices at each of these three levels of the covariate for each month. We see that at the mean covariate level there are differences between the treatments only at months three and four, while for high levels of baseline drinking there are also differences at month one. The substantive results for months three and four are very similar to the results presented in Table 8.2, so are not shown here (see the online materials for full information). At month one, and for levels of baseline drinking two standard deviations above the mean, the combination treatment is associated with significantly higher drinks per day (0.41, 95% CI: (0.18, 0.65) versus naltrexone; 0.34, 95% CI: (0.11, 0.57) versus CBI; and 0.25, 95% CI: (0.01, 0.49) versus neither) and the rest of the pairwise comparisons are not statistically significant. Thus, the beneficial effects of active treatment are not manifest until month three of the clinical trial. As indicated in the previous subsection, we can also calculate different slopes for the relationship of baseline intensity of drinking with outcome by treatment and time in order to explain the significant interaction, but these are of secondary interest, as the main purpose of the study is to assess treatment effects.

So far, we have considered only a time-independent covariate. In the next subsection, we focus on predictors that are time-varying.

8.4.3 Mixed-Effects Analysis of Depression Trajectories during Recent Unemployment with a Time-Dependent Covariate

In this study introduced in Section 1.5.9, 254 recently unemployed individuals were followed for up to 16 months after a job loss. At each of three interviews after the initial job loss (conducted at different times for different individuals), depression symptoms were measured using the CES-D questionnaire and unemployment status was recorded. More than half of the individuals remained unemployed until the end of the study. Some found work by the second or third interview, and some were re-employed and then lost their job again. We are interested in change in CES-D scores during the follow-up and how unemployment affects depression symptoms. Thus, the main predictor of interest is time. Strictly speaking, unemployment status here is a predictor in its own right, but we use it to illustrate different possibilities for incorporating time-varying covariates in the statistical model for change over time. The main predictor here is continuous (time) and the secondary predictor (unemployment status coded as 1 or 0) is binary.

TABLE 8.3

Tests of Effect Slices for the Treatment Effects by Time Period at Different Levels of Baseline Drinking Intensity

Month	Baseline Drinking Level	Test Statistic	P-Value
1	Two standard deviations below the mean	F(3,946) = 0.73	0.54
2	Two standard deviations below the mean	F(3,946) = 0.38	0.76
3	Two standard deviations below the mean	F(3,946) = 2.49	0.06
4	Two standard deviations below the mean	F(3,946) = 1.31	0.27
1	The mean	F(3,946) = 1.67	0.17
2	The mean	F(3,946) = 1.55	0.20
3	**The mean**	**F(3,946) = 3.95**	**0.008**
4	**The mean**	**F(3,946) = 4.04**	**0.007**
1	**Two standard deviations above the mean**	**F(3,946) = 4.54**	**0.004**
2	Two standard deviations below the mean	F(3,946) = 2.20	0.09
3	**Two standard deviations above the mean**	**F(3,946) = 3.31**	**0.02**
4	**Two standard deviations above the mean**	**F(3,946) = 6.62**	**0.0002**

Note: Significant effects at 0.05 level are indicated in bold.

The first model that we consider is a linear mixed model with CES-D as the response, time as a fixed predictor, and random intercept and slope in order to model individual variability around the average slope. The random intercept and slope are assumed to be correlated. Note that since this study has an unbalanced design (i.e., individuals are not observed at the same time points), the random effects approach is more appropriate than the covariance pattern approach. The second model adds time-varying unemployment status as a fixed main effect to the first model. Thus, unemployment status is assumed to shift CES-D scores by a fixed amount in the population. The third model adds a fixed-effects interaction between unemployment status and time. This means that how much CES-D scores are shifted depends on when during the study re-employment happens. We also considered models with random effects for unemployment status, but since these models either could not be fit or did not provide a better fit than models 1-3, they are not presented here.

Table 8.4 summarizes the results for the fixed-effects estimates from the three models and the model fit criteria. We do not present the random effects estimates here. The online materials present information on the variance components. The estimates in Table 8.4 vary considerably depending on which model is used. In particular, the slope estimate of the

TABLE 8.4

Estimated Slopes and Model Fit Criteria for the Association between Depression and Unemployment Study

Model	AIC	Estimated Slope over Time (95% CI)	Estimated Effect of Unemployment (95% CI)
Model 1: Main effect of time	5143.5	−0.42 (−0.59, −0.26)	—
Model 2: Main effects of time and employment (time-dependent)	5116.1	−0.20 (−0.39, −0.02)	−5.12 (−7.06, −3.17)
Model 3: Interaction of time and employment (time-dependent)	5112.8	Unemployed: 0.16 (−0.22, 0.54) Employed: −0.30 (−0.51, −0.10)	At month 2:−7.60 (−10.61, −4.59) At month 8:−4.81 (−6.77, −2.85) At month 14:−2.02 (−5.47, 1.43)

time effect is −0.40 when unemployment status is not considered, and this changes to −0.20 when unemployment status is considered. Thus, depression severity improves over time but the rate of improvement may be overestimated when we do not control for unemployment status. The main effect of unemployment in model 2 is sizeable (−5.12) which translates into a mean difference of more than five points on CES-D, with better scores for those employed at a particular time point compared with those unemployed. Since re-employment accounts for some of the improvement in depression scores with time after unemployment, it is not surprising that this diminishes the estimate of the time effect. Note, however, that the effects here do not have a causal interpretation since this is an observational study. Conceptually, unemployment may result in more depression symptoms, but depression may also lead to unemployment. A number of other unmeasured confounders may also affect the outcome.

From Table 8.4, we also see that model 2 fits significantly better than model 1. If we do not take unemployment into account we end up overestimating the time effect and might erroneously conclude that individuals recover naturalistically from depression triggered by recent unemployment.

Figure 8.3 shows the estimated mean trajectories from the main effects model 2 when employment status does not vary (employed versus unemployed throughout the study) and when employment status varies. Note that since everybody was unemployed at the first interview, the estimated depression score for employed individuals at the beginning is an extrapolation. Since there is no interaction, the lines are parallel, and change in employment has the effect of shifting estimated depression scores: downward in the case of re-employment and upward in the case of new unemployment.

Similarly, Figure 8.4 shows the estimated mean trajectories from the interaction model when unemployment status varies or does not vary. This time, the lines are not parallel because of the significant interaction ($F(1,425) = 4.55$, $p = 0.03$).

Based on the AIC (Table 8.3), the interaction model (i.e., Model 3) fits the best among the three considered models. The slope for change in depression levels over time is negative when employed (−0.30) and slightly positive (0.16) but non-significantly different from a slope of zero when not employed. Employment is generally associated with lower depression levels; however, there is an indication of converging lines toward the end of the study, which may at least partially be due to regression to the mean (see the three different

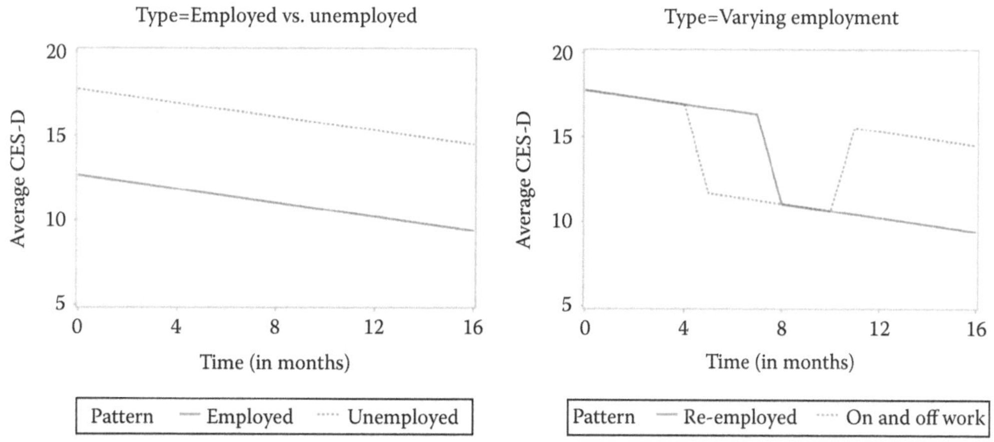

FIGURE 8.3
Estimated mean outcomes from the main effects model in the depression by unemployment status study.

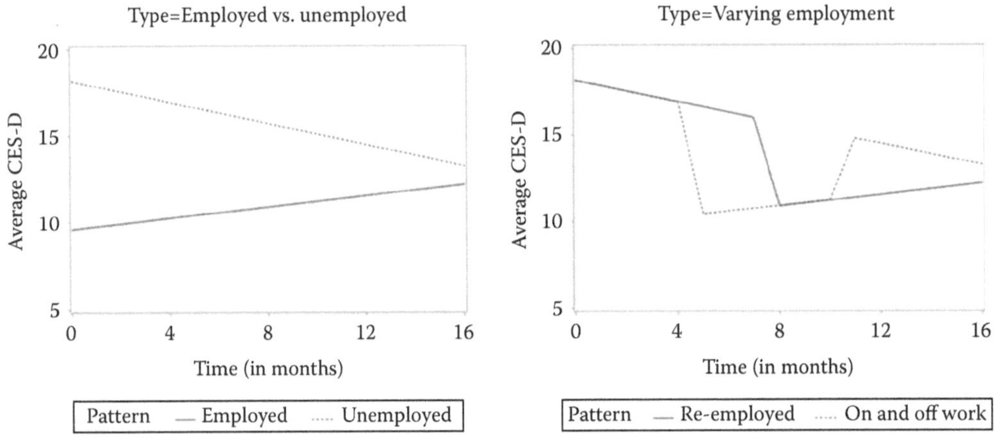

FIGURE 8.4
Estimated mean outcomes from the interaction model in the depression by unemployment status study.

estimates of the unemployment effects at months 2, 8, and 14 of the study). Because of the non-parallel lines, change in employment status has more of an effect on depression at the beginning of the study than toward the end. Note that because both time and employment status are time-varying covariates, interpretation is not as straightforward as in studies with time independent covariates only.

Furthermore, since this is a random effects model, there is inter-individual variability in change over time. Figure 8.5 shows the predicted trajectories for individuals with different patterns of transitions from unemployment to employment. As expected, individuals who remain unemployed tend to maintain their depression levels with only slight improvement. For those who are re-employed, depression scores are estimated to improve with employment and then potentially deteriorate if unemployment happens again.

Additional models and more detailed considerations of this data set can be found in Singer and Willett (2003).

8.4.4 Estimating the Effect of Transition to Retirement on Change in Self-Rated Health in the Health and Retirement Study

We use this analysis to illustrate the different versions of the propensity scoring approach of controlling for measured confounders. For simplicity, we focus on the first two waves of the study and evaluate the relationship between transition into retirement and a binary measure of change in self-rated health. The measure is equal to 1 if the self-rated health assessment worsened from wave 1 to wave 2, and 0 if it stayed the same or improved. A simple chi-square test indicates that retirement and change in self-rated health are indeed statistically significantly associated ($\chi^2(1) = 24.41$, $p < 0.0001$) with 35.9% of retirees compared with 27.5% of the individuals who do not retire in this period reporting worsening health. The estimated odds ratio is 1.48 (95% CI: (1.27, 1.73)); thus, individuals who retire are about 50% more likely to report worsening self-rated health.

The association between retirement and self-rated health may be confounded by a number of other predictors. For example, age is related to both retirement and health. Individuals who retire are older by about two years on average at baseline compared with those who do not retire. Also, older individuals in general report worse health. Other sociodemographic variables and previous self-rated health can also confound the relationship

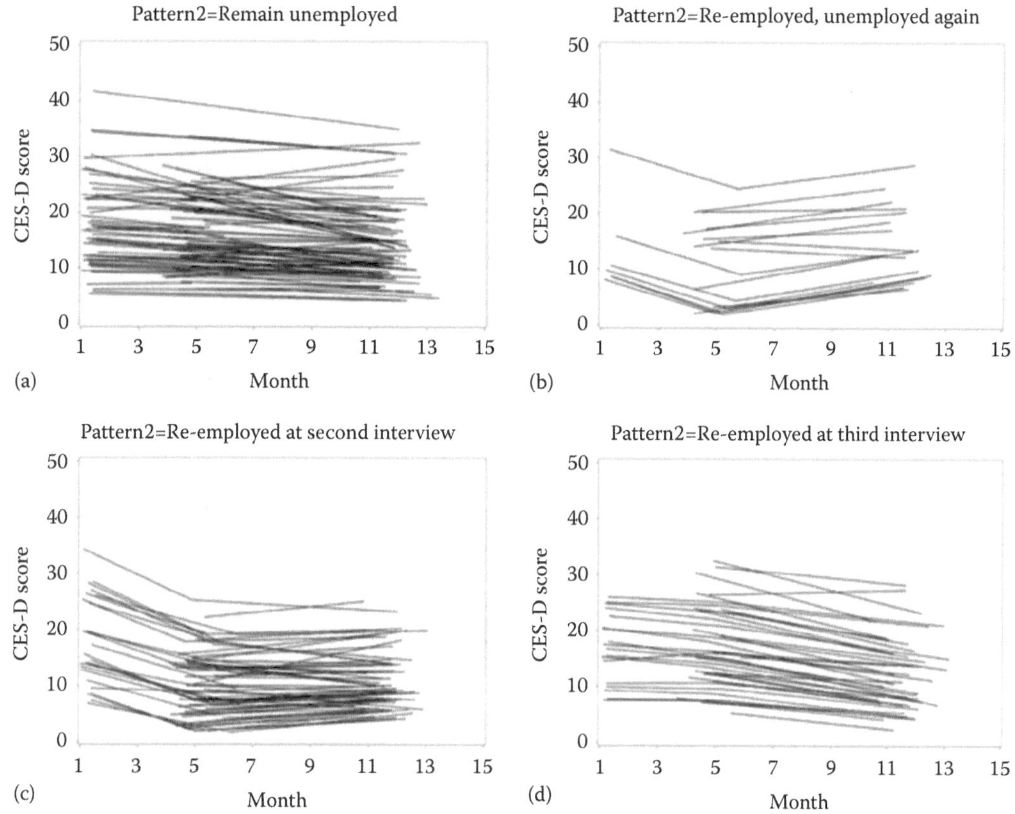

FIGURE 8.5
Estimated individual predictions from the interaction model in the depression by unemployment status study. The estimated individual trajectories are grouped as follows: those who remain unemployed for the duration of the study: (a) panel; those who were re-employed: (b) panel; those who were unemployed for the first interview and re-employed by the second interview: (c) panel; and those who were unemployed during the first and second interviews and re-employed by the third interview: (d) panel.

between retirement and health. Different health conditions can also affect both the decision to retire and the self-assessment of health. Table 8.5 lists variables that are available in the data set and that we considered as potential confounders. The second column of this table shows standardized differences in these variables between subjects who transitioned to retirement and subjects who did not transition. For quantitative variables, the standardized mean difference is the mean difference in the groups divided by the pooled standard deviation. For binary variables, it is the difference in proportions divided by the average of the standard deviations. Some authors prefer to use the standard deviation in the exposure group in the denominator rather than the average of the standard deviations, but both strategies are good as long as they are applied consistently. Standardized differences above 0.10 are considered problematic, especially if larger than 0.25, in variables that are prognostic of the outcome. In these data, the largest standardized differences prior to adjustment are in age, previous self-rated health, and some of the health condition variables (arthritis, heart disease, diabetes). A few other standardized differences are higher than 0.10 as well. Thus, the propensity scoring approach should be used to balance on these potential confounders. Note that the health conditions reflect lifetime prevalence.

TABLE 8.5

Potential Measured Confounders for the Relationship between Transition to Retirement and Change in Self-Rated Health with Standardized Differences between Groups (Retired versus Not Retired) before and after Propensity Score Matching

Variable	Standardized Difference before Adjustment	Standardized Difference after Adjustment
Age	0.59	−0.02
Previous self-rated health	0.34	0.04
Total non-housing wealth	0.04	−0.07
Gender	0.01	−0.01
Smoking (yes, no)	0.06	0.00
Race (white, non-white)	0.05	0.03
Obesity (yes, no)	0.11	0.03
Diabetes (yes, no)	0.23	0.02
High blood pressure (yes, no)	0.19	0.01
Heart disease (yes, no)	0.26	0.03
Stroke (yes, no)	0.20	0.01
Lung disease (yes, no)	0.16	−0.01
Arthritis (yes, no)	0.27	0.03
Cancer (yes, no)	0.06	0.04
Depression at baseline (yes, no)	0.14	−0.01
Ever had depression (yes, no)	0.21	0.03
Psychiatric conditions (yes, no)	0.17	−0.01

We use logistic regression to estimate the predicted probability of retirement (i.e., the propensity score) based on these variables. The distributions of the estimated propensity scores by retirement status are shown in Figure 8.6. There is substantial overlap between the two distributions but, as expected, the propensity scores of those who retire are shifted toward larger estimated probabilities and there is more variability. Thus, adjustment of the propensity score is expected to shift the estimates for the relationship between retirement and change in self-rated health.

We consider all four methods for propensity score adjustment and briefly present the results here. Detailed results are available in the online materials. The propensity score matching is done using a caliper approach, where each observation in the retirement group is matched to two observations in the control group with propensity scores within 0.05 of the target propensity score. The resulting data set is analyzed using conditional logistic regression for matched groups with change in self-rated health as the response and retirement indicator as the predictor. The balance on propensity scores after matching is checked by calculating standardized differences in the matched sample. Balance is excellent, with no standardized differences above 0.10 (see third column of Table 8.5). The adjusted analysis shows a statistically significant association between retirement and change in self-rated health that is stronger than the unadjusted association (see Table 8.6 for the comparison of results across methods).

Propensity score analysis with stratification is performed after dividing the propensity scores into five equal bins and running stratified logistic regression to obtain an overall estimate of the group differences across strata. This adjustment is not as precise as the matching adjustment, but is easier to apply, and in cases when there is good overlap of the propensity score adjustments it works fairly well. The adjusted odds ratio using this

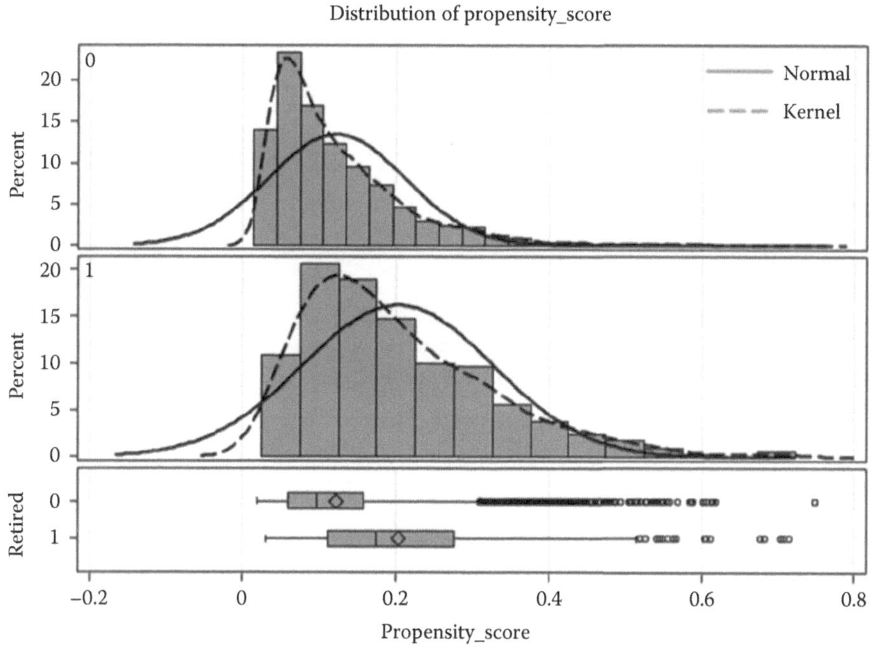

FIGURE 8.6
Distribution of estimated propensity scores for those who do not retire (top histogram) and those that do retire (bottom histogram) in the Health and Retirement Study.

method is in between the odds ratios from the matched propensity score analysis and for the unadjusted analysis.

The propensity score analysis with regression adjustment where the propensity score is simply included as a covariate in the logistic regression model gives very similar results to the stratified approach. Regression adjustment is also very easy to apply but is the least preferred approach, especially when propensity score distributions in the two groups are shifted with respect to one another.

Finally, the propensity score analysis with inverse probability weighting gives a similar result to the propensity score analysis with matching. It is applied by fitting weighted logistic regression. This approach is also easy to use and results in good adjustment except in cases when the probabilities are close to 0 or 1, thus resulting in large weights. In such cases, calibration of the weights can be done.

Although the results differ somewhat when using the propensity score method of adjustment, the general conclusion remains the same—namely, that in this sample, retirement is associated with significantly higher odds of worsening self-rated health which cannot be explained by age, sociodemographic, or health differences between groups. Note that it is still possible that the results are biased due to the effect of unmeasured confounders. In addition, we focused on relatively early retirement (in wave 2, when most individuals are younger than 65). The analysis can be extended to consider retirement in any of the remaining waves, but the analysis will become necessarily more complex as both the main predictor of interest and covariates may be time-varying. The basic idea of the propensity score approaches for time-dependent exposure and covariates is to match individuals based on their entire covariate history during the study. Such models are beyond the scope of this book but interested readers are referred to Lu (2005), Ertefaie and Stephens (2010), Tleyjeh et al. (2010), and Leon et al. (2012).

TABLE 8.6

Odds Ratios for the Association between Retirement and Change in Self-Rated Health in the Health and Retirement Study

Method	Model	Estimated Odds Ratio (95% CI)
Unadjusted association	Unadjusted logistic regression	1.48 (1.27, 1.73)
Propensity scores with matching	Conditional logistic regression for matched groups	1.70 (1.43, 2.01)
Propensity scores with stratification	Stratified logistic regression	1.59 (1.35, 1.87)
Propensity scores with regression adjustment	Logistic regression controlling for the propensity score	1.58 (1.34, 1.86)
Weighting by the inverse of the propensity scores	Weighted logistic regression	1.74 (1.61, 1.88)

8.5 Summary

In this chapter, we reviewed traditional ANCOVA methods and the propensity scoring approach which are used to control for potentially confounding variables. We clarified that the main strength of ANCOVA methods is in improving power and precision in randomized studies rather than in correcting for bias. We cautioned against improper uses of ANCOVA to control for unbalanced covariates in observational studies. The proper steps in performing ANCOVA analysis in cross-sectional and longitudinal studies with time-independent and time-dependent covariates were detailed and illustrated on data examples.

Controlling for covariates in observational studies received special attention. Contrary to popular belief, ANCOVA is rarely appropriate for observational studies, as it generally gives biased results. The propensity scoring approach of achieving balance on observed confounding variables provides estimates of causal effects under strong assumptions. The four different techniques for propensity score adjustment were illustrated on a data example with a single time-independent exposure. Detailed references on adjustments using propensity scoring and related approaches are D'Agostino (1998), Joffe and Rosenbaum (1999), and Rosenbaum (2010).

A limitation of the propensity scoring approach is that we can control only for observed confounders. It is possible that unobserved variables are confounding the observed relationship, in which case one could consider instrumental variable approaches. This is beyond the scope of this book and interested readers are referred to Angrist et al. (1996), Hogan and Lancaster (2004), and Hernan and Robins (2006). In general, methods for causal inference in longitudinal studies are a fast-developing field for statistical research. Useful references are Winship and Morgan (1999), Robins et al. (2000), Robins and Hernan (2009), and Morgan and Winship (2015).

9

Assessment of Moderator and Mediator Effects

In Chapter 8, we reviewed methods of controlling for potentially confounding variables in clinical trials and observational studies. We considered both main and interactive effects of the covariates but we did not posit a particular relationship between the potential covariate and the main predictor of interest. In this chapter, we focus on two particular types of variables—*moderators* and *mediators*—and detail how they clarify the relationship between the main predictor of interest (treatment or exposure) and the outcome. We first focus on randomized experiments and then indicate the additional challenges in assessment of moderator and mediator effects in observational studies.

In general, *moderators* are unrelated to and interact with treatment, and thus indicate for whom or in what circumstances treatment effects are more pronounced. On the other hand, mediators are changed by treatment and some, or all, of the effect of treatment is realized through the effect of the mediators on the outcome. Thus, moderators show for *whom* a treatment works, and hence play an important role in the recent wave of research targeted at personalized interventions or precision medicine. Mediators, on the other hand, show *how* a treatment works, and can provide important information on how to optimize treatment effects.

Assessment of moderator effects is fairly straightforward, and there is general consensus that moderation is present when there is an interaction between the moderator and the main predictor of interest. On the other hand, assessment of mediator effects is still subject to considerable debate, with somewhat different methods and/or differing assumptions offered in the statistics, epidemiology, and psychology literature. In this chapter, we provide an overview of the most commonly used methods at a non-technical level and provide information about recent publications that explain the methods in detail. We place most attention on methods justified from a causal inference perspective with clear assumptions under which the mediator effects have causal interpretation. Interested readers are referred to the recent books of MacKinnon (2008), Jose (2013), Hayes (2013), Hong (2015), and VanderWeele (2015) for more detailed and complete description of methods for moderator and mediator analysis. Important publications that introduce or review the concepts of moderation and/or mediation and describe methods for assessment of such effects are Baron and Kenny (1986), Robins and Greenland (1992), Kraemer et al. (2002), Pearl (2003), Frazier et al. (2004), MacKinnon and Luecken (2008), Imai et al. (2010), Ten Have and Joffe (2012), Hayes (2013), VanderWeele (2015), and Preacher (2015). A good overview of methods used in the psychology literature is MacKinnon et al. (2007). A fairly non-technical overview of causal inference methods for mediation is provided by VanderWeele (2016).

The chapter begins with a description of analysis of moderator effects (Section 9.1), followed by data examples in Section 9.2. Mediation effects are presented with emphasis on the importance of the assumptions required to claim mediation in Section 9.3, and illustrative data examples are provided in Section 9.4. The chapter concludes with a summary and reiteration of the challenges in moderation and mediation analyses in Section 9.5.

9.1 Moderators

Traditionally, clinical trials and observational studies have focused on average treatment or exposure effects. However, in recent years more and more emphasis is placed on identification of subgroups of individuals for whom treatments may be most effective or circumstances under which treatment or exposure effects might differ. Thus, there is an increased effort to identify moderators of treatment effects.

A *moderator* is a variable that affects the strength of the relationship between the main predictor of interest and the outcome. A common moderator in clinical trials is baseline severity of illness. Individuals with more severe illness may benefit to a greater extent from treatment since there is more room for improvement. Age and gender are other commonly explored moderators of treatment effects. A particular treatment may be more effective for younger individuals compared with older individuals, for females compared with males, or vice versa.

9.1.1 Assessment of Moderator Effects

The moderator can be categorical (qualitative) or dimensional (quantitative). We first consider a simple linear model to assess the effect of a dichotomous treatment on an outcome at the end of treatment, and a single moderator where the moderator is unrelated (i.e., independent) to treatment assignment. The latter assumption is crucial in order to be able to claim that moderation has occurred. This independence assumption is usually quite reasonable in randomized studies but not necessarily in observational studies. The model that is used to assess the potential moderating effect is as follows:

$$Y_i = \beta_0 + \beta_1 T_i + \beta_2 M_i + \beta_3 T_i M_i + \varepsilon_i$$

Here, T_i indicates experimental versus control treatment, M_i is the moderator (dimensional or dichotomous), and the interaction between treatment and the moderator is included in the model. The statistical test of the significance of the interaction coefficient, β_3, indicates whether statistically significant moderation is present. If moderation is present, the effects of treatment need to be evaluated at different levels of the moderating variable in order to understand the nature of the moderation. For categorical moderators, the treatment effects are estimated at each of K levels ($K \geq 2$) of the moderator. For continuous moderators, the approach described in Chapter 8 of evaluating treatment effects at the mean, and at values of the moderator one or two standard deviations above and below the mean, should be adopted.

Figure 9.1 shows several hypothetical scenarios illustrating different interaction effects between a dichotomous treatment and a dichotomous moderator on a quantitative outcome. In scenario one, there is a treatment effect at the "high" but not at the "low" level of the moderator. In this scenario, the experimental treatment compared with the control treatment is associated with a larger mean response at the high level of the moderator. In scenario two, there is a treatment effect at the "low" but not at the "high" level of the moderator. In scenario three, the treatment effects are in the opposite direction at the two levels of the moderator. The experimental compared with the control condition has a higher mean response at the "low" level of the moderator, but has a lower mean response at the "high" level of the moderator. In scenario four, there are treatment effects in the same direction at both levels of the moderator, but the magnitude of the effect is larger

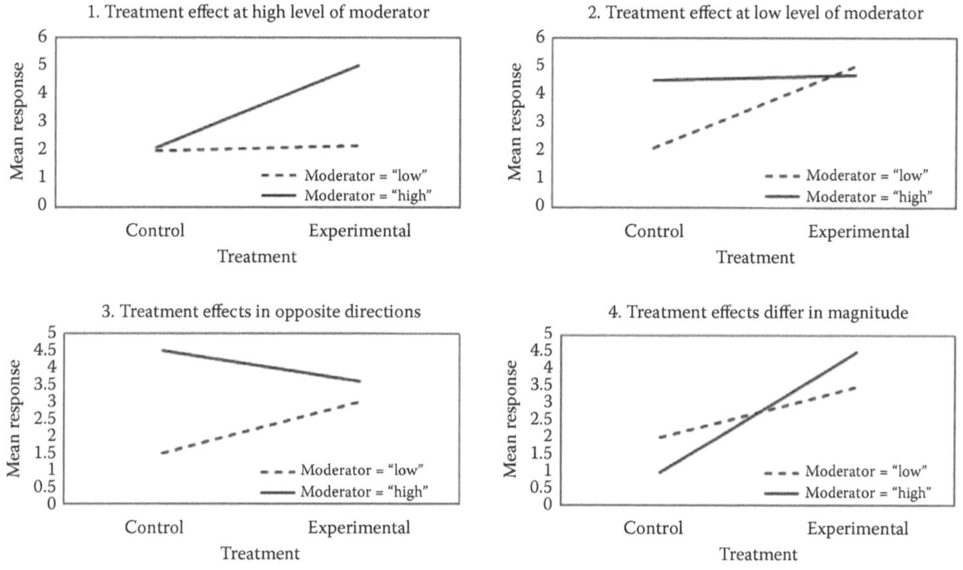

FIGURE 9.1
Four hypothetical scenarios of effects of dichotomous treatment on quantitative outcome moderated by a dichotomous variable.

at the "high" level of the moderator. Note that whether the effects depicted in this figure are statistically significant depends not only on the magnitude of the effect and the variance of the outcome variable but also on the available sample size. It is important to point out that the nature of interactions may change when transformations are applied to the outcome variable, so it is possible that there are moderating effects before, but not after, a transformation, or vice versa. That is, lines may be intersecting before transformation, but not after, or vice versa. Thus, moderator effects need to be interpreted only with respect to the chosen metric and in the context of the available sample size.

Assessment of the nature of the moderating effect is done by evaluating the simple effects of treatment at different levels of the moderator. As usual, it is much more informative to present effect sizes and associated confidence intervals for the simple effects than simply report p-values. Evaluation of simple effects was explained in more detail in Chapter 2. As an example, we used the endpoint data on log-transformed drinks per day in the COMBINE clinical trial to assess the effects of treatment. A significant naltrexone by CBI interaction was identified, and post hoc tests of simple effects were used to illustrate the nature of the interaction. Figure 2.1a showed the simple effects of naltrexone (active versus placebo naltrexone) at each level of CBI (CBI and no CBI) and Figure 2.1b showed the simple effects of CBI (CBI versus no CBI) at each level of naltrexone (active and placebo). These graphs illustrated that active naltrexone significantly lowered drinking compared with placebo for subjects not on CBI, but did not have a significant effect for subjects who received CBI. Thus, if our focus is on naltrexone effects, then we can consider CBI to be a moderator of naltrexone effects since it defines in what circumstance (when no CBI is given) or for whom (subjects who do not get CBI) naltrexone is effective. On the other hand, if we are interested in the effect of CBI, then naltrexone can be considered a moderator of its effect, because CBI is effective in reducing drinking only in the absence of naltrexone. The assumption of independence of the moderator and the main predictor of interest is satisfied in this case because both treatments are randomly assigned. However, in factorial designs such as this one, it is rather unusual to consider one treatment as a moderator of another treatment since we are equally interested in both randomized treatments. More often, moderators are third variables such as baseline characteristics (e.g., gender, initial disease severity) that are not treatments themselves but rather precede treatment. In this sense, there is no ambiguity as to which variable(s) moderates treatment. This is a basic premise of the MacArthur approach to moderation advocated by Kraemer (2011).

We next consider the situation when the outcome is not normally distributed and hence a non-linear link function is used to relate the outcome to the predictors. In this case, assessment of moderator effects can be done according to the following generalized linear model.

$$g(E(Y_i)) = \beta_0 + \beta_1 T_i + \beta_2 M_i + \beta_3 T_i M_i$$

where:

g is an appropriate link function

If Y_i is binary, then the logit function

$$\log \frac{P(Y_i = 1)}{1 - P(Y_i = 1)}$$

is most often used. For ordinal data, the cumulative logit

$$\log \frac{P(Y_i \le k)}{1 - P(Y_i \le k)}$$

is the preferred choice. If Y_i is a count, then $\log(E(Y_i))$ is most commonly used. For simplicity, we assume a binary treatment and a binary moderator. Note that in these cases, the effects (including the moderating effects) are multiplicative rather than additive. This is most readily seen from the model equation. We illustrate this with a count outcome Y_i and log link where we have

$$\log(E(Y_i)) = \beta_0 + \beta_1 T_i + \beta_2 M_i + \beta_3 T_i M_i$$

We can re-write this as

$$E(Y_i) = \exp(\beta_0 + \beta_1 T_i + \beta_2 M_i + \beta_3 T_i M_i) = \exp(\beta_0)\exp(\beta_1 T_i)\exp(\beta_2 M_i)\exp(\beta_3 T_i M_i)$$

Thus, at all possible combinations of the dichotomous treatment and moderator (i.e., substituting 0 and 1 for treatment and the moderator, 1 indicating experimental treatment or "high" level of the moderator, 0 indicating control treatment or "low" level of the moderator) we obtain

$$E(Y_i \mid T_i = 0, M_i = 0) = \exp(\beta_0)$$

$$E(Y_i \mid T_i = 1, M_i = 0) = \exp(\beta_0)\exp(\beta_1)$$

$$E(Y_i \mid T_i = 0, M_i = 1) = \exp(\beta_0)\exp(\beta_2)$$

$$E(Y_i \mid T_i = 1, M_i = 1) = \exp(\beta_0)\exp(\beta_1)\exp(\beta_2)\exp(\beta_3)$$

The simple effects of treatment are the ratios of the means for experimental and control treatment (i.e., when $T_i=1$ compared with when $T_i=0$) at the two levels of the moderator (i.e., when $M_i = 1$ and when $M_i=0$). Thus, the simple effect of treatment at $M_i=0$ is $\exp(\beta_1)$, and at $M_i=1$ is $\exp(\beta_1)\exp(\beta_3)$. The ratio of these simple effects is $\exp(\beta_3)$. When $\beta_3=0$, the two simple effects are the same, and hence there is no indication of a moderation because the treatment effect is the same at both levels of the moderator. When $\beta>0$, the simple effect of treatment at the "high" level of the moderator is $\exp(\beta_3)$ times higher than at the "low" level of the moderator. Similarly, when $\beta_1<0$, the simple effect of treatment at the "high" level of the moderator is $\exp(\beta_3)$ times lower than at the "low" level of the moderator. Note that the interpretation of the ratio (which indicates the strength of the moderator effects) depends on the magnitude of the effect at the "low" level of the moderator. For example, if there is no effect of treatment at the "low" level of the moderator (i.e., the mean ratio for the treatment effect is 1) and at the "high" level the treatment effect is increased 1.5 times (i.e., $\exp(\beta_3)=1.5$, an increase of 50%), then we might have a significant treatment effect at the "high" level of the moderator (i.e., a mean ratio of 1.5) but not at the "low" level of the moderator (i.e., a mean ratio of 1). But in another scenario, with $\exp(\beta_3)=1.5$, if at the "low" level of the moderator the treatment effect is below 1 (e.g., the mean ratio is 0.7), then a 50% increase ($0.7\times1.5=1.05$) brings this effect to the neutral range around 1, where there is almost no difference in outcome between the treatment levels. This means that there is no effect at the "high" level of the moderator, but there is an effect at the "low" level of the moderator. Thus, the interpretation of the magnitude and significance of the β_3 parameter (i.e., the log-mean ratio in the log-linear model) needs to be supplemented by interpretation of the magnitudes and significance of the simple effects. Plots of simple effects can be very helpful in such a situation. We present a data example to illustrate this point in Section 9.2.1.

Note that there is no guarantee that either the assumption of additive effects made in the linear model or the assumption of multiplicative effects made in the log-linear model is correct. If there are concerns about the model assumptions in the model used to assess moderation, non-parametric approaches or less restrictive models (e.g., General Additive Models [Hastie and Tibshirani, 1987; Hastie et al., 1990]) can be used. A non-technical reference is Wang and Ware (2013).

9.1.2 Moderator Effects in Experimental and Observational Studies

In experimental studies such as clinical trials the effect of treatment has a causal interpretation. That is, whatever differences occur in outcome between treatment groups can be interpreted as treatment effects, since the treatment groups are balanced on measured and unmeasured confounders (including the potential moderators) at baseline due to randomization. In this context, a moderator variable indicates how the causal treatment effect changes depending on the value of the moderator. In observational studies, however, the potential moderator and treatment\exposure can be related, in which case it is difficult to claim causality. That is, individuals can receive a particular treatment more often, or could be more often exposed at a particular level of the potential moderating variable, than at another level. For example, more severely ill patients may receive treatment A rather than treatment B in non-randomized studies. In such a case, assessing the moderating effect of baseline illness severity is problematic because the moderator and treatment are statistically associated.

In randomized studies, such as COMBINE, the moderating effects have causal interpretation because randomization ensures that the moderator and treatment are unrelated and there should be no residual confounding of the treatment with other variables. However, note that unchecked exploration of moderator effects (i.e., testing of every potential moderator one at a time) may still lead to spurious results because of the multiple testing issue, and because chance imbalances on covariates at baseline may lead to confounding between treatment and moderator effects, especially in small studies. In general, the gold standard for assessment of moderator effects is to pre-specify the moderator(s) and to stratify the randomization on the moderator(s), thus ensuring that treatments are balanced within each level of the moderator(s). Some of the most commonly explored moderators in clinical trials are gender, site (in multisite studies), and illness severity at baseline (often described with a categorical variable). It is frequently of interest to assess whether treatment effects are stronger/weaker in males versus females, at urban versus rural sites, or for subjects with more severe versus less severe illness.

In observational studies, assessment of moderator effects is more complicated, since exposure may be related to the potential moderators. For example, in Chapter 8 we used data from the Health and Retirement Study to assess the effect of the transition to retirement on self-rated health. As a further analysis, we might be interested whether age moderates the effect of retirement on health, since the transition from working life to retirement may be different for those who retire early and for those who retire late. However, age and retirement are not independent. Thus, even if there is an interaction between age and retirement, we cannot claim moderating effects, as alternative explanations may be as plausible: transition to retirement may be a mediator of age effects, and both can be proxy predictor factors (i.e., they stand in for other direct predictors of health). To assess whether the moderator and treatment are related, one can use chi-square tests of association for categorical moderators and treatment, correlations for continuous moderators and treatment, and t-tests or ANOVAs when one variable is categorical and the other is continuous. Propensity scoring approaches should be used for observational data in order to balance the treatment\exposure groups on levels of the moderator to be able to interpret interactions as moderating effects (see Chapter 8 for a description of the propensity scoring approaches).

In conclusion, in both experimental and observational studies, the potential moderator should be unrelated to the treatment or exposure. If treatment or exposure affects the potential moderator, or treatment is selected partly based on the level of the moderator, we may not have moderating effects. Rather, different relationship among the variables may exist—we might have mediation, partial mediation, proxy predictor factors, or overlapping predictors. See Kraemer et al. (2001) for a classification of predictors in observational studies.

9.1.3 Moderator Effects in Longitudinal Studies

Our discussion of moderating effects has so far applied to both cross-sectional and longitudinal studies. Note that assessment of moderator effects in longitudinal studies is often no more complicated than in cross-sectional studies. Since the moderator and the main predictor of interest (treatment or exposure) need to be independent of one another, moderators are often measured before treatment. Thus, in order to assess moderating effects, we simply assess interactions between the moderator and treatment. These interactions may be time-independent or time-dependent. When they are time-independent (i.e., there is no three-way interaction between the potential moderator, treatment and time), post hoc testing of simple effects proceeds as with cross-sectional data but is done within the mixed model or GEE model that takes time into account. The three-way interaction between the moderator, treatment and time could be removed from the model for ease of interpretation. In this case the simple effects of treatment by moderator level will be averaged across time.

On the other hand, when the interaction is time-dependent (i.e., when there is statistically significant interaction between the moderator, treatment, and time), tests of simple effects of treatment by level of the moderator need to also be performed by time point (in the case of categorical time and/or balanced designs). The relationship between treatment and time (e.g., differences in slopes of change over time between treatment groups) need to be evaluated by values of the moderator when time is treated as a continuous predictor and/or the design is unbalanced. Although this entails more comparisons, ultimately moderation can be claimed when the direction and/or magnitude of treatment effects varies by levels of the moderator (whether in a time-independent or time-dependent fashion). As long as the metric for assessment of moderator effects is correct, and there is indeed no relationship between the moderator and treatment, we can interpret significant interactions as moderating effects and follow up with tests of simple effects. We show some examples in Section 9.2.

9.1.4 Moderator Effects in Studies with Clustering

When data are clustered (e.g., individuals clustered within schools, patients within providers), moderators may be measured at the level of the individual or at the level of the cluster. In both cases, the interaction between the moderator of interest and the primary treatment or exposure variable needs to be considered to assess moderation. Interpretation is not problematic once the moderator and the predictor of interest are not related, but one needs to take into account the correlation of the observations within clusters in the analysis.

9.1.5 Multiplicity Corrections for Moderator Analyses

In addition to the requirement of no relationship between treatment and the moderator, a cautionary note must be made regarding "fishing" for moderator effects. Moderator analyses are often considered exploratory, and a large number of potential moderators are sometimes evaluated. Correction for multiple comparisons should be used in this situation. Depending on the number of moderators and the desired trade-off between power and the potential for a type I error, FWER or FDR corrections should be applied for all interaction tests as described in Chapter 6. Usually, for many simultaneous exploratory analyses, especially including multiple genotypes, an FDR correction is preferred. For confirmatory moderator analyses, FWER is more appropriate.

9.2 Data Examples of Moderator Analysis

9.2.1 Moderation of Treatment Effects on Number of Drinking Days in the COMBINE Study

In previous chapters, we outlined how interactive effects are used to assess the combined effects of treatments in linear models. In Section 9.1, we also described multiplicative rather than additive interactions in generalized linear models. Herein, we continue the COMBINE example to illustrate assessment and interpretation of moderator effects in log-linear models where the interactions are multiplicative on the original scale. We focus on the count outcome number of drinking days during the treatment period and use a log-linear GEE model to relate the outcome to naltrexone, CBI, and their interaction. Abstinence from drinking (dichotomized into less than two weeks and two weeks or more) in the 30 days prior to randomization is hypothesized to be a moderator of treatment effects based on prior research (Gueorguieva et al., 2014). Thus, we include interactions among the treatments, abstinence, and time (month in treatment) to evaluate moderator effects. The highest order interaction in this model involves four factors (naltrexone, CBI, pre-randomization abstinence, and time), and for simplicity, we eliminate non-significant interactions one at a time (first the four-way, then the three-way non-significant interactions, then non-significant two-way interactions). Table 9.1 shows the significant effects remaining in the model together with lower-order terms that make the model hierarchically well-formulated (e.g., the naltrexone main effect is retained, although non-significant, because the naltrexone by CBI interaction is statistically significant).

Herein, we focus on the significant interaction between baseline abstinence and CBI since it suggests that the effect of CBI varies for individuals who were able to remain abstinent for two weeks or more compared with those who were not. Simple effects are used to explain the interaction.

The estimate of the interaction parameter β_3 is −0.39 (SE = 0.16). Thus, the log rate ratio of CBI versus no CBI in the longer abstinence group is 0.39 units lower than in the shorter abstinence group. Bringing the estimate back to the original scale by exponentiating, we get

$$\exp(\beta_3) = \exp(-0.39) = 0.68$$

Thus, the rate ratio for the CBI effect in the longer abstinence group is 0.68 times that in the shorter abstinence group. However, without knowing what the effect is in the shorter abstinence group (i.e., whether it is beneficial, detrimental, or neutral) we cannot fully interpret this information. We need to look at the rate ratios for the effect of CBI for each abstinence group. We estimate that the rate ratio is 1.00 (0.87, 1.16) in the shorter abstinence group and 0.68 (95% CI: (0.52, 0.89)) in the longer abstinence group. Thus, CBI treatment does not affect the outcome in the shorter abstinence group, but there is a significant protective effect of CBI on number of drinking days in the longer abstinence group. This makes pre-randomization abstinence a moderator of the effect of CBI irrespective of the

TABLE 9.1

Tests of Main Effects and Interactions in the Final Model Evaluating Moderation by Pre-Randomization Abstinence of Treatment Effects on Number of Drinking Days in the COMBINE Study

Effect	Test Statistic	P-Value
Pre-randomization abstinence	$\chi^2(1) = 52.96$	<0.0001
Naltrexone	$\chi^2(1) = 1.94$	0.16
CBI	$\chi^2(1) = 5.78$	0.02
Time	$\chi^2(3) = 46.99$	<0.0001
Abstinence × CBI	$\chi^2(1) = 6.05$	0.01
CBI × Time	$\chi^2(3) = 11.13$	0.01
Naltrexone × CBI	$\chi^2(1) = 4.68$	0.03

level of naltrexone, and the results indicate for what type of individuals CBI is most effective. At the same time, pre-randomization abstinence is not a moderator of the effect of naltrexone as there are no significant interactions between naltrexone and abstinence in the final model. The other significant interactions in the model should also be interpreted, but they do not represent moderating effects of pre-treatment abstinence. Moderation in this example is described by multiplicative, rather than additive, effects because we are basing inferences on the log-linear model.

9.2.2 Type of Cigarettes Smoked as a Moderator of Nicotine Effects in Smokers

The human laboratory study of the effects of menthol on nicotine reinforcement in smokers introduced in Section 1.5.7 has a two-level cross-over experimental design with three different levels of menthol (high, low, placebo) administered on three different test days in random order. Within each test day, again in random order, three different nicotine concentrations (saline, low dose, high dose) were infused and effects of nicotine were measured using the Drug Effects Questionnaire scale. The design of the study is shown in Figure 1.12. In Chapter 5, we used these data to illustrate the non-parametric approach to the analysis of repeated measures data. We looked at menthol and nicotine effects and their interactions on drug liking effects. Herein, we focus on the entire sample of subjects and on a different outcome; namely, maximum stimulatory effects during each infusion. The sample consists of two types of individuals: those who smoke mentholated cigarettes and those who smoke non-mentholated cigarettes. The question of interest here is whether nicotine and menthol effects vary depending on the preferred type of cigarettes smoked. Thus, we are investigating whether preference for mentholated cigarettes is a moderator of nicotine and menthol effects. Note that the potential moderator in this study is pre-specified and randomization is stratified on it, thus guaranteeing that there is no relationship between the moderator and the treatments.

To assess the moderator effect, we fit a linear mixed model with maximum stimulatory effects during each test session (square root transformed to deal with positive skewness) as the repeatedly measured outcome, nicotine and menthol as within-subject factors, and type of cigarettes smoked as a between-subject factor. We also control for session and period effects since there might be systematic changes in individual responses from the first to the third test session as subjects adjust to the experimental setting, and from the first to the third period within each test session as subjects might be getting tired. The model with random effects for subject, menthol dose, and nicotine dose within subject fits the best according to the AIC and BIC. Table 9.2 shows the results from the tests of statistical significance of all interactions and main effects in the model.

We focus on the statistically significant interaction between mentholated cigarettes and nicotine because it indicates a moderating effect; that is, nicotine effects vary for smokers of mentholated cigarettes compared with smokers of non-mentholated cigarettes. Figure 9.2 shows the pattern of least square means that describes the nature of the interaction. Dose-dependent nicotine effects are highly statistically significant in both groups ($p < 0.0001$); thus, the moderating effect of type of cigarette is one of magnitude, not direction and significance. Additional post hoc testing shows that smokers of non-mentholated cigarettes acknowledge, on average, significantly greater stimulatory effects than smokers of mentholated cigarettes at high and low nicotine doses ($p = 0.0008$ and $p = 0.025$, respectively) but not when saline is infused ($p = 0.88$). Stimulating effects are significantly higher during the first session compared with the second session ($p = 0.0007$). All code and results can be found in the online materials.

TABLE 9.2

Tests of Main Effects and Interactions in the Study of Type of Cigarettes Smoked (Mentholated or Non-Mentholated) as Moderator of Menthol and Nicotine Stimulatory Effects in Smokers

Effect	Test Statistic	P-Value
Mentholated cigarettes	F(1,163) = 5.27	0.02
Menthol	F(2,85) = 2.33	0.10
Nicotine	F(2,105) = 70.30	< 0.0001
Mentholated × Menthol	F(2,163) = 0.41	0.66
Mentholated × Nicotine	F(2,163) = 6.51	0.002
Menthol × Nicotine	F(4,163) = 1.88	0.12
Mentholated × Menthol × Nicotine	F(4,163) = 1.99	0.10
Session	F(2,163) = 5.99	0.003
Period	F(2,163) = 1.05	0.35

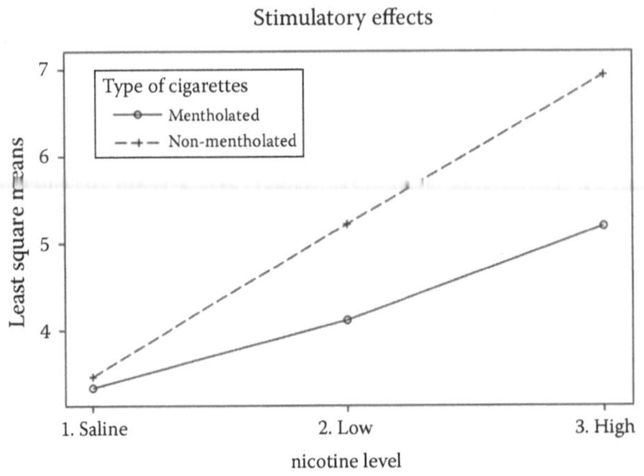

FIGURE 9.2
Estimated least square means for the moderating effect of types of cigarettes smoked on nicotine effects in the human laboratory study of menthol's effects on nicotine reinforcement in smokers.

9.3 Mediators

Mediation analyses assess how a particular treatment or exposure works. A mediator is a variable that is affected by treatment or exposure and reflects a mechanism through which all or part of the treatment/exposure effect on the outcome is produced. Treatment can have a direct effect on the outcome and/or an indirect effect via the mediator variable. Mediational analysis is focused on estimating the direct and indirect effects with the ultimate goal of making inferences about the causal effect of treatment via the mediator.

As an example, consider a medication treatment for alcohol dependence that is expected to reduce drinking by reducing craving. In this situation, the predictor is treatment, the potential mediator is craving, and the outcome is a measure of drinking, such as number of drinking days or drinks per drinking day. Treatment can have a direct effect on drinking behavior or an indirect effect via reduction of craving. In mediation analysis, the goal is to evaluate the direct and indirect effects and assess whether there is evidence to support pre-specified mechanistic hypotheses.

Unlike moderator analysis, where there is consensus among researchers about methods of assessment, assumptions, and limitations, the literature is not all in agreement regarding the approaches, assumptions and caveats of mediator analysis. In this section, we first provide a short overview of the most popular approach used in the psychology literature, then focus on the causal inference approach to mediation and carefully describe assumptions that are necessary to infer causality.

9.3.1 Assessment of Mediator Effects: The Baron and Kenny Approach

The basic idea of mediation analysis with a single mediator, presented in the influential article by Baron and Kenny (1986) and used widely in the psychology literature (see also Judd and Kenny, 1981), is illustrated in Figure 9.3. Mediation effects are typically assessed when there is an effect of the main predictor of interest (X, often called a *causal variable*) on the outcome (Y) as shown in Figure 9.3a. The total effect of X on Y is denoted by $\mathbf{c}_1$. Mediation occurs if the causal variable (X), affects the outcome (Y), X affects the mediator (M), M affects Y, and part or all of the effect of X on Y is via M. Figure 9.3b shows the effect of the predictor on the mediator (denoted by $\mathbf{a}_1$), the effect of the mediator on the outcome (denoted by $\mathbf{b}_2$) adjusted for the main predictor of interest, and the remaining *direct effect* of the predictor on the outcome (denoted by $\mathbf{b}_1$). The *indirect effect* of the predictor on the outcome is defined as the product of $\mathbf{a}_1$ and $\mathbf{b}_2$ (i.e., the product of the effects of X on M and the effect of M on Y), or it can be calculated as the difference between the total and the direct effect ($\mathbf{c}_1-\mathbf{b}_1$). The former definition is obtained using *the product method* (as originally proposed by Baron and Kenny). The latter definition has been more widely used in the epidemiology and biomedical literature. The two definitions coincide when linear models for a continuous outcome and a continuous mediator are used to estimate the relationships between the outcome, mediator and treatment. In such a situation, the *total effect* of the causal variable on the outcome is the sum of the direct and indirect effects ($\mathbf{c}_1=\mathbf{b}_1+\mathbf{a}_1.\,\mathbf{b}_2$). In other cases (e.g., non-linear models such as logistic regression and survival analysis), this simple decomposition of the total effect does not hold and the formulae need to be modified (to be discussed later).

Baron and Kenny (1986) suggested using regression models to ascertain these statistical relationships and described the following four steps for establishing mediator effects.

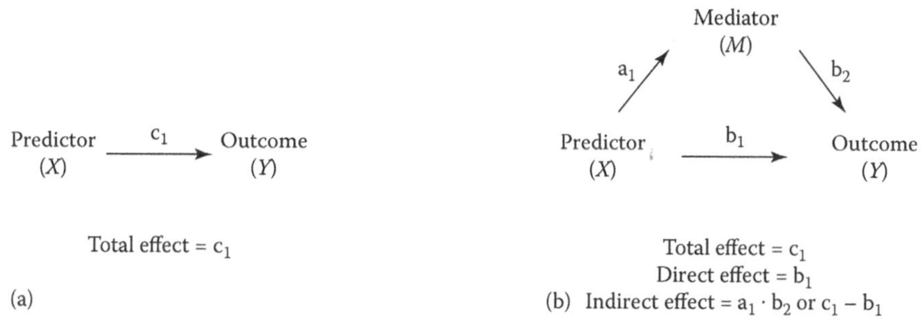

FIGURE 9.3
Total, direct, and indirect effect of predictor X on outcome Y via mediator M.

Step 1: Establish whether there is an effect that can be mediated. That is, assess the regression relationship between Y and X and evaluate whether effect $\mathbf{c}_1$ is different from zero.

Step 2: Establish that X is related to M. That is, establish a regression relationship between X and M, treating M as the outcome (effect $\mathbf{a}_1$).

Step 3: Establish that M is related to Y (effect $\mathbf{b}_2$) when X is controlled in a regression model.

Step 4: From the same equation used in the preceding step, evaluate whether the direct effect of X on Y (effect $\mathbf{b}_1$) is zero. If it is, declare that full mediation has occurred. If not, partial mediation has occurred.

Several cautions to this algorithm apply. First, statistical significance was originally required to be present at all steps to claim mediation, but statistical significance depends largely on the sample size and, hence, it is possible for mediation to occur even if some of the effects are not statistically significant. In addition, it can be the case that there is a statistically significant indirect effect but no total effect because the direct and indirect pathways are in opposite directions and are cancelling each other out. In this situation, when following the four-step approach described, one would stop at the first stage and not proceed. Thus, the modern interpretation of this approach is to focus only on steps two and three and to skip step one.

Second, even when the conditions in all four steps above are satisfied, mediation may not be present since alternative models may also be consistent with the data. This is especially true if *reverse causation* is present between the mediator and the predictor. That is, the mediator is effecting a change in the predictor and not the reverse. This may well appear as a statistically significant effect in step two, but the direction of the arrow is from M to X rather than from X to M. Some researchers (e.g., Kraemer, 2011) require that there is a strict temporal ordering of treatment/exposure, change in the mediator, and change in the outcome. In particular, treatment should precede the change in the mediator which should precede the change in the outcome in order to be able to claim that the effects are in the required direction for mediation. The causal inference approach discussed in the next section requires temporal precedence too, but this follows from the more general assumptions of that method.

Third, other variables may confound the mediation relationship. There may be variables that affect both the mediator and the outcome, both the predictor and the mediator, or all three variables. In this case, following the Baron and Kenny approach without additional adjustment for such confounders leads to biased and often uninterpretable results. Proper control for confounding is a focus of much current research and is the basis for many of the developments in causal inference and mediator analysis.

Fourth, the Baron and Kenny approach does not allow for an interaction between the treatment/exposure and the mediator. Other researchers (e.g., Kraemer et al., 2001; Kraemer et al., 2002; Valeri and VanderWeele, 2013; VanderWeele, 2013) consider interactive effects to be necessary for proper assessment of mediator effects, because mediator effects may be present only for certain levels of the predictor or can vary by treatment level. We focus on this issue when describing mediation analysis from a causal inference perspective in Section 9.3.2.

Fifth, there may be multiple mediation variables through which treatment or exposure effects are produced. It is possible to examine multiple mediators in the same model (see e.g., Preacher and Hayes 2008), but the models and assumptions become necessarily more complex.

As a last note of caution, when a parametric model is considered in the four steps, the results regarding mediation are valid only if the model is correctly specified. This applies to distributional assumptions; causal ordering of the predictor, mediator, and outcome; and no confounding by other variables (to be discussed in more detail in the causal inference subsection). We now consider the linear regression models most commonly used in the four-step approach for a continuous outcome and a continuous mediator.

The linear regression model equations are as follows:

$$\text{Step 1}: Y_i = c_0 + c_1 X_i + \varepsilon_{1i}$$

$$\text{Step 2}: M_i = a_0 + a_1 X_i + \varepsilon_{2i}$$

$$\text{Steps 3 and 4}: Y_i = b_0 + b_1 X_i + b_2 M_i + \varepsilon_{3i}$$

The usual assumptions of normality and independence of the errors apply. In particular, the errors ε_{2i} and ε_{3i} are assumed to be independent, which may very well not be the case. That is, there may be residual confounding between the outcome and the mediator due to unmeasured variables or failure to include interaction effects. Baron and Kenny's approach can be used when potentially confounding covariates are added to these models. However, the simple decomposition of total effect into direct and indirect effect as defined earlier no longer holds when there are interactions between treatment and the mediator. We show an extension of the Baron and Kenny approach from a causal inference perspective in Section 9.3.2.

As an additional note to the model definition described, generalized linear models, rather than linear models, can be used when the outcome and/or mediator are non-normal. However, since the relationship between outcome, mediator, and treatment are no longer linear (e.g., logit or log is used to relate the mediator and the outcome to treatment when the response is binary, log is used for count mediator and/or outcome), the total effect is not equal to the sum of the direct and indirect effects. In general, the Baron and Kenny approach does not generalize easily and naturally to non-linear models. In contrast, the causal inference approach presented in the next section is more general and can apply to both linear and non-linear models.

9.3.2 Assessment of Mediator Effects: The Causal Inference Approach

We now present the causal inference approach based on counterfactual logic, which extends the Baron and Kenny approach and clarifies the assumptions necessary to claim mediation. This approach can be used even in situations when there is an interaction between treatment and the mediator and when there are non-linearities in the effects. Many authors provide detailed descriptions with somewhat differing notation and the presentation is often technical (see e.g., Robins et al., 2000; Little and Rubin, 2000; Rubin, 2005; Imai et al., 2010; Pearl, 2010; Ten Have and Joffe, 2012; Valeri and VanderWeele, 2013; Muthen and Asparouhov, 2015). A recent publication that provides a good overview at a non-technical level is VanderWeele (2016).

The causal inference approach to mediation is based on the notion of *counterfactual outcomes*. We introduced counterfactual outcomes in Chapter 8 in the context of the propensity scoring method of adjustment for measured confounders when estimating treatment or exposure effects in observational studies. We continue this line of thought here to justify methods for assessment of mediator effects in experimental or observational studies.

Our focus is on a simple situation with a binary treatment (exposure) in a parallel design setting (i.e., each individual gets one of the treatments). For simplicity, our main predictor of interest, X, is a treatment with values 1 and 0, with 1 indicating experimental and 0 indicating control treatment. We observe only the outcome of the individual on the assigned treatment. The outcome on the alternative treatment is called a *counterfactual outcome* as it is unobserved. The causal effect of treatment for each individual is the difference between the outcome of the experimental and the control treatment (denoted by $Y_i(1) - Y_i(0)$). Since we observe only $Y_i(1)$ for subjects on the experimental treatment and $Y_i(0)$ for subjects on the control treatment, we cannot estimate the causal effect at the individual level for any of the individuals. However, the *average causal effect* is defined as the average of the individual causal effects over all individuals in the population $E\{Y_i(1) - Y_i(0)\} = E\{Y_i(1)\} - E\{Y_i(0)\}$. This effect can be estimated in randomized studies because the expected outcome in the population on each treatment can be estimated by the average of the outcomes of the individuals assigned to that treatment. Due to randomization, subjects in each treatment group are representative of the entire population; hence, their average response is a good estimate of the average response in the population. In observational studies, however, the causal interpretation is more problematic, since individuals in the exposed and non-exposed groups may differ on a variety of characteristics and there may be many variables that affect both exposure and treatment and thus act as *confounders* of the causal relationship of interest.

In causal mediation analysis, the idea is to define direct, indirect, and total effects of treatment on the outcome using counterfactual outcomes, under very general conditions, and to make clear the assumptions that are being made in order to claim mediation. To do this, we consider factual and counterfactual values of the mediator. Let $M_i(1)$ and $M_i(0)$ be the values of the mediator for subject i if this subject were to receive the experimental or control treatment, respectively. As with the outcome, only one of the two mediator values is observed for each subject. To define direct and indirect effects, we consider the outcome under different combinations of levels of the treatment and the mediator $Y_i(t,m)$. Treatment t can be 1 or 0 (experimental or control) and m denotes any value of the mediator. Of specific interest are the cases when $m = M_i(1)$ or $m = M_i(0)$ that reflect the value of the mediator under experimental and control treatment, respectively. The following outcomes are of interest:

$Y_i(0,M_i(0))$—outcome on the control treatment when the mediator value is fixed to what it would be if the control treatment was given

$Y_i(1,M_i(1))$—outcome on the experimental treatment when the mediator value is fixed to what it would be if the experimental treatment was given

$Y_i(1,M_i(0))$—outcome on the experimental treatment when the mediator is manipulated to reflect the effect of the control treatment on the mediator.

With this notation, the total causal effect of treatment for an individual is $Y_i(1,M_i(1)) - Y_i(0,M_i(0))$ and the *average total causal effect* (*TCE*) in the population is

$$\text{TCE}: E\{Y_i(1, M_i(1)) - Y_i(0, M_i(0))\}$$

The total causal effect is the effect of treatment when the mediator is allowed to take its natural value under experimental or control treatment.

The *natural direct effect* (NDE, also known as *pure/total direct effect*) is the effect of treatment when the mediator is fixed at the value it would take under the control treatment.

Thus, the direct effect is interpreted as the effect of treatment when the mediator is not allowed to be influenced by treatment and, therefore, the effect that is measured is occurring either directly or through other unspecified pathways. The population-averaged NDE is

$$\text{NDE}: E\{Y_i(1, M_i(0)) - Y_i(0, M_i(0))\}$$

The *natural indirect effect* (NIE) is the effect of the mediator on the outcome under the experimental treatment. It measures the effect that is transmitted through the mediator, not allowing treatment to directly influence the outcome. The population-averaged NIE is

$$\text{NIE}: E\{Y_i(1, M_i(1)) - Y_i(1, M_i(0))\}$$

There is another useful definition in the causal inference literature; namely, the *controlled direct effect* (CDE). The CDE measures the effect of treatment when the mediator is controlled at a particular value m:

$$\text{CDE}: E\{Y_i(1, m) - Y_i(0, m)\}$$

In the model formulation of the Baron and Kenny approach, the CDE is the direct effect, $\mathbf{b}_1$, that is estimated in the third step (rather than the NDE, which fixes the mediator at the value achieved under the control treatment). The CDE and the NDE coincide when there is no interaction between treatment and the mediator in the linear model as then the effect of treatment is the same for any fixed value of the mediator. However, when there is an interaction between treatment and the mediator, the CDE and NDE are not the same.

Note that as long as no assumptions of a particular model are made to define the direct and indirect effects, the formulae are valid for all kinds of outcomes (continuous, categorical) and there are no restrictions on what interactions are present. However, parametric models are often considered for assessment of mediator effects and hence more specific expressions appropriate for the particular types of outcomes (e.g., continuous, dichotomous, count) are defined.

We first focus on the situation with a continuous mediator, a continuous outcome, and a binary treatment and follow the approach of Valeri and VanderWeele (2013) in order to illustrate the similarities and the greater flexibility of the causal inference mediational analysis compared with the Baron and Kenny approach. The formulae extend to the situation when the main predictor of interest (treatment or exposure) is measured on a continuous scale.

We again assume linear models for the mediator and the outcome but this time allow for interactive effects between the treatment and mediator and adjust for potential covariates that might confound the effect of treatment on the mediator and outcome. It may be necessary to include interaction effects because the effect of the mediator on the outcome may vary by treatment level. In addition, observed covariates may confound the relationship between the mediator and outcome, and even between treatment and the outcome in observational studies; thus, ignoring them may produce bias in the estimates. Under these assumptions, the model equations for mediational analysis are as follows:

$$\text{Equation 1}: M_i = a_0 + a_1 X_i + a_2' C_i + \varepsilon_i$$

$$\text{Equation 2}: Y_i = b_0 + b_1 X_i + b_2 M_i + b_3 X_i M_i + b_4' D_i + \delta_i$$

The errors in the two equations are assumed uncorrelated once we have accounted for the potential confounders. The coefficient for the interactive effect of treatment and the mediator, which is also added to the model in Equation 2, is b_3. C_i are covariates that affect the mediator, while D_i are covariates that affect the outcome.

Based on this model, the formulae for the CDE, NDE, and NIE (obtained by replacing the mediator value in Equation 2 with the expression from Equation 1 and taking an expectation) are as follows:

$$\text{CDE} = b_1 + b_3 m$$

$$\text{NDE} = b_1 + b_3(a_0 + a_2'C)$$

$$\text{NIE} = (b_2 + b_3)a_1$$

To clarify how these are obtained, let us consider CDE and NIE. From the general formula for CDE, we need to evaluate $E\{Y_i(1,\text{m}) - Y_i(0,m)\}$ based on the assumed model. From Equation 2, we have

$$E\{Y_i(1,m)\} = b_0 + b_1 + b_2 m + b_3 m + b_4' D_i$$

and

$$E\{Y_i(0,m)\} = b_0 + b_2 m + b_4' D_i$$

Therefore, the difference is $CDE = b_1 + b_3 m$ because the rest of the terms cancel out.

Similarly, for NIE we evaluate $E\{Y_i(1,M_i(1))\}$ and $E\{Y_i(1,M_i(0))\}$. From Equation 1, we have

$$M_i(1) = a_0 + a_1 + a_2 C_i' + \varepsilon_i$$

and

$$M_i(0) = a_0 + a_2 C_i' + \varepsilon_i$$

Substituting these in Equation 2 and taking expectations gives

$$E\{Y_i(1, M_i(1))\} = b_0 + b_1 + b_2(a_0 + a_1 + a_2 C_i') + b_3(a_0 + a_1 + a_2 C_i') + b_4' D_i$$

and

$$E\{Y_i(0, M_i(0))\} = b_0 + b_1 + b_2(a_0 + a_2 C_i') + b_3(a_0 + a_2 C_i') + b_4' D_i$$

When we take the difference, we obtain the formula for the NIE given previously. In the same way, we can obtain the formula for NDE.

The expressions for CDE, NDE, and NIE are generalizations of the expressions for the direct and the indirect effects in the Baron and Kenny approach. The NDE is calculated at the mean values of the confounders of the treatment–mediator relationship, C, while the CDE depends on the value of the mediator but does not depend on the values of the confounders. If the interaction is not present (i.e., $b_3 = 0$), the CDE and NDE are simply b_1, which is exactly the direct effect in the Baron and Kenny approach. Without interaction, the NIE also reduces to $b_2 a_1$, the expression for the indirect effect in the Baron and Kenny approach.

In all linear models, TCE = NDE + NIE, but in the presence of an interaction CDE cannot replace NDE in this expression; hence, the total effect is not equal to the sum of the CDE and NIE. There is mediation when the TCE—NDE, or equivalently the NIE, is different from zero. A measure of *percent mediated effect* (PME) is often used to assess what proportion of the total effect is mediated via the specific pathway hypothesized in the model. PME is defined as the ratio of the natural indirect effect to the total effect: NIE/(NDE + NIE). The larger the value, the greater portion of the effect of the predictor is via the mediator rather than directly or via other mechanisms.

In non-linear models, a complication arises so that the total causal effect is generally not the sum of the natural direct and natural indirect effects. For example, this is true for binary outcomes when logistic models are used to relate the outcome to treatment and the mediator. With binary treatment, binary mediator, and binary outcome the models are

$$\textbf{Equation 1}: \text{logit}\{P(M_i = 1)\} = a_0 + a_1 X_i + a_2' C_i$$

$$\textbf{Equation 2}: \text{logit}\{P(Y_i = 1)\} = b_0 + b_1 X_i + b_2 M_i + b_3 X_i M_i + b_4' D_i$$

When the outcome is rare (about 10% prevalence or below), the CDE, NDE, and NIE are expressed as odds ratios (ORs). The CDE is the OR of positive response ($Y = 1$) when comparing experimental with control treatments ($X = 1$ versus $X = 0$) and controlling the mediator at a value m (either 0 or 1). The NDE is the OR for $Y = 1$ when comparing the experimental and control treatments and assuming the mediator is at the value it would take under the control treatment $M(0)$. The NIE is the OR for $Y = 1$ when comparing $M(1)$ to $M(0)$ for the experimental treatment (i.e., when $X = 1$). The second and third expressions that follow are approximately true (see Valeri and VanderWeele, 2013):

$$OR_{CDE} = \exp(b_1 + b_3 m)$$

$$OR_{NDE} \cong \frac{\exp(b_1)\{1 + \exp(b_2 + b_3 + a_0 + a_2' C)\}}{\{1 + \exp(b_2 + a_0 + a_2' C)\}}$$

$$OR_{NIE} \cong \frac{\{1 + \exp(a_0 + a_2' C)\}\{1 + \exp(b_2 + b_3 + a_0 + a_1 + a_2' C)\}}{\{1 + \exp(a_0 + a_1 + a_2' C)\}\{1 + \exp(b_2 + b_3 + a_0 + a_2' C)\}}$$

These formulae also describe the direct and indirect effects when the outcome is not rare, in which case a log-linear rather than logistic model needs to be used for the outcome (i.e., the probability of 1 is related to the predictors via log link rather than logit). In this case, the effects are risk ratios (i.e., ratios of probabilities) rather than ORs (i.e., ratios of odds). In addition, when the outcome is count rather than binary and a log-linear model is used the same expressions for the risk ratios hold. We show a data example in Section 9.4.2.

In these cases, in the absence of an interaction between treatment and the mediator, TCE is approximately equal to the product of the NDE and NIE. We demonstrate how the causal inference approach works with non-normal data on a data example in Section 9.4.2. Interested readers are referred to Valeri and VanderWeele (2013) for more general expressions, including for different combinations of outcomes, mediators, and treatments. Formulae for standard errors are available for all the effects described, and a SAS macro is available for calculation of the effects with associated p-values and confidence intervals at https://www.hsph.harvard.edu/tyler-vanderweele/tools-and-tutorials/.

Since the validity of model-based inference relies on the model being correctly specified, models should be selected carefully using model diagnostics to indicate possible issues with lack of fit (see Chapter 3). Non-parametric approaches to estimation of causal effects are available when one is not willing to make strong assumptions about the distributions of the mediator and/or the outcome (see e.g., Ten Have and Joffe (2012) for a review); however, these are generally more difficult to implement.

Regardless of whether parametric or non-parametric approaches are used for estimation of causal effects, general assumptions under which the causal approach provides valid estimates of mediation effects need to be carefully considered. The conditions for a causal interpretation of the direct and indirect effects are as follows:

For the CDE, we make the assumptions that there is *no unmeasured confounding of the treatment–outcome relationship* (Assumption One, A1) and *no unmeasured confounding of the mediator–outcome relationship* (Assumption Two, A2). That is, there are no third variables (other covariates) that have not been included that would affect both treatment and the outcome, and both the mediator and the outcome. The first two panels of Figure 9.4 indicate violations of these assumptions when the potential confounder variable E is not included in the models. Note that identifying and measuring all potentially confounding variables for inclusion in statistical mediation models is a very complicated task. Randomization of treatment usually assures that Assumption One is satisfied but not that Assumption Two is satisfied.

Assumption Two may be satisfied if randomization of the mediator occurs. As an example, consider a study such as the one in Ten Have and Joffe (2012), in which depressed subjects are randomized to cognitive behavioral therapy (CBT) or treatment as usual. Subjects are encouraged to seek outside treatments in addition to the primary study treatment. The outcome is improvement in depression. Because subjects are randomized to CBT, there is no unmeasured confounding of the treatment–outcome relationship, and thus Assumption One is satisfied. If outside treatment (the potential mediator) is also randomized, then Assumption Two of no unmeasured confounding of the mediator–outcome relationship will also be satisfied. If the second intervention (i.e., the potential mediator) is not randomized, then we are not guaranteed that Assumption Two holds. *Manipulation-of-mediator*

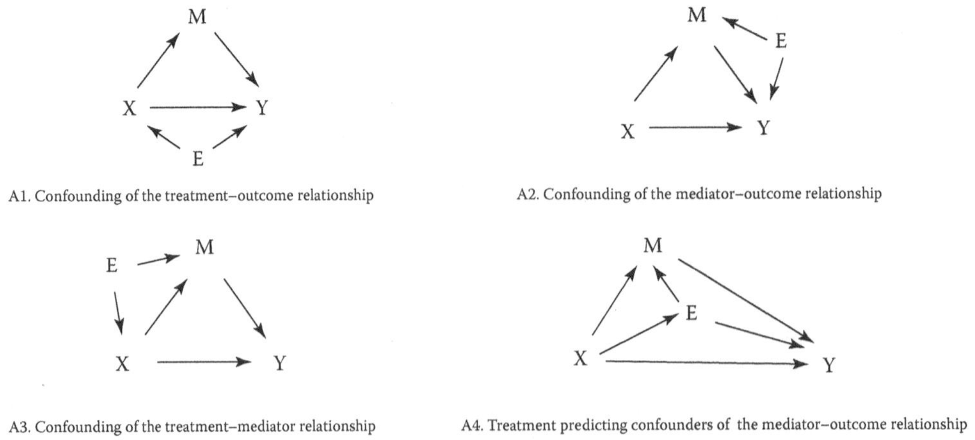

FIGURE 9.4
Examples of violations of different assumptions for casual interpretation of mediation effects.

designs (Pirlott and MacKinnon, 2016) that use double randomizations (i.e., randomization of both the treatment and the mediator) or experimental manipulations of the mediators are tools to ensure that the second assumption is satisfied, but such designs are rarely utilized and often impractical.

When it is not possible to manipulate the mediator, one needs to include all common causes for the mediator and the outcome being covariates in Equation 2 to adjust for potential confounding of the mediator–outcome relationship. In the CBT example, all factors that increase the likelihood of seeking additional treatments and may also be related to improvements in depression (e.g., economic support and stress factors) should be included in Equation 2. As the equation gets more complicated, this task becomes more challenging and requires substantial theoretical support.

For the NDE and NIE formulae to be valid for causal inference there are two additional conditions: *no unmeasured confounding of the treatment–mediator relationship* (Assumption Three, A3) and *no treatment effects on confounders of the mediator-outcome relationship* (Assumption Four, A4). Assumption Three implies that all variables that affect both the treatment and the mediator are included in Equation 1, while Assumption Four requires that treatment be independent of the covariates in Equation 2 that are confounders of the mediator–outcome relationship. Note that in randomized designs, both Assumption Three and Assumption One are directly satisfied. In the CBT example, there is no unmeasured confounding of the randomized CBT treatment and additional out-of-study treatments due to the randomization of CBT. However, in observational studies, unmeasured confounders may lead to violation of this assumption as shown in the third panel of Figure 9.4.

In both randomized and observational studies, it is difficult to ensure that Assumption Four is satisfied. A violation of this assumption in the context of the CBT example occurs if economic support and stress factors (potential confounders of the relationship between the additional interventions and the outcome) are affected by CBT treatment. Having all such variables independent of treatment is a very strong assumption indeed. The fourth panel of Figure 9.4 shows a violation of the fourth assumption.

If Assumptions Three and Four are violated, estimates of the NDE and NIE can be substantially biased. Note that it is not possible, based on the observed data, to assess whether the assumptions are satisfied or not. The determination of whether they are reasonable should be based on theoretical (subject-matter) considerations. Sensitivity analyses can be performed to assess the effects of violations of assumptions (see e.g., Imai et al., 2010). Estimation methods such as marginal structural models and structural nested models are available to estimate controlled direct effects when the predictor of interest affects the confounders of the mediator–outcome relationship (e.g., VanderWeele et al., 2014).

A very important point is that the set of four assumptions implies that the treatment, mediator, and outcome are temporarily ordered (i.e., treatment precedes the mediator which in turn precedes the outcome). If this is not the case, then associations cannot be interpreted as causation.

9.3.3 Mediators in Experimental and Observational Studies

As mentioned in the preceding paragraphs, randomization of treatment ensures that the assumptions of no unmeasured confounding of the treatment–mediator (Assumption Three) and treatment–outcome (Assumption One) relationships are satisfied. For example, since treatments in the COMBINE clinical trial are randomized, we can safely assume that there is no unmeasured confounding of the treatment–mediator and treatment–outcome relationship. That is, there are no third variables that affect both treatment and the mediator, or both treatment and the outcome.

In manipulation-of-mediator designs, the other two assumptions (no unmeasured confounding of the mediator–outcome relationship and no treatment effects on confounders of the mediator–outcome relationship) are also automatically satisfied. Thus, experimental studies with randomization of both treatment and the mediator can safely be used for causal inference. However, commonly, in situations such as the COMBINE study, the potential mediator (craving) is not randomized; thus, we are not guaranteed that there is no mediator–outcome confounding. Designs in which only the treatment is randomized require inclusion of all confounders of the mediator–outcome relationship in Equation 2. Thus, all variables that can potentially influence both craving and drinking post-randomization should be included. If potential confounders are omitted the effects may not have causal interpretation.

Observational studies are the least desirable for causal inference, as all common causes of the exposure and the mediator need to be included in Equation 1, and all common causes of the exposure and the outcome, and of the mediator and the outcome, need to be included in Equation 2. This is virtually impossible to do if we do not know the temporal ordering of the exposure, the mediator, and the outcome since simple association studies cannot be interpreted as causal. Thus, cross-sectional studies in which there is no clear temporal ordering should not be used for causal inference. Observational studies in which the temporal ordering can be ascertained with a reasonable degree of certainty (e.g., subjects recall accurately the sequence of events, measures are extracted from time-stamped sources, or studies are prospective), then mediational analyses may proceed, but with caution, since the possibility of unmeasured confounding remains.

9.3.4 Multiple Mediators

Quite often, there are multiple mechanisms that account for how or why a treatment works. Considering mediators one at a time is not a good approach, as it does not take into account the potential relationships among the mediators. The single-mediator causal approach is extended to handle multiple mediators by VanderWeele and Vansteelandt (2014). Ideally, mediators should be identified *a priori* rather than in a post hoc fashion, as the chance of ambiguous results increases.

Another approach used to deal with potential multiple mediation mechanisms is *structural equation models* (SEM), which allow simultaneous modeling of multiple pathways. However, such models make assumptions regarding linearity, normality, and lack of confounding on all considered sets of variables. Such assumptions are very strong and are rarely satisfied in their entirety. Thus, SEMs should be used with great caution and most likely as hypothesis-generating, not confirmatory, analyses (VanderWeele and Tchetgen, 2016).

9.3.5 Mediator Effects in Longitudinal Studies

Due to the requirement for temporal precedence of treatment, mediator, and outcome, all mediation analyses that have the goal of assessing causal effects should be based on studies with measurements over time. Although, technically, the equations in Section 9.3.2 are valid with cross-sectional data when the assumptions are satisfied, in practice one needs to measure the mediator and outcome (and potentially treatment) longitudinally in order to be sure that there is temporal ordering. This is true both for experimental and observational studies. Longitudinal data offer unique opportunities to test causal hypotheses because they allow one to determine when changes in variables occur and how to attribute these changes to treatment and/or mediator effects. However, they come with their own set of challenges, including measurement times that may not be optimal and vary from subject to subject, missing data, difficulties in specifying models, and mechanisms of action among many others.

There are three different types of longitudinal mediation models that have been considered in the psychological literature: *autoregressive models* (Cole and Maxwell, 2003), *latent growth models* (Muthen and Asparouhov, 2015) and *latent difference score models* (Ferrer and McArdle, 2003; McArdle, 2009).

Autoregressive models specify contemporaneous relationships and/or relationships between variables one measurement occasion apart. For example, exposure at one occasion may effect change in the mediator at the next occasion which in turn may affect the outcome at the next assessment time point. Repeated evaluations over time can be used to assess stability of the mediational relationship. That is, whether the mediational relationship between treatment/exposure, mediator, and outcome is the same throughout the study period and is stronger/weaker as time progresses.

Latent growth models examine whether the predictor (or the change in the predictor) affects the growth trajectory of the mediation variable, which in turn affects the growth trajectory of the outcome variable. The predictor can also have a direct effect on the growth trajectory of the outcome.

In the *latent difference score* approach, changes in the mediator values, and changes in the outcome values, between repeated occasions are subjected to methods for simple mediational analysis with a single measurement of each variable.

Different combinations of models are also possible (Bollen and Curran, 2004). Each of these approaches has advantages and disadvantages, but the most glaring drawback is that the effects are most often not derived from a causal inference perspective and the assumptions under which causal interpretation can be made are not clear.

In order to deal with the interpretability issue and to formalize conditions under which causal inference can be performed, a few publications in the statistical literature have considered mediation analysis with time-varying exposures and repeated assessments of the mediator (VanderWeele, 2010; Bind et al., 2016). An approach that has gained popularity in the statistical and epidemiology literature to assess mediation effects when treatment is not randomized and there may be time-varying confounders and exposures is *marginal structural models* (MSM, see e.g., Moodie and Stephens (2011) for a non-technical description). These models are marginal because they assess population-averaged effects of the treatment and the mediator on the outcome, and structural because they focus on causal rather than associational effects. There are different methods for estimation: *inverse probability weighting* (Robins et al., 2000), *g-estimation* (van der Wal et al., 2009), or *targeted maximum likelihood* (Rosenblum and van der Laan, 2010). These methods have not yet gained popularity in the subject-matter literature.

To provide a more specific example of mediation analysis with longitudinal data, we focus on the approach of Bind et al. (2016), as it is very general and justifies effects from a causal inference perspective. The authors suggest using generalized linear mixed models (GLMM) to specify relationships among exogenous exposure variables, repeatedly measured mediators, and the outcome. They derive definitions of direct, indirect, and percent mediated effect from a causal inference perspective. Interactions between the exposure and the mediator are allowed. The approach can handle multiple mediators and different types of mediators and outcomes. Thus, Bind et al. (2016) extend and formalize some of the methods that have been previously used in the psychological literature. We outline their approach here, consider an example in Section 9.4, and refer the interested reader to the original publication for more information.

Briefly, the approach involves specifying a GLMM, with the mediator as the outcome and treatment and covariates as predictors, and a second GLMM for the outcome of interest with the mediator, treatment, and covariates as predictors. Individual-level random intercepts and slopes for the treatment (and mediator in the second GLMM) effects are included, thus allowing for subject-specific differences in the strength of treatment–mediator and mediator–outcome relationships. All random effects in both models are allowed to be correlated. If there are positive correlations between the slopes of the treatment and mediator effects, individuals who are more likely to experience exposure effects on the mediator are also more likely to experience mediator effects on the outcome. Negative correlations imply the opposite.

The assumptions under which the derived direct and indirect effects have causal interpretation are similar to those for single measurements of the exposure, mediator, and outcome, but in the longitudinal case these assumptions are defined to be conditional on the random effects. There is also the added assumption of *no time-varying confounding* with respect to both the exposure and the mediator variables. What this means is that the mediator and the outcome, measured up to a particular time point, depend only on recent values of the exposure and confounders, and not on previous values of the outcome or mediator. Future values are also assumed not to affect current and past values. An example illustrating this approach is shown in Section 9.4.

9.3.6 Mediator Effects in Studies with Clustered Data

A multitude of papers in the psychological literature have proposed mediational analyses in hierarchical (multilevel) models (e.g., Krull and MacKinnon, 1999; Kenny et al., 2003; Bauer et al., 2006; Tofighi et al., 2013) that can be used in studies with clustered data. In nested designs, predictor and mediators can be measured at the cluster or individual level, and mediation mechanisms may vary depending on the level of measurement. That is, different variables may mediate the relationships at the cluster level (e.g., group-based intervention) and others at the subject level (e.g., individual-level response to treatment).

When clustering is present, performing a mediation analysis at the individual level, ignoring potential clustering of individuals within groups, inflates the probability of type I error and underestimates standard errors of effects. Random effects are typically used to allow for correlations among observations within clusters and often the direct and indirect effects themselves are represented as random effects (e.g., in Figure 9.3 we allow $\mathbf{a}_1$, $\mathbf{b}_1$, and $\mathbf{b}_2$ to be random). This is quite appropriate when we expect direct and indirect effects to vary from cluster to cluster. For example, individuals in different families may respond in systematically different ways to an intervention and the strength of the mediating effect may vary from family to family. Random coefficients for the effects of treatment on both the mediator and the outcome, and for the mediator on the outcome allow for this flexibility. Any valid estimation of the effects, however, needs to take into account inter-cluster variability and covariance among the various random effects.

A word of caution applies when using approaches for multilevel mediational analysis. Most publications do not justify the proposed estimates of direct and indirect effects as contrasts of counterfactual outcomes and the assumptions under which the effects have causal interpretation are often not clear. Exposure–mediator interactions are also often not considered. Note, however, that the approach of Bind et al. (2016) can be used with clustered data and allows for exposure–mediator interactions.

9.3.7 Moderated Mediation and Mediated Moderation

Moderators can often impact the relationships in mediation models. Two situations are particularly relevant: *moderated mediation* (Preacher et al., 2007) and *mediated moderation* (Muller et al., 2005). In *moderated mediation*, the mediation effect depends on the level of a moderator. That is, whether there is mediation of the relationship between X and Y via M, its direction, and the magnitude of the indirect effect depends on a third variable, Z (a moderator). Such a situation can be handled by including the moderator and its interactions with treatment and the mediator in the models for mediation analysis. Assessing the magnitude and the significance of the interactions involving the moderator shows how much the treatment and/or mediator effects vary depending on the level of the moderator. Interpretation of moderated mediation effects is more straightforward with categorical moderators. See MacKinnon (2008) for more information.

In *mediated moderation*, there is an interactive effect of X and the moderator, Z, on the outcome, Y, and M mediates this effect. Models for such a situation include main and interactive effects of the predictor and the moderator on the mediator, and on the outcome. Morgan-Lopez and MacKinnon (2006) describe such models but further methodological developments are needed.

Note that the interactive effects of treatment and the mediator inherently suggest moderation such that treatment assignment moderates the effect of the mediator. That is, the effect of the mediator varies by level of treatment. As discussed previously, the calculation of NDE and NIE effects becomes more complicated in such situations, but is appropriately handled via the causal inference approach.

9.4 Data Examples of Mediation Analysis

9.4.1 Improvement in Sleep as Mediator of the Effects of Modafinil on Cocaine Use in Cocaine-Dependent Patients

In this study, patients were randomized to modafinil treatment or placebo during a period of inpatient treatment and then were followed up for six weeks as outpatients (Morgan et al., 2016). The treatment goal was to reduce cocaine use, and it was hypothesized that the anticipated reduction would be at least partially mediated through improvements in slow-wave sleep. The outcome of interest was percent negative urine samples during the six weeks of outpatient treatment. Improvement in slow-wave sleep was the hypothesized mediator, and it was measured during the inpatient phase when subjects were abstaining from cocaine use. Due to the schedule of the measurements we have clear temporal ordering of the treatment, the mediator, and the outcome; thus, we can perform causal inference mediation analysis. We consider models with and without an interaction between the treatment and the mediator. The outcome and the mediator are assumed normally distributed, hence the total treatment effect is represented as the sum of the natural direct and indirect effects (TCE = NDE + NIE). Since this is a linear model, the controlled direct effect is the same as the natural direct effect (CDE = NDE) when there is no interaction between the treatment and the mediator. Thus, the Baron and Kenny approach and the causal mediation approach without an interaction are expected to produce the same results. We do not control for potential confounders between the mediator and the outcome, although it is possible to include such variables in the equations.

The two fitted models are as follows:

$$\text{Equation 1: Sleep\_duration} = -2.48 + 18.76\text{treatment}$$

$$\text{Equation 2: Percent\_negative\_urine\_tests} = 27.29 + 12.15\text{treatment} + 0.70\text{sleep\_duration}$$

From Equation 1, we see that slow-wave sleep duration is on average about 20 min (18.76 to be precise) longer in subjects on modafinil than for subjects on placebo, which is statistically significant ($a_1 = 18.76$, $SE = 5.53$, $p = 0.002$). Thus, there is evidence of a statistically significant effect of treatment on the mediator. From Equation 2, we see increased sleep is associated with increased percent negative urine samples. An increase of 10 min is associated with an average increase of seven points in percent negative urine samples. The effect of sleep is statistically significant ($b_2 = 0.70$, $SE = 0.26$, $p = 0.01$), while the effect of treatment is no longer statistically significant ($b_1 = 12.15$, $SE = 11.27$, $p = 0.29$). The estimates of the direct, indirect, and total causal effects with 95% confidence intervals are as follows:

$$\text{CDE} = \text{NDE} = 12.15,\ 95\%\ \text{CI}:\ (-9.94,\ 34.24)$$

$$\text{NIE} = 13.12,\ 95\%\ \text{CI}:\ (0.88,\ 25.37)$$

$$\text{TCE} = 25.27,\ 95\%\ \text{CI}:\ (4.35,\ 46.20)$$

Although the confidence intervals are quite wide (possibly due to the small sample size), the intervals for the NIE and TCE are entirely above zero, thus indicating statistically significant indirect and total effects. The percent mediated effect is 51.3 (obtained as approximately 13.12/(13.12 + 12.15)), thus about half of the effect of treatment on outcome is explained via improvement in sleep.

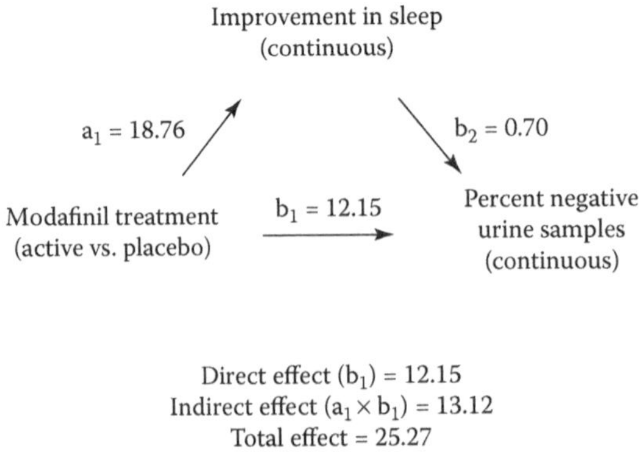

FIGURE 9.5
Total, direct, and indirect effect of modafinil treatment on percent negative urine samples via improvement in sleep.

The results are obtained using the %mediation macro in SAS (Valeri and VanderWeele, 2013; see online materials). Figure 9.5 shows a diagram of the mediation analysis and the estimated magnitudes of the direct, indirect, and total effects. The indirect effect is obtained as the product of the coefficients of the effect of treatment on the mediator and of the mediator on the outcome.

We next include an interaction between treatment and the mediator in Equation 2:

$$\text{Equation 2: Outcome} = 27.20 + 10.71\text{treatment} + 0.66\text{sleep\_duration} + 0.13\text{treatment} * \text{sleep\_duration}$$

Based on this model, the following causal estimates of the effects are obtained:

$$\text{CDE} = 10.71,\ 95\%\ \text{CI}:\ (-14.82,\ 36.25)$$

$$\text{NDE} = 10.39,\ 95\%\ \text{CI}:\ (-16.57,\ 37.36)$$

$$\text{NIE} = 14.71,\ 95\%\ \text{CI}:\ (-2.06,\ 31.48)$$

$$\text{TCE} = 25.11,\ 95\%\ \text{CI}:\ (3.78,\ 46.43)$$

In this case, the CDE and NDE are slightly different, the NIE is no longer statistically significant (the 95% CI includes zero), and all confidence intervals are wider. Hence, evidence of a mediation relationship is not as strong.

To decide between the two models, we check the significance of the interaction between treatment and sleep. The p-value is highly non-significant ($p = 0.82$), and thus there is no need to include the interaction and we can use the simpler main effects model. We conclude that the effect of modafinil on cocaine use is partially mediated through improvements in sleep.

9.4.2 Intent-to-Smoke as a Mediator of the Effect of a School-Based Drug Prevention Program on Smoking

The second example uses a data set from a longitudinal school- and community-based drug intervention program analyzed by MacKinnon et al. (2007). Middle schools were randomly assigned to experimental or control conditions. The outcome was measured at the student level and was a dichotomous indicator of cigarette use (1 = yes, 0 = no). The potential mediator was intention to use tobacco, measured several months after the program

TABLE 9.3

Data from the Study of the Effects of a School-Based Drug Prevention Program on Smoking

	Experimental Treatment		Control Treatment	
Intent-to-Smoke	**Cigarette Use**		**Cigarette Use**	
	No	**Yes**	**No**	**Yes**
No	396	43	265	43
Yes	24	30	23	40

was initiated and before the outcome assessment. Table 9.3 presents the number of individuals by treatment group, intent-to-smoke (dichotomous), and cigarette use.

We consider a logistic regression model to estimate the effect of treatment on the mediator, and in two separate analyses, logistic and log-linear regression, the effect of treatment and the mediator on the outcome. The outcome here has an overall prevalence of about 22% (larger than the 10% cutoff for rare outcomes), so the log-linear model is more appropriate, but we fit both logistic and log-linear models in order to illustrate both approaches. As in the previous example, we considered models with and without an interaction between treatment and the mediator, but since the interactions were not statistically significant, the results herein are presented based on the main effects models. The complete results are available in the online materials.

The fitted logistic models are as follows:

$$\text{logit}\{P(M_i = 1)\} = -1.59 - 0.51T_i$$

$$\text{logit}\{P(Y_i = 1)\} = -1.83 - 0.38T_i + 2.41M_i$$

where:

- T_i indicates the treatment prevention program (1 is for experimental, 0 is for control)
- M_i indicates the intent of the individual student to smoke (1 corresponds to "yes," 0 corresponds to "no")
- Y_i is the outcome (1 corresponds to smoking, 0 corresponds to not smoking)

The estimated odds ratios describing the CDE, NDE, NIE, and TCE based on these models obtained by substituting the regression coefficient estimates in the approximate formulae of Valeri and Vanderweele (2013), shown in Section 9.3.2, are as follows:

$$\text{OR}_{\text{CDE}} = \text{OR}_{\text{NDE}} = 0.68,\ 95\%\ \text{CI}:\ (0.46,\ 1.00)$$

$$\text{OR}_{\text{NIE}} = 0.78,\ 95\%\ \text{CI}:\ (0.63,\ 0.95)$$

$$\text{OR}_{\text{TCE}} = 0.53,\ 95\%\ \text{CI}:\ (0.34,\ 0.82)$$

The OR for the total effect shows that the odds of smoking for students in the experimental prevention program are only about half of those on the control treatment, a statistically significant effect ($p = 0.004$). The OR for the total effect (0.53) factors out approximately into the product of the OR for the natural direct effect (0.68) and the OR of the natural indirect effect (0.77) (TCE = NDE × NIE). Both the NDE and the NIE are statistically significant ($p = 0.05$ and $p = 0.01$, respectively). Thus, we conclude that there is statistically significant partial mediation of the effect of the prevention program via the intention to smoke acknowledged by individual students. The prevention program reduces the intent to smoke, which in turn leads to reduced odds of smoking. There is also a direct effect of the program on smoking.

Since the outcome is not rare, we prefer to use log-linear regression rather than logistic regression to relate the outcome to the treatment and the mediator. Thus, the second fitted equation is changed to:

$$\log\{P(Y_i = 1)\} = -2.04 - 0.22T_i + 1.61M_i$$

Based on this model (together with the logistic regression for the mediator above), the estimated risk ratios of the CDE, NDE, NIE, and TCE are as follows:

$$\text{RR}_{\text{CDE}} = \text{RR}_{\text{NDE}} = 0.81,\ 95\%\ \text{CI}:\ (0.63,\ 1.03)$$

$$\text{RR}_{\text{NIE}} = 0.86,\ 95\%\ \text{CI}:\ (0.76,\ 0.97)$$

$$\text{RR}_{\text{TCE}} = 0.69,\ 95\%\ \text{CI}:\ (0.53,\ 0.90)$$

In this scenario, the risk ratio for the TCE is estimated to be 0.69; thus, individuals who receive the experimental program are estimated to have a 31% lower probability of smoking, which is a statistically significant decrease ($p=0.007$). The risk ratios for the NDE and NIE are 0.86 and 0.81, respectively, which correspond to about 14% and 19% decreases in the probability of drinking, while the NDE is not statistically significant ($p=0.09$), the NIE is ($p=0.01$).

In the log-linear model TCE = NDE × NIE, as was the case in the logistic model. Both approaches indicate that there is a statistically significant NIE, and thus the effect of treatment on the outcome is partially mediated via the considered intention-to-smoke variable. The difference in the estimates and associated confidence intervals arise because we are estimating odds ratios in the logistic model and risk ratios in the log-linear model. For rare outcomes, the two sets of estimates will be approximately the same.

9.4.3 Mediator Effects in a Simulated Repeated Measures Data Set

We use the simulated data from Bauer et al. (2006) with eight repeated occasions per individual to illustrate causal mediational analysis with repeated measures data. On each occasion, a continuous predictor variable, X, a continuous mediator, M, and a continuous response variable, Y, are available. All variables, including the predictor, are time-varying. The question of interest is whether the effect of X on Y is mediated through M. We apply the approach of Bind et al. (2016) to assess direct and indirect effects in this scenario. Linear mixed models are assumed for 1) the effect of X on M with random intercept and random slope of X and 2) for the effect of X and M on Y with random intercept and random slopes of X and M. The random effects are assumed to all be correlated, which takes into account the variance–covariance structure of the data. The fitted models, with the random effects indicated by alphas and betas, are as follows:

$$\text{Equation 1}: M_{it} = 0.09 + 0.61X_{it} + \alpha_{i0} + \alpha_{i1}X_{it}$$

$$\text{Equation 2}: Y_{it} = -0.10 + 0.22X_{it} + 0.61M_{it} + \beta_{i0} + \beta_{i1}X_{it} + \beta_{i2}M_{it}$$

Since the predictions for subject-specific random effects vary from individual to individual, we are not showing them here. SAS code to fit the models and estimate the effects is available in the online materials. Similar code is also available at http://www.ats.ucla.edu/stat/sas/faq/ml_mediation2.htm, with standard errors obtained by the delta method rather than by bootstrapping. Although the approach of Bind et al. (2016) allows for an interaction between the treatment and mediator variables, we do not consider it here since the data were generated according to a main effects model only. The estimated effects and confidence intervals are as follows:

$$\text{CDE} = \text{NDE} = 0.22,\ 95\%\ \text{CI}:\ (0.18,\ 0.30)$$

$$\text{NIE} = 0.47,\ 95\%\ \text{CI}:\ (0.35,\ 0.54)$$

$$\text{TCE} = 0.69,\ 95\%\ \text{CI}:\ (0.60,\ 0.79)$$

There is a statistically significant effect of X on Y such that a unit increase in X increases Y by 0.69 on average. Most of this increase is due to the change in the mediator (0.47), while the remaining effect (an increase of about 0.22) is not explained by this particular mediator and may be due to other pathways or to a direct effect of the intervention program on the outcome. The percent mediated is estimated to be 0.68, 95% CI: (0.58, 0.74) or about two-thirds of the total effect.

9.5 Summary

In this chapter, we focused on two special types of variables that affect the relationship between a predictor (treatment, exposure) of interest, X, and an outcome, Y. Moderators are unrelated to the predictor and describe for whom or under what conditions the treatment or exposure produces its effect on the outcome. Mediators explain how the effect of X on Y is produced, are affected by the predictor, and in turn affect the outcome.

While moderator analyses and interpretation are relatively straightforward, mediator analyses are challenging and a universally used approach is yet to emerge. The causal inference framework is very attractive in that it unifies different types of predictors, mediators, and outcomes under the same umbrella, provides clear definitions of direct and indirect effects, and is explicit about assumptions under which causality can be claimed. However, as of now, most causal inference analyses appear in the statistical literature, partly because most software packages do not yet provide convenient modules for such analyses and partly due to difficulties with positing and verifying assumptions (especially in longitudinal models). There is a complexing array of macros available for use, but they generally offer little user guidance and require some level of sophistication. In general, the assumptions underlying mediator analysis are difficult to assess, and in some studies, mediation cannot be properly tested (e.g., cross-sectional studies where temporal ordering cannot be established). Theoretical support is often needed in order to specify appropriate models.

Randomized studies provide much better frameworks than observational studies for evaluating moderation and mediation since they guarantee that the potential moderator and treatment are unrelated, and automatically satisfy some of the assumptions of mediation analysis. Designs that allow for randomizing the mediator in addition to treatment are the best for mediation analysis in terms of satisfying the assumptions for causal interpretation. However, they are logistically difficult to implement and not really an option in most situations. Designs without double randomization are vulnerable to the effects of unmeasured confounding. *Structural mean models* and *principal stratification* approaches are available to provide effect estimates in such scenarios (Robins and Greenland, 1992; Robins et al., 2000; VanderWeele and Vansteelandt, 2009).

Longitudinal studies provide unique opportunities for the assessment of mediator effects because the temporal ordering of the treatment, mediator, and the outcome can be ascertained, and treatment and mediator effects can therefore be more accurately attributed. However, they come with their own set of challenges. Despite some recent methodological advances, such as the approach of Bind et al. (2016) that was discussed and illustrated in this chapter, much research is still needed on general models and accessible modules need to be incorporated into software programs.

In addition to moderation and mediation, other types of relationships may exist between *X*, *Y*, and a third variable that can shed light on the relationship between the predictor and the outcome. Variables related to both the predictor and the outcome are confounding variables, and ignoring them can lead to incorrect inferences. Confounding variables can also be responsible for bias in mediator analysis, where confounders of the relationship between the treatment and the mediator, and/or the mediator and the outcome are ignored. The third variable can be an independent predictor of the outcome, in which case ignoring it will not lead to bias, but taking it into account may improve precision in estimating moderator and mediator effects, as it helps reduce the unexplained variability in *Y*. This is usually what is done in classical ANCOVA when there are no interactions among the predictors. A review of different types of relationships among risk factors is available in Kraemer et al. (2001).

More work is needed on effect sizes for mediation, improving power for testing mediation effects, and simultaneous assessment of multiple moderators and mediators. Non-parametric models and simulation-based approaches for estimation of direct and indirect effects can be quite useful when one is unwilling to make parametric assumptions or parametric assumptions are unlikely to hold (Imai et al., 2010). Thus, mediational analyses are going to continue presenting a multitude of challenges, including the need for more methodological development, better and more consistent software capabilities, careful assumption checks, and sensitivity analyses to assess the effects of violations of assumptions.

10

Mixture Models for Trajectory Analyses

Generalized linear mixed models (GLMM) for longitudinal data (described in Chapter 4) assume that individuals follow the same type of trajectory over time with random variability (in the form of random intercepts, slopes, or other effects) around the mean trends. Traditional generalized estimating equations (GEE) (also described in Chapter 4) do not allow for random effects, but also assume that all individuals with the same baseline covariates have the same trajectory over time. However, it is possible that there are categorically different classes of trajectories, with individuals having different chances of being in a particular class. This is especially common with categorical outcomes. For example, in studies such as COMBINE, some individuals abstain from drinking throughout the observation period while others increase or decrease their drinking. Developmental trajectories of substance use are often also heterogeneous with some individuals showing progression to substance abuse while others show an increase followed by recovery or no change at all. Such situations are difficult to capture with traditional models for longitudinal data and may be more suitably described by latent class-based approaches (Nagin, 1999; Muthén and Muthén, 2000). These approaches are focused on data-driven extraction of distinct trajectory patterns and use the available data to determine both the number of patterns (trajectory classes) and the shapes of response over time in each of these classes. Treatment and covariates typically affect the probability of following a particular trajectory pattern. Since the classes themselves are unknown and unobserved, they are referred to as *latent classes*.

Models with latent trajectory classes are useful when interest lies in categorizing patterns of response in treatment studies or types of developmental trajectories. If groups of individuals with similar trajectories can be identified in a data-driven way and we can identify predictors of trajectory membership and how it relates to future outcomes, interventions can be planned to prevent adverse outcomes.

In this chapter, we introduce two commonly used methods for latent class growth analysis: *latent class growth models* (LCGM) and *growth mixture models* (GMM). Both approaches aim to classify individuals into distinct groups (classes) based on the response patterns over time so that individuals within a group are more similar than individuals in different groups. The major difference between the two approaches is that GMM allows individuals to vary in their trajectories around the mean trend of the class they most likely belong to (much like GLMM allows for random intercepts and slopes in the entire population) while the LCGM approach does not (much like GEE posits that the expected trend is the same for all individuals). This makes the GMM approach more flexible, but also more prone to computational and convergence problems since individuals are not as easily classified in groups. In addition, from a conceptual perspective, GMM rely on the assumption that categorically different subgroups exist in the population, while LCGM are aiming to capture population heterogeneity simply by categorizing trajectories of response over time into a small number of groups. These groups may or may not correspond to different subpopulations. This is a fine distinction between the two approaches and one that not all researchers agree on. Since LCGM are a special case of GMM one can argue that they also rely on the assumption of the existence of distinct trajectory classes in the population. The differences and similarities of the two approaches are emphasized throughout the chapter.

The structure of the current chapter is as follows. Section 10.1 describes LCGM with their advantages and disadvantages while Section 10.2 does the same for GMM. Section 10.3 focuses on model fitting and model selection issues while Section 10.4 presents a couple of data examples. The chapter concludes with a summary (Section 10.5) and reiteration of the versatility and caveats of these approaches.

As always, we keep the presentation non-technical and focus only on the key aspects of the methods. Other non-technical presentations are available in Muthén and Muthén (2000), Nagin and Tremblay (2005), Jung and Wickrama (2008), Ram and Grimm (2009), Bauer and Reyes (2010), Berlin et al. (2014), Nagin (2014), and Frankfurt et al. (2016). More demanding technical overviews of the methods can be seen in Muthén and Shedden (1999), Muthén et al. (2002), Pickles and Croudace (2010), Vermunt (2010), and Muthén and Asparouhov (2015).

10.1 Latent Class Growth Models (LCGM)

LCGM aim to identify categorically different trajectory classes over time and investigate how membership of a particular class is affected by treatment, exposure, or covariates. These models are also commonly referred to as *trajectory models*, *semi-parametric group-based models*, and *group-based trajectory models* (GBTM). Our presentation here is based on the model definition of Nagin (1999). For more information at a non-technical level, we refer the interested reader to Nagin and Odgers (2010) and Frankfurt et al. (2016). A review of the similarity and differences with GMM is provided by Frankfurt et al. (2016).

Note that unlike the usual mixed-effects models for longitudinal data, where we can compare different *a priori* specified groups (i.e., individuals on different treatments or with different characteristics), in LCGM the trajectory groups (classes) are unknown. We are using the data to identify such classes, and the number of latent classes is decided based on the fit of models with different numbers of classes to the observed data. The repeatedly measured outcomes can be continuous, dichotomous, or counts and we use polynomial trends to describe change over time in each class. Other types of outcomes (e.g., ordinal) can also be considered.

Figure 10.1 shows a hypothetical situation with three distinct trajectories of a dichotomous outcome over time. We have observed similar trajectories when investigating medication adherence (Gueorguieva et al., 2013) and also when exploring trajectories of drinking in clinical trials (e.g., Gueorguieva et al., 2007). The outcome is a binary measure (e.g., taking prescribed medication or not; drinking or not), evaluated daily. To be specific, we consider the medication adherence outcome. In this context, the trajectory class at the top shows consistently high probabilities of taking the prescribed medication throughout the study and hence we call this the *adherence trajectory*. The trajectory class at the bottom shows consistently low probabilities of taking the prescribed medication and hence we call this the *non-adherence trajectory*. The third trajectory class is called the *progressive non-adherence trajectory* as initially high probabilities of taking the prescribed medication are followed by a gradual decrease, ending in almost zero probabilities of adherence. Treatment is expected to have some effect on the likelihood to follow a particular trajectory either alone or in combination with other predictors. For example, individuals who

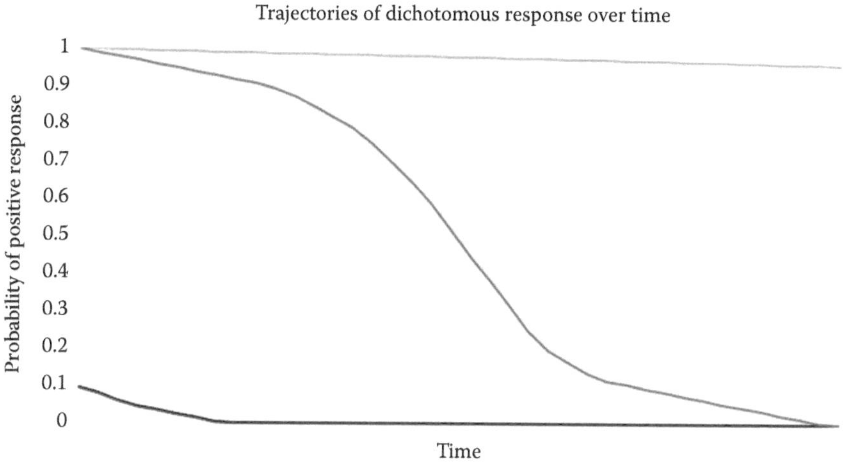

FIGURE 10.1
Hypothetical example of a latent class growth model with three trajectory classes.

experience side effects may stop taking their prescribed medication and thus follow the "non-adherence" or "progressive non-adherence" trajectory. On the other hand, treatment may have a true beneficial effect and thus increase the likelihood of following the "adherence" trajectory.

Such a situation is difficult to describe with traditional mixed models with random intercepts and slopes because individual trajectories tend to cluster at the end of the measurement scale (i.e., individuals are consistently complying or not complying with treatment, and some change their adherence behavior intermittently or progressively). Traditional mixed models assume normal distribution of the random effects which implies that the majority of trajectories are closer to the mean trajectory with some outliers. In contrast, LCGM assume that there are a number of trajectory types and individuals have a certain probability of falling into a particular class. Residual variability at each time point around the mean of the trajectory is allowed, but in LCGM no additional random effects (i.e., intercepts and slopes) are specified. Thus, all individuals in a latent class are expected to have the same starting point and rate of change over time, and LCGM also assumes that, given class membership, repeated measurements within a subject are independent. The goal in LCGM is to use the data to identify the classes and shapes of change over time within each class.

To specify a LCGM one needs to go through the following steps:

1. Decide how many classes of trajectories to estimate.
2. Specify a generalized linear model (GLM) for the repeatedly measured response in each class.

   For example, if the outcome is binary, we commonly use logistic regression to describe the change in response over time within the class. If the outcome is count, we use Poisson or negative binomial regression. Zero-inflated models can also be considered. For a normally distributed outcome, a GLM is preferred.

   Polynomial trends are used to describe change over time and one can choose whether to use linear, quadratic, or cubic effects in each class. Covariates other than time can be included in the linear predictor for each class.

3. Specify a generalized logistic regression model for the individual's odds of belonging to a particular class. One of the classes is selected as the reference class, and the log of the ratio of the probability of each of the other classes versus the probability of the reference class is related to treatment, exposure, or other baseline covariates.

As an example, consider the situation shown in Figure 10.1. The LCGM used to describe this scenario is specified by (1) assuming three trajectory classes, (2) formulating a logistic regression model to describe the time trend in the odds of positive response within each class, and (3) using a generalized logistic regression model for trajectory membership with treatment and other potential covariates as predictors.

The logistic regression model within class k could be

$$\log\left(\frac{p_{t|k}}{1-p_{t|k}}\right) = \beta_{k0} + \beta_{k1}t + \beta_{k2}t^2$$

where $p_{t|k}$ is the probability that the response at time t for an individual in the class is 1. This probability is conditional on membership in class k and the regression coefficients (betas) are specific to the class. In general, the form of the model is the same in all classes, although it is possible to have different polynomials in the different classes and additional covariates (e.g., starting or stopping other concurrent medications, life events).

The generalized logistic regression model relating treatment and baseline covariates to trajectory membership could be

$$\log\left(\frac{P_{ik}}{P_{iK}}\right) = \alpha_{k0} + \alpha_{k1}\ \text{treatment}_i + \alpha_{k2}\ \text{covariate}_i$$

Here, P_{ik} denotes the probability that individual i follows the trajectory of class k and K is the reference class. Note the difference between $p_{t|k}$ (the probability of the observed outcome at time t if the subject belongs to class k) and P_{ik} (the probability that the trajectory of individual i belongs to class k). In LCGM, we always have the generalized logit model for P_{ik} (even if there are no predictors, in which case we just estimate the class membership probabilities). In the generalized logistic regression model, treatment and a single covariate are shown to predict class membership. Thus, individuals who receive different treatments and have different levels of the covariate are expected to have different probabilities of membership in a particular trajectory class. Additional covariates can be added as needed.

The logistic regression model for $p_{t|k}$ is used when we have a binary outcome. Different types of outcomes can be considered by changing the models describing the trajectory within each class. That is, replacing the logistic model in step 2 with another type of GLM (e.g., Poisson or normal regression). Note that there are no random effects within each class. The only random variable (in addition to the repeatedly measured response) is class membership, a categorical latent class variable.

It is clear that for each situation there are a multitude of possible models that can be considered with different numbers of classes, forms of the GLMs within classes, and different predictors of class membership and outcome within classes. We defer consideration of the issues of model selection and assessment of model fit to Section 10.3, after we introduce GMM, since the issues are common for both approaches. Herein, we just emphasize several popular misconceptions regarding LCGM.

1. Individuals do not actually belong to a trajectory group. Their trajectories may be most consistent with a particular trajectory group, but individual time courses are not set at the outset and external factors could alter them.
2. The number of trajectory groups is not set in stone and does not necessarily represent distinct groups in the population. Thus, much care needs to be taken when interpreting treatment effects on trajectory membership.
3. The trajectories of individuals classified as most likely members of a particular group are not identical. There is still random variability allowed around the mean for each trajectory, but it is not a systematic deviation such as is modeled in random effects models.

LCGM are most commonly used for balanced designs (i.e., when individuals are observed at the same fixed time points) and are fit using a specifically designed SAS procedure (SAS PROC TRAJ) introduced by Jones et al. (2001), and reviewed and revised by Jones and Nagin (2007). However, theoretically, the approach is not limited to balanced designs and can be applied using other software (e.g., MPlus, Muthén and Muthén (1998–2015)).

There are a number of advantages of the LCGM approach, including (1) data-driven assessment of patterns over time; (2) data-driven identification of groups of subjects with similar trajectories over time; (3) estimation of effects of covariates and treatment on trajectory membership; (4) assessment of the proportion of the population whose treatment response corresponds most closely to each trajectory group; (5) accounting for time-dependent covariates; and (6) valid inference under missing at random assumptions (i.e., when observations from some of the fixed time points are missing on some individuals).

At the same time, there are disadvantages to this approach, including (1) the reliance of the analysis on the assumption that different classes of trajectories represent the population distribution well; (2) the tendency to over-extract latent classes under model misspecification (see e.g., Bauer and Curran, 2003); (3) the number and shape of trajectories are limited by sample size and number of fixed time points; (4) there is no allowance for systematic between-subject variability around the different trajectories; (5) there is no allowance for testing of interactions between treatment or baseline covariates and time-dependent covariates; and (6) the results may be biased if data are informatively missing.

Guidelines for the use of LCGM and presentation of results from LCGM can be found in Nagin and Odgers (2010), van de Schoot (2015), and Frankfurt et al. (2016), among others. Extensions of the LCGM approach to model trajectories of related behaviors over time are proposed by Nagin and Tremblay (2001).

10.2 Growth Mixture Models (GMM)

GMM (Muthén and Shedden, 1999) can be regarded as extensions of LCGM in that they allow for random variability in the form of random intercepts, slopes, or higher order terms in each trajectory class. They are also extensions of the GLMM, which are actually GMM with a single latent class. Thus, GMM provide incredible flexibility in modeling trajectories over time but the models become very complex. Model fitting and model selection is also very challenging. Note that, unlike LCGM, which are focused on grouping observed trajectories in latent classes that might or might not correspond to distinct subpopulations, GMM require the assumption that there are distinct trajectory classes in the population to yield interpretable results. Thus, it is not appropriate to fit GMM when there is no reason to believe that there are categorically different trajectories in the population. In such cases, spurious results can occur and erroneous conclusions can be reached.

Compared with LCGM, GMM are very flexible in accommodating inter-individual variability in trajectories within a latent class, which is a clear advantage of the approach, but at the same time it is more difficult to classify individuals in a particular class, and this may be regarded as a disadvantage of the approach. To clarify, we consider a simulated data example.

Figure 10.2 shows a hypothetical scenario with two trajectory classes: a flat trajectory class and a linearly decreasing trajectory class over time. Six individual trajectories (three per class) are also shown. The individual trajectories indicate that there is variability in the intercepts and slopes even within a class, and thus there is a very rich variety of longitudinal profiles that can be accommodated using such a model (especially if one considers also non-linear change over time). Since some of the variability in individual trajectories is contained within specific classes in GMM rather than across different classes, fewer classes are usually necessary in GMM in order to capture that variability of the data compared with LCGMs.

On the other hand, as can be seen from Figure 10.2, some individuals are clearly members of their corresponding classes (i.e., the two trajectories that end up with the lowest scores belong to the decreasing trajectory class, the two trajectories that end up with the highest scores belong to the flat trajectory class) but some individuals (i.e., the two trajectories in the middle) are not unequivocally members of either class. When a GMM is fit to the data, these individuals may have probabilities compatible with being classified in either class (e.g., 55% probability to be in one class versus 45% probability to be in the other). Thus, there may be quite a bit of uncertainty in classifying individuals; hence, the

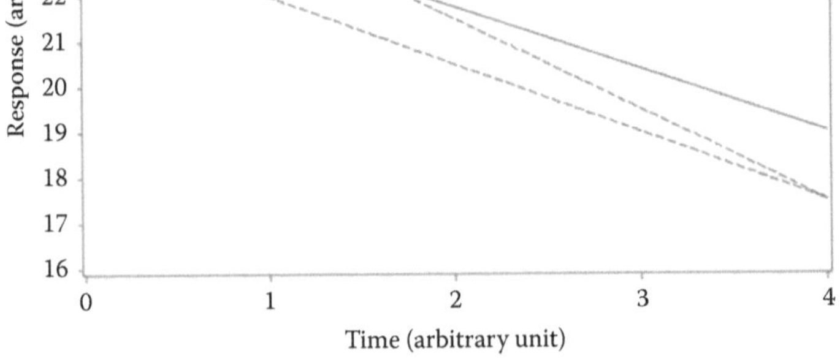

FIGURE 10.2
Profile plot of hypothetical data generated according to a two-class growth mixture model. The solid lines correspond to the average response over time in the two trajectory classes (black line—flat trajectory class, gray line—decreasing trajectory class). The black dashed lines correspond to individuals whose trajectories match that of the flat trajectory class more closely, the gray dashed lines correspond to individuals whose trajectories follow the decreasing trajectory class more closely.

classification accuracy of GMM is often lower than the classification accuracy of the corresponding LCGM.

To specify a GMM one needs to go through the following steps:

1. Decide how many classes of trajectories will be estimated.
2. Specify a GLMM (rather than GLM as in LCGM) for the repeatedly measured response in each class. That is, one needs to specify a response distribution (e.g., binomial, Poisson, negative binomial, normal), a link function (e.g., logit, log, identity), and the form of the linear predictor. Polynomial trends describe change over time, and one can choose whether to use linear, quadratic, cubic, or some other time effects (e.g., change-point) in each class. Random effects are included in the model in addition to fixed effects. Time-dependent covariates can also be incorporated in the model.
3. Specify a generalized logistic regression model for the individual's odds of belonging to a particular class. Treatment, exposure, or other baseline covariates can be included as predictors.

To illustrate, consider again the situation shown in Figure 10.1, with three medication compliance trajectories. A GMM for this scenario is specified by (1) assuming three trajectory classes, (2) formulating a logistic regression model with random effects within each class, and (3) using a generalized logistic regression model for trajectory membership.

The logistic regression model within class k could be

$$\log\left(\frac{p_{it|k}}{1-p_{it|k}}\right) = \beta_{k0} + \beta_{k1}t_i + \beta_{k2}t_i^2 + b_{ik0} + b_{ik1}t_i + b_{ik2}t_i^2$$

The fixed-effects portion of the model is the same as in the corresponding LCGM, but there are also class-specific random intercepts, slopes, and quadratic terms. The random effects b_{ik0}, b_{ik1}, and b_{ik2} are assumed to be normally distributed and are in general correlated within the class. The random effects in different trajectory classes are assumed to be independent of each other. The rest of the model formulation is exactly the same as in LCGM.

Note that compared with the corresponding GLMM with a single trajectory class there are many more parameters in GMM (k times as many to be precise). Thus, one needs a sizeable sample size in order to estimate GMM accurately. Empirical identifiability issues often arise so that, for example, some variances are not identifiable (cannot be estimated) from the data. Thus, restrictions are often imposed on some of the parameters in the model.

One possible restriction is to set all variances of the random effects in all classes to be equal to zero. That is, we assume that there is no between-subject heterogeneity of growth trajectories within the class. In this case, GMM reduce to LCGM.

Another possible restriction is to set the variances of only some random effects (e.g., the quadratic terms, or the quadratic and slope terms) to be equal to zero. Thus, we may assume that individuals have unique starting points for their trajectories but then the shape of change is the same across subjects within a trajectory class.

A third possible restriction is to assume that the variances of the random intercepts, the random slopes, and the quadratic terms are the same for all classes. That is, we assume that the variability in starting points, rates of change, or curvature of individual trajectories around the corresponding class means are the same for all trajectory classes. This may seem like a rather restrictive assumption, but it might otherwise be very difficult to identify the trajectory types, as a class with large variances of the random effects may partially or completely subsume a class with lower variances of the corresponding random effects.

Finally, another common restriction applied in the case of normally distributed outcomes in each trajectory class is that the residual variances (i.e., the variances of the errors) are the same across time points. That is, the amount of random variability beyond what is predicted by the mean trajectories within the class and the variability of random intercepts, slopes, and quadratic terms within the class is constant over time. Again, this may be a necessary assumption for stability of the estimates, but not necessarily a valid one, as there might be changes in variability over time in addition to changes in mean values.

The multitude of possible restrictions of the parameters presents additional challenges for model fitting and for identification of a best-fitting model. Inconsistent reporting of such aspects of model fitting in the scientific literature also hampers the use and interpretation of such models. Aspects of model specification that most commonly receive attention are selection of the number of trajectory classes and evaluation of classification accuracy. We present these in Section 10.3.

Herein, we briefly discuss the advantages and disadvantages of the GMM approach. Advantages include (1) data-driven assessment of patterns over time; (2) flexible characterization of variability within and between latent classes; (3) estimation of effects of covariates and treatment on trajectory membership; (4) assessment of the effects of time-dependent and time-independent predictors (including treatment) on growth factors (i.e., intercepts, slopes, quadratic terms) within trajectory classes; (5) accounting for time-dependent covariates; and 6) valid inference under missing at random assumptions.

Disadvantages include (1) the reliance of the analysis on the assumption that different classes of trajectories exist in the population; (2) potential problems with model non-identifiability, model non-convergence, or multiple solutions when different starting values for the fitting algorithm are used; (3) difficulties in identifying the best-fitting model as misspecification in one part of the model can affect estimates in other parts of the model; (4) potential problems with classifying individuals in trajectory classes; (5) the number and shape of trajectories are limited by sample size and number of time points; (6) potential biasing of results if data are informatively missing.

The most important potential drawback is that GMM is predicated on the assumption that distinct trajectory classes exist in the population. If there are no distinct classes, GMM can lead to spurious results, as skewed distributions can be approximated by mixtures of standard distributions (see e.g., Bauer and Curran, 2003). If non-existent classes are identified, then treatment effects on trajectory membership and on individual growth trajectories may be uninterpretable.

GMM are most commonly fit using MPlus (Muthén and Muthén (1998–2015)). Recently, a new R package (lcmm) has become available (https://cran.r-project.org/web/packages/lcmm/lcmm.pdf).

We now turn our attention to model fitting and model selection in GMM. Since LCGM are a special case of GMM, most of the issues discussed apply to LCGM as well. We devote special attention to model convergence issues and the decision of how many latent classes are supported by the data. Detailed reviews of this problem and solutions are provided in Tofighi and Enders (2008) and Nylund et al. (2007).

10.3 Issues in Building LCGM and GMM

10.3.1 Model Fitting

GMM and LCGM are estimated using maximum likelihood via an iterative algorithm. That is, initial estimates of all the parameters in the model are considered (or just some fixed starting values), and at each iteration of the algorithm those estimates are updated based on the fit of the model to the observed data. The algorithm guarantees that at each step the likelihood improves; that is, the new estimates provide a better fit to the data. The algorithm converges when estimates from subsequent iterations are virtually the same (within a certain precision).

However, unlike traditional linear mixed models, in mixture models the likelihood is not well-behaved in a sense that it is not like one smooth mountaintop, the top of which can eventually be reached if one keeps climbing. Rather, the likelihood surface is like a mountain range with many peaks and valleys, and hence there is a real danger that the algorithm will end at a peak away from the highest point, and that the achieved peak will be different depending on the starting point. Thus, the algorithm is likely to converge to a local, rather than to a global, maximum. To combat this problem, different sets of starting values are selected and the achieved maxima compared. With a sufficiently large number of starting points, the global maximum should be repeatedly achieved, but unfortunately this is not guaranteed. A measure of the convergence of the algorithm to the global maximum is whether the highest likelihood value is reached from multiple starting values. Another indicator of whether the global maximum has been achieved is how frequently the largest likelihood value is reached from different starting values. If the largest value is reached only in a small percentage of the runs, it is likely that there is a problem with model specification.

There are different recommendations regarding how many starting points are needed. In general, only about five to ten may be sufficient in LCGM, but, in GMM, hundreds of starting values are needed. Note that the number of starting values can always be increased if the best likelihood value is not replicated with the originally specified number of starting values. Some software packages (e.g., MPlus) automatically generate starting points and users just need to specify how many they want to consider. The limitation is the time needed for the algorithm to converge. The more starting points, the longer the run times. Users can always provide starting points that may be based on prior results or substantive considerations.

Note that algorithms may also fail to converge. This happens when consecutive iterations do not improve the likelihood and it is usually due to singularities in the likelihood function. Increasing the number of starting points can help, but sometimes there is no solution and a simpler model with parameter restrictions should be used instead.

Convergence problems are more likely to occur when more classes are considered because the number of parameters increases substantially as more classes are added. As mentioned in Section 10.2, restrictions on the parameters are often placed to avoid problems with convergence. In general, if there is suspicion that the algorithm has not converged to the right solution because the maximum likelihood value is not (or is infrequently) replicated, model restrictions should be imposed to stabilize the model fit. The most common solutions are to set the variances of the random effects in the latent classes to be the same or to fix some of these variances to zero. The first option is the default option in MPlus. The flip side of such constraints is that they may not be consistent with theory and can have a large impact on parameter estimates.

10.3.2 Model Selection

There are several aspects of model selection that need to be considered. Perhaps the most important is the selection of the number of classes, but other aspects involve identifying the best-fitting shapes over time (both fixed and random effects structure), inclusion of time-dependent or time-independent covariates within latent classes, and predictors of trajectory class membership. Note that misspecification of one aspect of the model can have substantial impacts on another part. For example, a two-class model with only linear trends over time may represent the data equally as well as a one-class model with quadratic effects.

Usually, the highest reasonable polynomial (depending on the number of time points, theoretical and prior considerations) is considered in each class, models with increasing number of classes are fit, and only essential covariates (e.g., treatment, exposure) are included as predictors. To decide on the best model, the fit of all considered models is compared. The Schwartz-Bayesian Information Criteria (BIC) is the most commonly used model fit criterion, with smaller values indicative of a better model fit. However, the BIC tends to favor models with too many classes. Thus, the BIC is used mainly to select from alternative predictor sets and polynomials of different degree within classes rather than the number of classes.

There are specific tests for the selection of number of classes: the *Lo-Mendell-Rubin likelihood ratio test* (Lo et al., 2001) and *the bootstrap likelihood ratio test* (Nylund et al., 2007). These tests compare the fit of a model with (k–1) classes to the fit of the corresponding model with k classes. Small p-values indicate that the model with k classes provides a better fit than the model with one fewer class. Usually, a significance level of 0.05 is used.

Another indication of whether a model fits the data well is the *entropy*, a measure of classification accuracy. To calculate the model entropy, posterior probabilities of class membership for each individual are calculated (based on the overall model and observed outcomes), and then individuals are classified in the most likely class (i.e., the class for which the posterior probability is the highest). If the model successfully identifies distinct patterns of responses over time, then subjects have probabilities close to one and zero to be classified in a particular class. Thus, we can fairly convincingly assign individuals to the most likely trajectory class. Roughly speaking, the entropy is calculated based on the average of the posterior class probabilities. The values are between zero and one, with one indicating perfect classification accuracy. Models with higher classification accuracy are preferred, with values exceeding 0.7 considered good.

Since there is no reliable test to "prove" that there are categorically different trajectories, one informal way to assess this assumption is to examine posterior probabilities that subjects belong to a particular trajectory class. In the case where there are no categorically different trajectories there will be a substantial percentage of subjects who cannot be reliably classified to any one trajectory. On the other hand, when there are different trajectories and the model fits the data well, then individuals should be classified in a particular trajectory more accurately.

Several additional aspects of model fit based on posterior probabilities should also be routinely evaluated:

- Whether there is good correspondence between the estimated probability of group membership and the proportion of individuals assigned to that group based on estimated posterior probabilities

- Whether the average of the posterior probabilities of individuals assigned to each group exceeds a pre-specified high threshold (e.g., 0.7)
- Whether group membership probabilities are precisely estimated, that is, the standard errors of the group membership probabilities are small

Additionally, trajectory classes with too few subjects (e.g., less than 1% of the sample in large samples, less than 5% of the sample in smaller samples) should be avoided, as they cannot be reliably estimated.

In general, there is a danger of idiosyncratic results if the final decision on a model rests on a single number (whether this is the BIC, the bootstrap likelihood ratio test, or entropy) and no attention is paid to the interpretation of obtained results. The model fit indices themselves can also contradict each other. Although this introduces an element of subjectivity, a more complex decision process is needed to select meaningful and well-fitting latent class models.

Note that sample size plays a role in identification of the best model. In general, the larger the sample size, the more classes one can reliably estimate. For GMM/LCGM, both number of individuals and number of observation points per individual are important. Simulation studies have shown that about 200–500 individuals are sufficient for reliable inference, even in the presence of trajectory classes with a relatively small number of subjects. Increasing the number of follow-up points usually leads to an increase in the number of trajectories.

10.3.3 Guidelines for Model Selection

Because of the complexity of the models, selection of the best model is difficult. Many reasonable models need to be considered and the final model should satisfy the following conditions:

- Stable solution achieved (i.e., maximum likelihood value replicated in a substantial proportion of the runs).
- Lower BIC value among models with different number of classes, fixed and random effects structures, and predictors (it is desirable for the final model to have the lowest BIC value, but sometimes other criteria and interpretability may lead to selection of a model with somewhat higher BIC than the best achieved).
- Significantly better fit according to the bootstrap likelihood ratio test or Lo-Mendell-Rubin's test than the same model with one fewer class. The model with one more class does not fit significantly better than the model in question.
- Good classification accuracy (usually above 0.7).
- No classes with few individuals per class (e.g., less than 1% in big samples, less than 5% in smaller samples).
- Parsimonious model (i.e., among different models that fit the data approximately equally well, the one with fewer parameters is selected).
- Interpretable results (consistent with existing theory). Classes are considered meaningful if they differ in relevant characteristics and outcomes.

A general recommendation is to include predictors of class membership directly in the model as well as to incorporate concurrent events and consequences. Concurrent events can be considered as time-varying covariates with class-varying effects, time-varying outcomes predicted by the latent classes, or as parallel growth processes. Consequences may be considered as distal outcomes predicted by trajectory classes.

Some residual diagnostics are available for GMM but are not widely used. For example, Wang et al. (2005) proposed residual diagnostics for number of classes, mean growth trajectories, and covariance structures.

More detailed guidelines on the use of GMM are provided in Muthén and Muthén (2000), Muthén et al. (2002), Hipp and Bauer (2006), and by Frankfurt et al. (2016). Detailed criticisms of LCGM and GMM, including the tendency to over-extract trajectory classes, run into computation problems, and to achieve unstable solutions, can be found in Bauer and Curran (2003), Sher et al. (2011), and Skardhamar (2010).

10.4 Data Examples

10.4.1 Trajectories of Heavy Drinking in COMBINE

To illustrate mixture models, we focus on the COMBINE study (introduced in Section 1.5.3 and repeatedly analyzed in subsequent chapters), in which we evaluate drinking outcomes and the effects of the randomized treatments over approximately four months in over 1000 alcohol-dependent individuals. The heavy drinking outcome considered herein is coded as 1 if 5 or more drinks are consumed on a day during each monthly interval during the treatment part of the study and 0 otherwise. If no data are available during a particular month, then the outcome is missing for that month. We first fit LCGM with two to four latent classes, a logistic regression model with linear and quadratic trends over time in each latent trajectory class, and trajectory membership predicted by naltrexone, CBI, and the interaction between naltrexone and CBI. The purpose of this analysis is to evaluate whether there are distinct trajectory patterns of heavy drinking over time, how they are described, and whether the treatments affect the chance of following a particular pattern. PROC TRAJ in SAS is used for the analysis, and the results are replicated using MPlus. The code for both can be found in the online materials.

Table 10.1 presents indices of model fit. Models with five classes do not converge to stable solutions so are not presented here. We select the model with linear time trends in four classes as the final model because it has the lowest BIC of the considered models, good entropy (0.73), and a highly significant p-value on the bootstrap likelihood ratio test when compared with the model with three classes ($p < 0.0001$).

Figure 10.3 shows the model-based and sample-based means by time point in the four trajectory groups. The four trajectories can be described as: (1) "abstinence from heavy drinking" (485 subjects out of 1220 with outcome data, or approximately 40% of the sample, are most likely to be classified in this trajectory class); (2) "decreasing probability of heavy drinking" (194 out of 1220, or 15.9%); and (3) "increasing probability of heavy drinking" (81 out of 1220, 6.6%). That is, the "decreasing probability of heavy drinking" description should be preceding the "increasing probability of heacy drinking". The numbers pertaining to each description go with the description. and (4) "heavy drinking" (460 out of 1220, 37.7%). The four trajectories are quite distinct, and the majority of individuals are classified in one of the extreme classes (either abstainers from heavy drinking or heavy drinking throughout the study). In addition, there is very good correspondence between the model-based probabilities of heavy drinking (i.e., the probabilities calculated based on the model) and the sample-based probabilities calculated when each individual's contribution is weighted by the estimated posterior probability of trajectory membership.

TABLE 10.1

Results from Fitting Six Latent Class Growth Models to the COMBINE Data

	BIC	Entropy	Bootstrap Likelihood Ratio Test P-value
Linear time trend			
Two classes	5054.33	0.83	<0.0001
Three classes	5002.71	0.78	<0.0001
Four classes	5002.15	0.73	<0.0001
Quadratic time trend			
Two classes	5026.44	0.84	<0.0001
Three classes	5011.12	0.71	<0.0001
Four classes	5019.62	0.76	<0.0001

Note: The outcome is a dichotomous measure of heavy drinking evaluated for each of the four months of the study.

In order to assess how well individuals are classified in trajectory classes, we examine the posterior probabilities of class membership. Table 10.2 shows the averages of the estimated posterior probabilities in each of the four classes by most likely class membership. We see that these averages are all quite high for the most likely class. For example, individuals most likely to be classified in the "abstinence from heavy drinking class" have, on average, a probability of 0.87 of falling within that class and much lower estimated probabilities of being classified in an alternative class (all probabilities less than 0.10). Similarly,

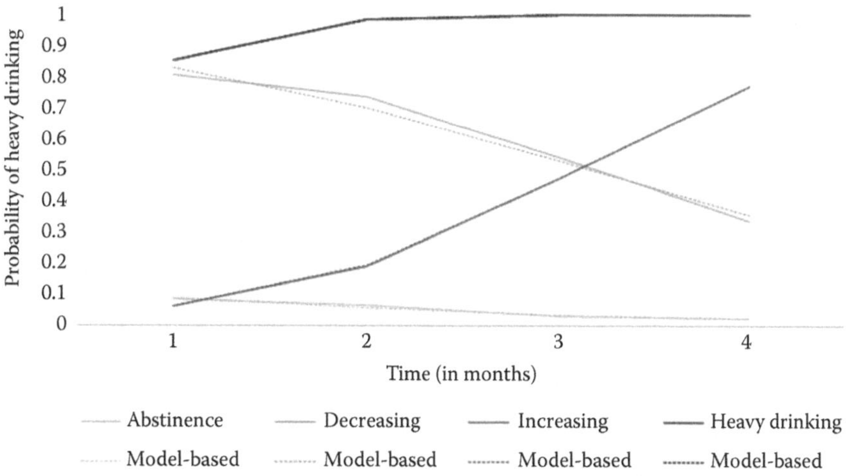

FIGURE 10.3
Sample-based and model-based probabilities of heavy drinking in the four trajectory classes during the treatment period of the COMBINE study. Solid lines represent sample-based probabilities of heavy drinking, based on all subjects weighted by the posterior probability of trajectory membership. Dotted lines represent model-based probabilities of heavy drinking. Dotted lines are not visible where solid and dotted lines overlap.

TABLE 10.2

Probabilities of Class Membership by Most Likely Latent Class in LCGM Applied to Monthly Heavy Drinking Measures in the COMBINE Study

	Average Probabilities of Class Membership				
Most Likely Trajectory Class	**Abstinence from Heavy Drinking**	**Decreasing Heavy Drinking**	**Increasing Heavy Drinking**	**Heavy Drinking**	**Sample Size**
Abstinence from heavy drinking	0.87	0.08	0.05	0.00	485
Decreasing heavy drinking	0.03	0.88	0.05	0.04	194
Increasing heavy drinking	0.10	0.09	0.80	0.01	81
Heavy drinking	0.00	0.10	0.02	0.88	460
Entire sample	0.36	0.21	0.09	0.34	1220

individuals most likely to be classified in the "heavy drinking" trajectory class have, on average, a probability of 0.88 of being classified in this trajectory class. The lowest average probability of membership in the most likely class is the one for "increasing heavy drinking," and even this probability is pretty high (0.80). Thus, this model appears to classify individuals quite well, which translates into a high overall measure of classification accuracy of 0.73.

Turning our attention to treatment as a predictor of trajectory membership, we evaluate the effects of naltrexone, CBI, and their interaction. Since there are four different trajectories and each pair can be compared, there are multiple tests that can be conducted and effect estimates that can be calculated. For a full list and results, refer to the online materials. Since the overall test of the interaction between naltrexone and CBI is not statistically significant ($\chi^2(3)=5.27$, $p=0.15$) we focus on the main effects of naltrexone and CBI and present odds ratios for the pairwise comparisons of the trajectories with associated 95% confidence intervals. Table 10.3 shows these results without any adjustment for multiple tests. Naltrexone significantly lowers the odds of following the "heavy drinking" trajectory compared with the "abstinence from heavy drinking" trajectory and the "decreasing heavy drinking trajectory." There are no significant pairwise comparisons for CBI.

We next consider GMM with linear trends over time and use the default assumptions in MPlus of equal variances and covariances of the random effects across different classes. The model with linear time trends in two latent trajectory classes converges and fits better than a model with only one class, as the bootstrap likelihood ratio test for the two-class GMM compared with a one-class model is highly statistically significant ($p<0.0001$). GMM with three trajectory classes does not converge to a replicable solution even with 500 random starts and imposing additional restrictions on the parameters. Thus, the GMM reliably identifies only two trajectory classes for these data.

The GMM with two latent classes had a slightly lower BIC than the LCGM with four trajectory classes (BIC = 4943.26 compared with 5002.15), but the entropy is 0.63, lower than the entropies of all considered LCGMs. This is a common finding, because the random effects within classes allow GMM to match the observed data more closely than LCGM, but, at the same time, it is harder to accurately classify individuals in latent classes.

TABLE 10.3

Odds Ratios and 95% Confidence Intervals for the Effects of Naltrexone and CBI on Trajectory Membership in Heavy Drinking Classes in COMBINE Based on the LCGM with Four Classes

Effect	Trajectory Comparison	Odds Ratio (95% Confidence Interval)
Main effect of naltrexone	"Decreasing heavy drinking" versus "No heavy drinking"	1.10 (0.74, 1.62)
	"Increasing heavy drinking" versus "No heavy drinking"	0.70 (0.34, 1.42)
	"Heavy drinking" versus "No heavy drinking"	0.68 (0.51, 0.92)
	"Increasing heavy drinking" versus "Decreasing heavy drinking"	0.64 (0.30, 1.34)
	"Heavy drinking" versus "Decreasing heavy drinking"	0.63 (0.42, 0.94)
	"Heavy drinking" versus "Increasing heavy drinking"	0.98 (0.49, 1.97)
Main effect of CBI	"Decreasing heavy drinking" versus "No heavy drinking"	1.22 (0.81, 1.84)
	"Increasing heavy drinking" versus "No heavy drinking"	0.68 (0.34, 1.36)
	"Heavy drinking" versus "No heavy drinking"	0.85 (0.63, 1.14)
	"Increasing heavy drinking" versus "Decreasing heavy drinking"	0.56 (0.27, 1.13)
	"Heavy drinking" versus "Decreasing heavy drinking"	0.69 (0.45, 1.07)
	"Heavy drinking" versus "Increasing heavy drinking"	1.25 (0.63, 2.49)

The two latent classes are shown in Figure 10.4 and can be regarded as a "heavy drinking" class and an "abstinence from heavy drinking" class. About 38.3% of the sample (467 out of 1220 individuals) are classified as most likely belonging to the "heavy drinking" class while the remaining 61.7% (753 out of 1220) are classified as most likely belonging to the "abstinence from heavy drinking" class. Of those most likely to follow the "heavy drinking" trajectory, the average probability of being assigned to this class is 0.75, while of those most likely to follow the "abstinence from heavy drinking" trajectory, the average probability of assignment to this class is 0.97 (Table 10.4). Both are fairly high, although

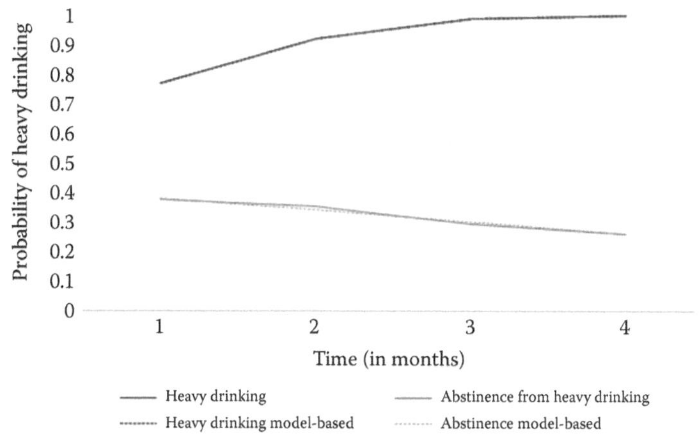

FIGURE 10.4
Sample-based and model-based probabilities of heavy drinking in the two trajectory classes during the treatment period of the COMBINE study identified using generalized mixture models. Solid lines represent sample-based probabilities of heavy drinking. Dotted lines represent model-based probabilities of heavy drinking. Dotted lines are not visible where solid and dotted lines overlap.

TABLE 10.4

Probabilities of Class Membership by Most Likely Latent Class in GMM Applied to Heavy Drinking in the COMBINE Data

	Average Probabilities of Class Membership		
Most Likely Trajectory Class	**Abstinence from Heavy Drinking**	**Heavy Drinking**	**Sample Size**
Abstinence from heavy drinking	0.97	0.03	753
Heavy drinking	0.25	0.75	467
Entire sample	0.69	0.31	1220

the overall entropy is lower than the one in the four-class LCGM. Compared with the four latent classes identified using LCGM, the two classes identified using GMM are the two extremes, with individuals who follow a heavy drinking trajectory identified accurately by both approaches. In the LCGM, the remaining individuals are split into three groups depending on whether they increase or decrease the probability of heavy drinking over time, while in the GMM these individuals are in the same class ("abstinence from heavy drinking"). They can be absorbed into the same class because their intercepts and slopes are allowed to vary within a class.

To compare the results from the LCGM and GMM further, we focus on the treatment effects on trajectory membership. Similar to the overall test in the four class LCGM, the interaction between naltrexone and CBI is not statistically significant in the two-class GMM ($\chi^2(1)=2.22$, $p=0.14$), there is a statistically significant main effect of naltrexone ($\chi^2(1)=7.61$, $p=0.006$), and no significant main effect of CBI ($\chi^2(1)=1.30$, $p=0.25$). Naltrexone significantly decreases the chance of following the "heavy drinking" class trajectory (OR = 0.62, 95% CI: (0.44, 0.87)).

Note that although GMM and LCGM identify different numbers of trajectory classes, most individuals are classified in the two extreme classes in LCGM, and the effects of treatment on trajectory membership are similar (i.e., naltrexone significantly reduces the chance of following a heavy drinking trajectory). In deciding which approach to use, one needs to consider conceptually whether the goal of the analysis is to categorize individuals in particular meaningful groups (in which case LCGM is arguably better because it has higher entropy) or discover underlying population structure (in which case GMM is preferable). In this particular application, and more generally with categorical data, LCGM often provides more useful and detailed descriptions of the responses over time.

In conclusion, for this example, we have evidence that most individuals are either heavy drinkers or not heavy drinkers throughout the study. A minority show a change in response over time. Naltrexone decreases the likelihood of following a heavy drinking trajectory. Further analyses incorporating predictors of trajectories, time-dependent covariates, and distal outcomes can be considered. Examples of the application of LCGM to daily drinking data from the COMBINE study can be found in Gueorguieva et al. (2010, 2011, 2012).

10.4.2 Trajectories of Depression Symptoms in STAR*D

Our second example focuses on identification of distinct trajectories during 12-week antidepressant treatment with citalopram using the data on more than 400 individuals from the STAR*D clinical trial (Section 1.5.2). As in the analysis of these data in Chapter 3, we focus on the three clusters of depressive symptoms (core, atypical, and sleep). Herein, we seek to identify distinct trajectory classes of all three clusters simultaneously. That is, each class is characterized by a particular combination of patterns on all three symptoms. Compared with the models with a single repeatedly measured outcome variable, a GMM with three repeatedly measured outcome variables requires specification of three GLMM in each latent class (one for each outcome), with different fixed and random effects. The random effects of the same and different outcomes measures on the same individual are assumed to be correlated within but not across latent classes. The default assumptions of equal variances and covariances across latent classes are used.

We focus on the scheduled visits at weeks 0, 2, 4, 6, and 9 and fit linear mixed models with random intercepts and slopes for each symptom within each trajectory class. Week 12 is excluded, since only about 20% of the individuals in the sample provide data at this time point. Time is log-transformed as in this case the response over time is well described by a straight line. Although it is theoretically possible to consider multiple outcomes in LCGM, PROC TRAJ in SAS can handle only two outcomes measures at a time, and hence we focus only on GMM that can be fit seamlessly using the MPlus software. All code, output, and graphs are available in the online materials.

Table 10.5 shows the results from the GMM with two, three, and four latent classes. We use the Lo-Mendell-Rubin (LMR) test rather than the bootstrap likelihood ratio test to test whether models with more classes fit the data significantly better, since the LMR test statistic is more easily calculated and performs well with continuous data. In all models, the variance of the random slope in all classes for the atypical symptom are fixed at zero in order to achieve model identifiability.

From Table 10.5, we see that the model with four classes has the lowest BIC and the highest entropy (0.60); however, it does not provide a better fit to the data than the three-class model according to the LMR test and its entropy is only slightly higher than the entropy of the three-class model (0.59). Neither entropy is particularly high (in general, entropies above 0.7 are preferred) so there is a fair amount of uncertainty when classifying individuals in latent classes.

Figure 10.5 consists of three panels and shows the estimated mean trajectories for each of the three symptom clusters. The three trajectories in each panel can be described as a "non-response," "rapid response," and "improvement" trajectories. The "non-response" trajectory class shows minimal decrease in core and sleep symptom severity and some deterioration of atypical symptom severity. The "rapid response" class shows marked and fast improvement in core symptoms and to a lesser degree in sleep symptoms and atypical symptoms. The "improvement" class shows improvement in all three symptom clusters but not as fast as in the "rapid response" group, and with residual symptoms remaining

TABLE 10.5

Results from Fitting Three Growth Mixture Models to the STAR*D Data. The Outcome is Cluster Severity Score Evaluated at Baseline and Weeks 2, 4, 6, and 9

			Lo-Mendell-Rubin test
	BIC	**Entropy**	**P-value**
Two classes	64118.18	0.47	<0.0001
Three classes	63728.93	0.59	0.02
Four classes	63562.30	0.60	0.21

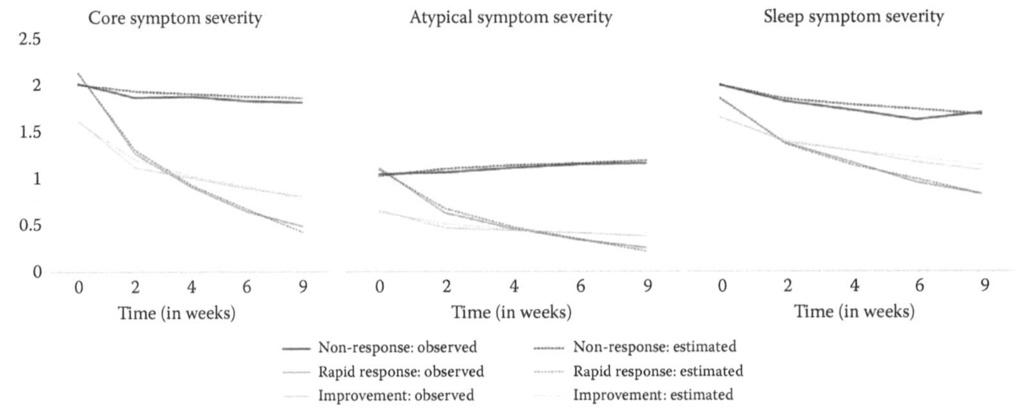

FIGURE 10.5
Sample-based and model-based symptom severity in the three trajectory classes fitted to the STAR*D data.

by nine weeks. Two-thirds of the individuals in the sample (2693 out of 4018, or 67%) have trajectories most consistent with the "improvement" class, while only about 10% (402 out of 4018) are most likely to show trajectories of "non-response" on all three symptom clusters. The remaining subjects are classified in the "rapid response" trajectory (923 out of 4018, or 23%). Table 10.6 shows that the average probabilities by most likely latent class are reasonably high.

Note that the trajectory classes differ not only in rate of improvement but also in baseline starting point. Individuals in the "non-response" and "rapid response" classes start with a higher average baseline severity than individuals in the "improvement" class. Comparing trajectories across clusters, we see that individuals acknowledge mostly core and sleep symptoms at baseline. Atypical symptoms are less frequently acknowledged, which at least partially explains the flatter slopes for this group.

In this data set, all individuals received citalopram treatment, so we cannot explore medication effects. However, an exploration of predictors of trajectories of improvement and the relationship between these trajectories and distal outcomes are of considerable interest. In a study of such large sample size as the STAR*D trial, state-of-the-art prediction models can be used (see e.g. Chekroud et al. (2016), who used machine learning methods for a prediction of a simpler outcome of clinical response within 12 weeks of treatment).

Note that we considered latent classes identified by the combination of patterns on the three different clusters of symptoms simultaneously. It is possible, although more

TABLE 10.6
Probabilities of Class Membership by Most Likely Latent Class in GMM Applied to Symptom Severity of Three Clusters in the STAR*D Data

	Average Probabilities of Class Membership			
Most Likely Trajectory Class	**Non-Response**	**Rapid Response**	**Improvement**	**Sample Size**
Non-response	0.80	0.03	0.17	402
Rapid response	0.04	0.77	0.19	923
Improvement	0.06	0.11	0.82	2693
Entire sample	0.13	0.25	0.61	4018

complicated, to define separate trajectory classes for each symptom and then relate these trajectory classes to each other. This was the approach taken by Nagin and Tremblay (2001) when studying related behaviors using LCGM.

10.5 Summary

In this chapter, we reviewed two types of latent class models for data-driven identification of distinct trajectory patterns over time. Such models have intuitive appeal for heterogeneous populations and when classifying patterns of change is of interest. Latent class growth models offer a semi-parametric group-based approach that allows for normal, censored normal, Poisson, zero-inflated, and binary outcomes. It assumes polynomial trends, can handle missing data, both time-dependent and time-independent covariates, and can model related behaviors over time. However, it does not allow for random variability in growth factors within each trajectory class, and thus is less flexible than the other latent class approach presented in this chapter; namely, growth mixture models. GMM share the advantages of the LCGM approach but are more prone to computational and identifiability problems. Also, philosophically, the aim of LCGM is to describe the population variability in patterns of response over time for a small number of distinct groups, while GMM relies on the assumption that there are underlying latent classes of individuals within the population in order to produce interpretable results.

Identifying a well-fitting model is challenging for both types of models, but more so for GMM, since there are too many possible combinations of numbers of trajectory classes, patterns of change over time, sets of fixed and random effects, and covariates. A systematic model selection approach has been recently proposed by Frankfurt et al. (2016). The initial step is to fit a single-class GMM without covariates (i.e., a GLMM with only time as a predictor) and examine the variances of the random effects. If there is no evidence of significant inter-individual variability (i.e., non-zero variances) then latent class models should not be fit to the data. On the other hand, if there is evidence of significant variability, then in step 2 , a latent class model (LCGM or GMM) should be specified. This involves specifying the patterns of change over time within classes. No covariates are included yet in the model. In step 3, the number of classes should be determined. In general, the bootstrap likelihood ratio test is preferred, but since it is computationally intensive, the BIC or Lo-Mendell-Rubin's can be used initially, and BLRT considered only for the final decision. Convergence issues need to be addressed in step 4. In the last step (step 5), covariates are added to the model. Although this is a very reasonable algorithm, there is disagreement among researchers as to the order of the steps, in particular whether models with or without covariates should be considered initially. Furthermore, different latent class models may be appropriate, and one may need to go repeatedly through the steps in order to identify a best-fitting model.

A complication in this process is that one cannot rely on a single decision rule to select the number of classes, patterns, covariates, and random effects. When there is contradiction among commonly used fit statistics, such as the BIC, the LMR or BLRT, and the entropy, one needs to consider the research question of interest, model parsimony, theoretical justification, and interpretability. The entire process of model selection needs to be transparent and accurately described so that results can be reproduced.

Methodological research in GMM is ongoing. Some recent developments include using GMM for causal inference (Haviland and Nagin, 2005; Brown et al., 2008; Muthén et al., 2002) and GMM to account for non-random attrition (Havilandet al., 2011; Muthén et al., 2011). An alternative approach to GMM to handle non-normal variability is to consider GLMM with random effects that are not normally distributed (e.g., Verbeke and Lesaffre, 1996).

In conclusion, LCGM and GMM are useful in identifying different trajectories over time and potentially in characterizing individuals following a particular trajectory. Predictors of trajectory membership and distal outcomes are useful in providing substantive justification of the latent classes. However, due to the potential for identifiability and convergence issues, model selection and assessment of model fit are critical. Sensitivity analysis may also need to be performed. GMM have mostly been used as an exploratory tool but have potential as a confirmatory tool. Both LCGM and GMM have been used to classify individuals in latent trajectory classes and then to use these assignments as response variables in regression modeling. This two-stage approach is problematic when the uncertainties of trajectory classifications are not accounted for in the second-stage models. One can allow for the uncertainty by using the posterior membership probabilities to construct weights that reflect the uncertainty of classification.

11

Study Design and Sample Size Calculations

The emphasis of the first ten chapters of this book has been on analysis methods for clustered and longitudinal data. However, an equally important aspect of studies with repeated measures is the study design. At the design stage, decisions are made about the primary goals of the investigation (i.e., what questions should the study answer), type of study most suited to the goals (e.g., experimental or observational), study design (e.g., parallel group versus cross-over clinical trial), the population for which inferences should be valid, sampling scheme in order to obtain a representative sample, response variable(s), assessment schedule, specific analysis plan, and adequate sample size to achieve the study goals.

If crucial mistakes are made at the design stage, then even the best statistical analysis will not be able to correct for fatal flaws. For example, if one is interested in evaluating treatment efficacy but does not include a control group in the study, it is not possible to disentangle the effect of treatment from the effect of time. Changes may occur over time due to regression to the mean or other phenomena that have little to do with treatment. Similarly, if treatments A and B are compared to each other within individuals but treatment A always precedes treatment B, the effect of treatment B may be confounded with the residual effects of treatment A. A common flaw of many studies is that they are not sufficiently powered to detect the effects of interest. This is sometimes a flaw at the design stage when overly optimistic measures of effect size are used in order to calculate the necessary sample size. At other times, inadequate power reflects a problem with recruitment as the study cannot achieve its recruitment goals. Higher than expected rates of missing data often result in bias and increased probability of type II error (i.e., failure to find effects when effects exist).

This chapter reviews design considerations for studies with correlated data and focuses specifically on sample size estimation. Section 11.1 reviews the importance of careful study design for experiments and observational studies with repeated measures and lists key aspects that need consideration. Section 11.2 describes the most commonly used repeated measures designs and weighs in on their advantages and disadvantages. Section 11.3 introduces methods for sample size calculations for cross-sectional data. Section 11.4 focuses on sample size calculations for clustered and longitudinal data with emphasis on mixed regression and GEE models. Methods based on traditional ANOVA-based approaches and power calculations based on summary measures are also briefly discussed. Common randomization approaches for experimental studies are reviewed in Section 11.5, and the chapter concludes with a summary and discussion (Section 11.6). Data examples are presented throughout the chapter with code and results included in the online materials. Useful references regarding study design and/or sample size calculations are Lachin (1981), Fleiss (1986), Kraemer and Blasey (1987), Cohen (1988), Bailar and Mosteller (1992), and Borenstein (1997). A reference for power analysis for longitudinal and clustered data that includes many recent developments is Ahn et al. (2015).

11.1 Study Design Considerations

11.1.1 Study Objectives

At the design stage, the first and most important question is to define clearly the *goals of the study*. In clinical trials, most commonly, the goal is to establish whether an experimental treatment is better than or as good as a control treatment. In observational studies, most commonly, the goal is to evaluate whether individuals with a particular exposure have different outcomes than individuals without that exposure. The size of the effects needs to be estimated precisely in both types of studies.

11.1.2 Target Population

Another important decision concerns the *target population*; that is, the population to which the results should apply. Do we want to know how individuals with a particular disease respond to a particular treatment? Should we place any restrictions on the population? For example, should we exclude from the study individuals with certain co-morbidities? Below or above a certain age? What other inclusion/exclusion criteria should we consider? These questions become very complex, as one wants to balance the need for generalizable results with the feasibility of recruitment, and the potential benefits with the potential risk to the individuals participating in the study. If the target population is very diverse, then the results will be applicable to a wider range of individuals; but, on the other hand, the variability in measures may be so high that an unrealistically large sample is needed in order to estimate treatment or exposure effects precisely. In addition, certain individuals in the population may be more likely to suffer adverse effects, and hence it is an ethical dilemma whether to include them in a study. If higher-risk individuals are excluded, then results may not generalize to such individuals in the population. On the other hand, if they are included, they might be exposed to unnecessary risk.

11.1.3 Study Sample

Once the goal of the study and the target population are defined, a decision needs to be made on how to obtain a *representative sample* of the population. Practicality and generalizability are again at odds here. For clinical studies, individuals are often selected when they seek contact with a health care professional. However, this may lead to a biased sample, as sicker individuals may seek help and may be more likely to be selected. In addition, different types of health centers may have different mixtures of individuals.

In observational studies, such as longitudinal surveys, individuals are often selected based on their residence. Ideally, one would want to capture a wide variety of individuals and settings. Sometimes, it is necessary to oversample from certain sociodemographic groups in order to be able to generalize to the entire population. There are a variety of sampling schemes that could be used in order to obtain representative samples. Sampling strategies are beyond the scope of this book, but the interested reader is referred to Levy and Lemeshow (1999). The sampling scheme needs to be taken into account in the analysis. Most national surveys provide special weights in order to adjust estimates for the sampling process.

11.1.4 Outcome Measures

In addition to the goals of the study, target population, and methods for obtaining a representative sample, one needs to identify the measure of interest and choose the most appropriate design for the study. We focus on the *measure(s) of interest* first. The goals of the study are often defined in a general way. For example, the aims may be to assess whether depression severity decreases more with treatment A than with treatment B in the target population, or whether working memory in schizophrenic patients is worse than in healthy controls when performing certain tasks. In order to formulate an actionable statistical plan for the study, we need to specify the outcome measure. In the depression example, one has the choice of several rating scales of depression severity. Which one should be chosen? This may depend on the population of interest (some measures may be validated or more appropriate in populations of younger individuals, some in populations of older individuals). Additionally, some variables may have lower variability, which may make it easier to detect change. Measures can also be selected based on the participant burden they place. A lengthy questionnaire may be more precise but more burdensome to complete.

Note that multiple outcome measures may be of interest in a particular study. They may capture the same aspect of the response (e.g., the Hamilton Depression Rating Scale and a simpler ordinal measure of depression severity, such as the Clinical Global Severity Scale; time to response or relapse and repeated measures of severity) or different aspects of interest (e.g., measures of efficacy and safety). A decision then needs to be made about primary versus secondary outcomes, and about adjustments for multiple testing. When few outcomes are of equal interest, a simple Bonferroni-based adjustment is often appropriate. On the other hand, when there are many simultaneous hypotheses tests or effect size estimations that are of interest, adjustments based on the false discovery rate may be more appropriate (see Chapter 6).

11.1.5 Study Design

There are many different *design choices* for longitudinal data studies: parallel group designs (see e.g., Figure 1.1), cross-over designs (e.g., Figure 1.2), cluster-randomized trials, stepped-wedge and other practical designs, and adaptive designs that sequentially assign or randomize participants to different treatments. We describe the most common designs in more detail and focus on their advantages and disadvantages in Section 11.2. In general, the choice of the design is based on feasibility, ability to achieve the study goals, and sample size requirements. Evaluation of several alternatives is usually performed at the design stage and the best choice agreed on by the study planners.

11.1.6 Data Collection, Management, and Monitoring

Design considerations in longitudinal studies also include decisions about the *assessment schedule* (e.g., number of occasions the outcome variables are evaluated; whether individuals will be followed up at the same or different time points; by whom and how the data will be collected), methods for preventing and *minimizing the impact of missing data*, and plans for data collection, *data management*, and *statistical analysis*. Data also need to be continually monitored in order to identify issues with data collection, outliers, or other problems with data capture.

11.1.7 Statistical Analysis Plan

A mark of a well-designed study is the presence at the onset of a detailed *statistical analysis plan.* In order to be able to formulate such a plan, one needs to have gone through all the steps mentioned previously. The analysis plan includes details about the *modeling approach,* the *level of uncertainty* allowed in the statistical inference, and what results will be considered *supportive of the study aims.*

We first focus on the *modeling approach.* A basic question in any study with repeated measures data is whether a simple baseline-to-endpoint comparison is sufficient to address the aims of the study or whether a more sophisticated mixed model or GEE approach is needed. The latter is preferred if one hopes to obtain information and perform inference about the pattern of change over time. Simple baseline-to-endpoint comparison may be appropriate if the study is of short duration or if it is expensive or impractical to measure the outcome repeatedly. If a more sophisticated modeling approach is selected, one needs to consider what assumptions will be made about the correlation structure of the data and the mean trends. For example, would a linear trend be adequate to describe change over time or would higher order polynomials be needed? If the rate of change over time is expected to be different at the beginning of the study compared with the end of the study, a curvilinear trend or a time transformation may be more appropriate.

Another very important question in the analysis plan is what distributions will be used to model the study outcomes. If the outcome is continuous and expected to be bell-shaped, normal distribution should be used. For skewed continuous data, alternative distributions (such as gamma) may be preferred, or one may transform the data prior to using models for normally distributed data. For discrete outcomes such as counts, one may consider Poisson or negative binomial distributions. When the outcomes are not conforming to the chosen distributions, transformations or non-parametric methods should be considered.

One also needs to specify if any covariates will be included in the statistical model. Ideally, these should be pre-specified and balanced across groups. This is achieved with stratified randomization in experimental studies (see Section 11.5) and matching in observational studies.

Another very important question is how missing data will be handled in the analysis approach. As described in Chapter 7, two gold standard approaches are available to deal with missing data—full information maximum likelihood and multiple imputation. However, with informatively missing data, even those approaches may produce biased results. Thus, sensitivity analyses under different conditions should be considered in the analysis plan.

It is also very important to specify what *level of statistical significance or confidence* will be used for hypotheses testing and effect estimation. Traditionally, the 0.05 significance level and corresponding 95% confidence level for confidence intervals are used for primary outcomes. However, when there are multiple primary analyses, this may prove to be too liberal and corrections should be considered. Depending on the goals of the study, family-wise error rate corrections or false discovery rate corrections can be used (see Chapter 6).

In the statistical analysis method, one needs to be very clear what results will be considered consistent with the study aims. For example, in clinical trials with multiple groups, one often focuses on the group by time interaction. However, it is not sufficient to state that one expects to observe a significant group by time effect. It is important to indicate also what pattern of follow-up tests will be consistent with the study hypothesis. For example, the expectation may be that there is greater rate of change from baseline to endpoint in the experimental group compared with the control group. If the goal is to estimate effect sizes, a successful outcome would be to estimate those with a good precision (i.e., with a narrow confidence interval).

11.1.8 Sample Size Estimation or Power Analysis

All components of the design mentioned so far have a bearing on the *sample size estimation*, which is the most widely recognized component of the study planning process. Sample size calculations are described in detail in Sections 11.3 and 11.4. Herein, we just emphasize the main purpose and ideas behind this process. Traditionally, sample size calculations are performed for simple hypotheses tests and the sample size calculation is intended to guarantee with a particular level of confidence that the study will not miss a meaningful effect and will not falsely identify a non-existent effect, if conducted as planned. In recent years, there has been a movement away from hypothesis testing and toward effect size estimation, and hence, the goal of the sample size calculation has become to estimate within a certain precision the effect of interest from the study data. This has the advantage that an interval is achieved that captures the true effect with a certain level of confidence, but is sometimes impractical when there are multiple groups that are being compared. Sample size calculations need to take into account corrections for multiple testing if there are multiple study hypotheses and/or outcome measures.

Note that, often, rather than estimating sample size, *reverse sample size calculations* are performed, in which a feasible sample size is assumed and then the detectable effect size of interest for the outcome is calculated. If such a detectable effect size of interest is deemed reasonable, the study can proceed, otherwise alternatives need to be considered.

Similarly, for a particular sample size and effect size, the available power to declare the effect as statistically significant could be calculated. If power is high enough (usually 80% or above), the study proceeds, otherwise an alternative need to be considered.

Sample size/power calculations are a very important part of the study planning. If properly performed and described, they give credence to the results. However, such calculations are often missing from study descriptions, are performed in a post hoc fashion, or do not correspond to the study design or outcome measures. Scientific journals in recent years have become increasingly rigorous about requesting this information and holding authors responsible for gaps and discrepancies between power calculations, *a priori* analysis plans, and final analyses. Furthermore, more sophisticated and flexible software programs have become available to perform power calculations, thus simplifying the study planning process.

Note that although the design of the study and the analysis plan need to be pre-specified, one can allow for pre-specified modifications depending on the data generated from the trial. For example, the sample size can be adjusted based on interim analysis or randomization allocation can be adjusted depending on the outcomes of individuals already enrolled in the trial. Such clinical trials are called *adaptive* and are the topic of very intensive research in recent years. Reviews of adaptive designs are provided by Schaefer et al. (2006), Coffey and Kairalla (2008), Chow (2014), and Bauer et al. (2016).

Guidelines for study design in epidemiological studies and/or clinical trials are provided by Fleiss (1986), Woodward (1999), Katz (2006), Parfrey and Barrett (2009), and Friedman et al. (2010) among others.

11.1.9 Reporting Guidelines

In recent years, detailed *reporting guidelines* for different types of studies have been developed. The most popular ones are the CONSORT (**CON**solidated **S**tandards **O**f **R**eporting **T**rials) guidelines for randomized controlled trials and the STROBE (**ST**rengthening the **R**eporting of **OB**servational Studies in **E**pidemiology) guidelines for epidemiological studies. The EQUATOR (**E**nhancing the **QUA**lity and **T**ransparency **O**f health **R**esearch) network has been established with the goal of promoting transparent and accurate reporting of health research studies (Simera et al., 2010) and has put together a comprehensive list of reporting guidelines, including CONSORT and STROBE. Altman and Simera (2016) provide a historical overview of the development of the guidelines and outline future challenges. Following established guidelines ensures higher quality of studies and their reporting, and thus, investigators should be familiar with, and whenever possible follow, the guidelines. Furthermore, publishing study protocols prior to carrying out the study serves to prevent scientific misconduct associated with post hoc changes in outcomes measures, presented analyses, and sample size calculations. We now turn our attention to specific aspects of study planning and consider those in more detail.

11.2 Repeated Measures Study Designs

In this section, we briefly review some of the most popular study designs for repeatedly measured outcomes and emphasize their advantages. We first focus on experimental studies and on designs with a single randomization.

11.2.1 Commonly Used Experimental Designs

The most commonly used design is the *parallel group design* presented in Chapter 1 (Figure 1.1), with individuals randomized to different groups and followed up over a specified period of time. The advantages of this design are its simplicity and in the case of randomization, the ability to obtain causal treatment effects. When repeated measures are collected on each individual, one can measure the change over time and compare the average change between groups.

Another commonly used design (also introduced in Chapter 1, Figure 1.2) is the *cross-over design*, in which individuals receive different treatments in a sequence. The order is randomized between individuals. This design has the advantage over the parallel group design in that the treatment comparisons can be performed within individuals, which increases power for statistical testing and precision for effect size estimation. However, it is not appropriate when carry-over effects are expected or when treatments are of long duration.

In many situations, randomization is performed not at the individual level but at the provider level. For example, a study might be focused on evaluating the effect of specific training of medical personnel on individual outcomes, or different behavioral interventions may be provided in group settings. The training is given at the provider level and the interventions are simultaneously administered to a group of individuals. Such designs are *cluster-randomized*, and since clustering introduces correlations between observations at the individual level, these correlations need to be taken into account for proper inference. In general, cluster-randomized trials require a larger sample size than the corresponding parallel group designs. The stronger the correlation between outcomes on individuals within a cluster, the larger the increase in the sample size. We discuss adjusting for such correlations in Section 11.4.

Another type of design that is more naturalistic and appropriate for the evaluation of service delivery-type implementations is the *stepped-wedge design* (see e.g., Hemming et al.

[2015]). This is a cluster-randomized design in which clusters sequentially cross over from control to an intervention condition until all clusters have crossed over. This design is pragmatic and is often chosen because of logistical constraints (i.e., it may not be possible to randomize at individual or provider level within a center). However, the effect of the intervention may be confounded with underlying temporal trends and lack of blinding is often an issue. Sample size calculations and the analysis plan must account for both clustering and the confounding effect of time.

In recent years, more and more attention has focused on designs with multiple randomization stages. This allows researchers to assess the effect of sequences of treatment assignments or to limit the potential for placebo effects. The simplest such design is a *two-stage parallel group design*, in which two completely independent randomizations occur at stage one and then at stage two. The treatments can be the same or different at the two stages. A variation of this design that is focused on optimizing treatment outcomes performs different randomizations at the beginning of stage two in responders and non-responders to the assigned treatment at stage one. Responders could be randomly continued or discontinued on their current treatment in order to assess duration of treatment response. Non-responders could be offered alternative treatments in order to improve their outcomes.

A variation of this design is the *sequential parallel design* (Fava et al. 2003), which has been proposed in order to deal with the issue of placebo response, particularly in trials with antidepressant medications. When a number of individuals are expected to respond to placebo, treatment differences are harder to detect. Some trials of antidepressant medications include a placebo lead-in period in order to reduce the number of potential placebo responders from the actual clinical trial and thus increase power to detect true treatment effects. However, this increases the duration of clinical trials and may bias the study sample. The sequential parallel design offers another alternative so that randomization of the treatments occurs at two stages, and at the second-stage treatment effects are evaluated only among placebo non-responders at stage one. Individuals can either receive active treatment in both phases, placebo in both phases, or placebo followed by active treatment. This type of design has been proven more efficient than a parallel group design when a substantial proportion of placebo responders is expected.

There are a number of other modifications of the basic clinical trial designs and many adaptive designs. This is a rapidly developing area of statistical investigation, mainly in the area of pharmaceutical statistics where more efficient design for evaluating novel drugs and treatments are needed. A good current reference for clinical trial designs is Chow and Liu (2013).

11.2.2 Observational Study Designs

While randomized experiments are the gold standard for evaluation of causal effects, in many instances it is impossible, impractical, or unethical to randomize individuals. For example, it would be unethical to randomize individuals to a harmful exposure such as smoking. In addition, when long-term effects of exposure or treatment are evaluated, it is impractical and not feasible to randomize individuals and follow them up for a long period of time. Similarly, when studying rare diseases, it may not be possible to recruit a sufficient number of individuals for an experimental study. Finally, when treatment effects are expected to be small, an unrealistically large sample size may be needed for a randomized study.

In such cases, observational studies are the only alternative. Although they do not provide such good control of potentially confounding factors as randomized studies, they do have the advantage of being able to recruit a more representative and larger sample of the population. Two basic types of epidemiological studies are used for evaluating longitudinal effects: *cohort* and *case-control studies.*

Cohort studies follow up a group of individuals over a period of time. Individuals in the cohort are selected based on exposure or a characteristic of interest that is measured at baseline, and then the outcome measure is (repeatedly) evaluated over time and compared between groups with different exposures. Cohort studies can be *prospective* or *retrospective,* depending on how the information is collected (i.e., by following up individuals over time or performing a chart review or an interview in order to retrospectively collect information). Retrospective cohort studies are susceptible to recall or information bias. Prospective cohort studies may require long durations of follow-up, are prone to the effects of missing data, and may be expensive to conduct. However, both types of studies gather information regarding the sequence of events, are good for investigating patterns of change over time, and are well suited to studying rare exposures.

Case-control studies select individuals based on the measured outcome. Typically, cases (i.e., individuals with a particular disease or outcome of interest) are selected first and then controls (i.e., comparable individuals from the same population who do not have the outcome of interest) are also identified. Data about the exposure or risk factor(s) of interest are collected retrospectively by record review, interview, or survey on both groups of individuals. Often, controls are matched to cases on a number of characteristics (e.g., age, gender, other potentially confounding factors) in order to decrease the potential for bias and increase power for statistical inference regarding the effects of the exposure on the outcome. Case-control studies are less expensive than cohort studies and are well suited to investigating rare outcomes or outcomes that take a long time to occur (e.g., long-term survival). However, they are susceptible to recall or information bias and do not allow determination of rates of disease in exposed and unexposed individuals. More information about observational study designs for longitudinal studies can be obtained in Rothman et al. (2008).

11.3 Sample Size Calculations for Traditional Methods

We first consider sample size/power calculations when there is a single outcome measure per individual. This is the case for cross-sectional data and may be the case in longitudinal data if we consider endpoint analysis or analysis of summary measures as described in Chapter 2. Initially, we consider sample size calculations for hypothesis testing. Further, we extend our presentation to confidence interval estimation. We conclude this section with an example. More information about sample size calculations is provided in Altman (1982).

11.3.1 Power Calculations for Simple Hypothesis Tests

All power calculations for hypotheses tests link four elements according to the design of the study. If any three of the elements are specified, the fourth can be calculated. The four elements are as follows:

- The sample size (overall and in each group if groups of different sizes are compared)

- The effect size (magnitude of effect that is not to be missed)
- The significance level (the maximum allowed probability of committing a type I error, i.e., to reject the null hypothesis when it is in fact true)
- Power to detect the effect size of interest (the probability of declaring a particular effect to be statistically significant, i.e., to reject the null hypothesis when it is indeed false).

To formalize the presentation, let us consider a comparison of means of two independent groups. This may be the focus of analysis if we are performing an endpoint comparison of outcomes in two independent groups of individuals. The main hypothesis of interest in such a scenario is that the means are the same versus that they are different. This is formally expressed as follows:

$$H_0 : \mu_1 = \mu_2 \text{ versus } H_a : \mu_1 \neq \mu_2$$

We want to calculate the needed sample size per group, so that we have at least the target level of power, $(1-\beta)\times 100\%$, to detect a particular clinically meaningful mean difference when performing a two-sample t-test of these two hypotheses at a pre-specified significance level, α. Remember that power is the probability of rejecting the null hypothesis when the alternative is true. Power is equal to one minus the probability of committing a type II error, with the latter being the failure to reject the null hypothesis when it is false. Power is usually set at 80% or 90% with corresponding type II error probabilities of 20% or 10%, respectively.

Significance level is the allowed rate of type I error (i.e., probability of rejecting the null hypothesis when it is in fact true) and it is usually set at 5%, but may be reduced if the consequences of type I error are drastic or multiple hypotheses are tested. For example, if five hypotheses tests are to be performed, we might want to use a 1% significance level in each hypothesis test in order to limit the familywise error rate to 5% (see Chapter 6).

The meaningful effect size for the comparison of two means is expressed as a standardized mean difference; that is, $d = |\mu_1 - \mu_2|/\sigma$. The effect size, d, is the absolute difference between the means of the two groups that is considered clinically meaningful and is not to be missed, expressed in terms of standard deviations of the measurements (which are assumed to be equal in the two groups). This effect size has come to be known as Cohen's d (Cohen, 1988). As a rough guide, effect sizes are referred to as small ($d=0.2$), medium ($d=0.5$), and large ($d=0.8$); however, what effect size to use in sample size calculations is study dependent. The effect size is the element of power calculations with the largest effect on sample size or power, and is often the most difficult to specify. We explain its role and impact in the next couple of paragraphs.

The formula H_0: $\mu_1=\mu_2$ for the sample size calculation for the comparison of two means, assuming equal sample sizes, n, per group and equal standard deviations is as follows:

$$n = \frac{2\left(z_{1-\alpha/2} + z_{1-\beta}\right)^2}{d^2},$$

where $z_{1-\alpha/2}$ is the z-score such that the probability of a value from a standard normal distribution (i.e., normal distribution with mean 0 and variance 1) smaller than that is $1-\alpha/2$, and similarly $z_{1-\beta}$ is the z-score such that the probability of a value from a standard normal

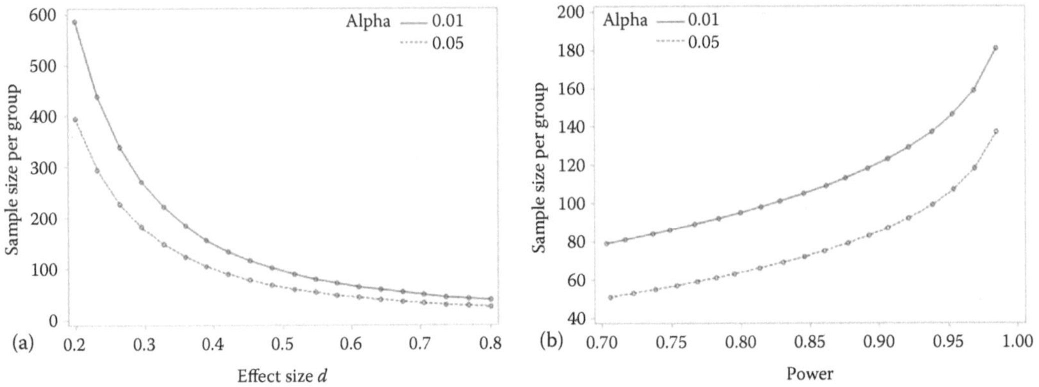

FIGURE 11.1
Sample size per group for a two independent samples t-test as a function of effect size (a) and power (b). Power in panel (a) is fixed at 80%. Standardized mean difference effect size in panel (b) is fixed at $d = 0.50$.

distribution smaller than that is $1 - \beta$. For the most common values $\alpha = 0.05$ and $\beta = 0.20$, $z_{1-\alpha/2} \approx 1.96$ and $z_{1-\beta} \approx 0.84$. The effect size d is study-specific.

This formula shows that as the effect size, d, increases (keeping the type I and type II error rates α and β constant), the required sample size, n, decreases as it is inversely proportional to the square of the effect size. Indeed, if we want to be adequately powered to detect a particular difference between groups, the larger the difference, the fewer individuals we need. Conversely, to detect smaller differences between the two groups, we need larger sample sizes.

It is a little bit harder to see, but as either of the error rates decrease (keeping the other one and the effect size constant), the sample size increases. This is logical, since if we want to detect the same difference between groups with lower probability of committing type I or type II error, we need larger sample sizes. Figure 11.1 illustrates how the sample size requirement changes as we vary the effect size, the significance level, and power one at a time.

Figure 11.1a shows that as the effect size increases, the sample size decreases. To detect a small effect size ($d = 0.2$) with 80% power at a two-sided alpha level of 0.05 one needs close to 400 individuals per group, whereas for a large effect size ($d = 0.8$) one needs fewer than 30 individuals per group. If the significance level is decreased from 0.05 to 0.01, sample size requirements increase by about one-third at the fixed power level. Figure 11.1b shows that for a fixed-effect size (medium effect size $d = 0.5$), higher power is associated with increased sample size. Whereas a little over 60 individuals are needed to achieve 80% power to detect a medium effect size at a two-sided significance level of 0.05, close to 80 are needed in order to achieve 90% power. Again, sample size requirements increase substantially as the alpha level is decreased.

A few notes of caution should be emphasized regarding sample size calculations. We illustrate these with a hypothetical sample size planning experiment.

1. The selected effect size should be specified *a priori* and should reflect a clinically meaningful effect. Thus, it needs to be selected based on substantive considerations and not estimated using pilot studies. As an example, consider planning a clinical trial of a new medication. Suppose individuals improve, on average, by five points on standard treatment, and the standard deviation of the improvements is four

points (these estimates are obtained from prior data, hopefully from a large sample of individuals from the same target population). More improvement is expected with the experimental medication. Clinicians are willing to use that medication if, on average, it improves the outcome by at least two more points (i.e., by a total of at least seven points compared with five points on the standard medication). This corresponds to half a standard deviation difference between groups; that is, to a medium effect size $d = 0.5$. Thus, the study needs to be powered for a medium effect size.

2. The significance level should be based on the tolerance for type I error. If the 0.05 level is selected in the hypothetical example, this means that we are willing to allow up to a 5% probability of declaring statistically significant differences between the experimental and standard medication when such differences do not exist.
3. Power should be based on the tolerance for type II error. If power of 0.8 (i.e., 80%) is selected, then this means that we are willing to tolerate up to a 20% probability of failing to find statistically significant differences when such differences exist and are of the magnitude of the considered effect size. Note that as type I error increases, type II error decreases, and vice versa, so unfortunately we cannot keep both of them very low. Usually, type II error is allowed to be larger since it is more risky to adopt a new experimental treatment with unknown side effects than to continue using the proven treatment. However, there is no reason why the hard-ingrained defaults of 5% for type I and 20% for type II error rates should not be broken. If, in a particular application, it is more costly to miss a true difference, the type II error rate may be decreased to 10% or even 5% (corresponding to 90% or 95% power, respectively) and type I error could be increased to 10%, or even 15%. This might be the case if there are no good treatments, and any potential improvement may have the potential to change clinical practice.
4. Often, one-sided rather than two-sided tests are used because they require a smaller sample size to detect the same effect size. In the hypothetical example, if we expect the mean improvement on the experimental treatment to be more than on the control treatment, we could choose to use a one-sided test (i.e., H_a: $\mu_1 > \mu_2$. However, if the difference is in the opposite direction (i.e., $\mu_1 < \mu_2$), we are going to miss such an effect and may potentially expose future individuals to an ineffective treatment if the two treatments are mistakenly declared not to be significantly different from one another. Note that the sample size needed to detect a particular effect size at a fixed level of power at the α one-sided significance level is the same as the sample size needed to detect the same effect size at the same power level at a 2α two-sided significance level.
5. When comparing different groups, the best power (smallest sample size) is usually achieved when the number of individuals in the two groups are equal. However, sometimes, for ethical or other considerations, the size of one of the groups may need to be smaller than the size of the other group (e.g., there might not be a sufficient number of individuals with a particular disease available for study, individuals may be less likely to participate in a placebo-controlled trial unless they have a higher chance of being assigned to an active medication).
6. The variances of the groups in the two-mean comparison example are assumed to be the same. A modification of the calculations is necessary when variances are widely different.

7. Although, most often, sample size calculations estimate the sample size needed to detect a target effect size at particular significance and power levels, feasibility constraints sometimes require that the calculations are performed in reverse. That is, for a particular sample size (e.g., maximal number of individuals that could be recruited under feasibility constraints), significance level, and effect size, power is calculated. This is achieved by solving the preceding equation for the parameter β, since power is equal to $(1-\beta) \times 100\%$. If power is satisfactory (i.e., above at least 80%, usually), then the experiment can be performed and will have a good chance of delivering a clear-cut answer to the research question of interest. If not, then alternatives must be considered (e.g., a different design, including an additional center that could recruit more individuals, using a measure with lower variability so that one could power for a larger effect size). In rare instances, power calculations are performed with a fixed sample size, power, and significance level in order to obtain a minimum detectable effect size. In this case, one needs to evaluate the minimum detectable effect size and decide whether it is clinically meaningful. If it is, then the experiment or study may proceed. If it is not, alternatives should be considered.
8. Power calculations should be performed prior to study initiation. Sometimes, researchers perform *post hoc power calculations* with the available sample size, using the observed effect size instead of the minimum clinically significant effect size that should not be missed. This is often done when study results are negative (i.e., no significant effects are found), in the mistaken belief that such a calculation would help distinguish between studies that are truly negative and those that are simply underpowered. However, such post hoc power calculations not only fail to achieve this goal but do not provide any additional useful information compared to the p-value of the statistical test. In fact, post hoc power (also referred to as *observed power*) is directly determined by the p-value, regardless of sample size and effect size. In particular, a p-value of 0.05 corresponds to post hoc (observed) power of 50%. This issue is discussed in more detail and further arguments are provided against its use by Hoenig and Heisey (2001).

Note that we considered the simplest hypothesis, comparing two means, in which we aim to establish *superiority* of one of the treatments over the other. Other types of tests that can be performed are *equivalence* or *non-inferiority* tests. To test the equivalence of two treatments, one needs to specify the bounds around the two means within which the treatments will be assumed to be equivalent. Similarly, for non-inferiority, a lower (or upper) bound needs to be specified so that if the experimental treatment is, at most, that much worse than the control treatment, it will be considered non-inferior. Testing of equivalence and non-inferiority and sample size calculations for these scenarios are beyond the scope of this book. We refer the interested reader to Wang et al. (2008) for details.

Similar to testing the equality of means, sample size can be calculated for a two-sample test comparing *two independent proportions*. For example, the number of individuals needed for a clinical trial can be based on having sufficient power to detect certain differences in proportions of responders in the two treatment groups at a pre-specified alpha level. The basic principles of sample size estimation are the same, but the proportion in the control group needs to be specified, together with a measure of the effect size comparing the experimental to the control group. Unlike the test of the means, where there is a clear-cut measure of effect size (i.e., the standardized difference, d), there are different options for proportions. One can define the effect as an odds ratio, relative risk, or difference in proportions. Furthermore, there are slightly different formulae that one could use depending on whether the sample size is large or small, and exactly what test is used. Details can be found in Wang et al. (2008).

When there are more than two groups to be compared, the hypothesis test of interest is the overall F-test in ANOVA, which indicates whether there are statistically significant differences among the group means. The effect size for this test is Cohen's f, and it is defined as the ratio of the standard deviation of the group means over the standard deviation of the individual observations. In the case of two groups, Cohen's d and Cohen's f are equivalent, in particular $f = d/2$. Small, medium, and large effects for differences among group means are $f=0.1$, $f=0.2$, and $f=0.4$, respectively.

There are a number of other hypotheses for which sample size or power calculations can be performed (e.g., correlations, regression analysis). We refer the interested reader to Cohen (1988) and Wang et al. (2008) for detailed information. A review of sample size calculations at a fairly non-technical level with advice on how to proceed is provided in Lenth (2001).

11.3.2 Power Calculations for Confidence Intervals

Hypotheses tests have been the backbones of statistical inference, especially in clinical trials where decisions regarding efficacy and safety need to be reached. However, they have the major disadvantages of failing to provide an estimate of how large differences are, and are dependent on sample size. With a sufficiently large sample size, any statistical test is significant, but statistical significance often does not translate into clinical significance. Thus, in recent years, more and more emphasis has been placed on effect estimation using confidence intervals. Sample size can be calculated so that effect sizes are estimated within a certain precision.

To illustrate, consider again the scenario of comparing two means of independent populations. Rather than powering the study so that a certain effect size is detected with good power at a reasonable significance level, we can estimate the sample size needed to construct a confidence interval for the mean difference within a certain width at a pre-specified level of confidence. The half-width of the confidence interval is often referred to as the *margin of error* or *precision* and needs to be small enough so that the confidence interval is informative. For example, suppose that a 95% confidence interval for the difference in mean improvement on two antidepressant medications is constructed, and the obtained confidence interval is (−5; 10) for a scale such as the Hamilton Depression Rating Scale. This is quite a wide range that does not even show which treatment is better. In comparison, a confidence interval from 2 to 6 is tighter and provides important information about which treatment is better, with a good degree of confidence in the magnitude of superiority. Likewise, an interval from −1 to 3 is just as tight, and although it does not show which treatment is better, from it, one can fairly confidently say that the two treatments are similarly effective.

To estimate the sample size for a confidence interval, one needs to specify the required confidence level $(1-\alpha) \times 100\%$ (usually 90% or 95%), the half-width (this is study dependent and should be based on clinical considerations), and the standard deviation(s) (usually estimated based on prior studies). When two means are compared, the two standard deviations are often assumed to be equal and the estimated sample size is equally divided between groups. Alternative formulae are available when the sample sizes are unequal.

There are two versions of power calculations for confidence intervals. One assumes that the future standard deviation is equal to the one used in the power calculation, and the sample size is calculated so that the expected width of the confidence interval is within the specified margin. The other takes into account the uncertainty when estimating the standard error(s) from the future data and requires the specification of a *tolerance probability*. This is the probability that the constructed confidence interval's length will be within the specified half-width. For example, we may want 90% tolerance probability that a 95% confidence interval for the quantity of interest (e.g., difference in two means) will have a half-length within the specified margin. The tolerance in confidence interval calculations corresponds to the power in the hypotheses test calculations. The effect size is more clearly separated into mean difference and standard error in confidence interval sample size estimation compared with hypothesis testing sample size estimation. A specific data example is included in the next section to illustrate how this is done.

Note that, as in sample size calculations for hypothesis testing, calculations for confidence intervals could be performed in reverse. For example, one might fix the sample size based on feasibility and then estimate what margin of error could be achieved given the assumed standard deviation, the desired confidence level, and tolerance probability. If the margin of error is meaningful, that is, an informative confidence interval can be obtained, then the study can proceed; otherwise, alternatives should be considered.

The estimated sample size for confidence interval estimation increases as the confidence level increases, the tolerance probability increases, the desired margin of error decreases, or the standard deviation increases (keeping all other elements of the calculation fixed). A one-sided confidence bound can be constructed rather than a two-sided confidence interval, but similar to hypotheses testing, caution needs to be applied in order not to miss differences in the opposite to the hypothesized direction.

Note that confidence intervals are quite useful when the study is focused on a particular simple contrast: for example, difference between two means or proportions, evaluation of average change from pre- to post-treatment, comparison of a proportion to a particular value (e.g., 50%). However, more complicated designs require testing of more complicated hypotheses (e.g., differences among multiple groups, evaluation of group by time effects) and, in such cases, the confidence interval approach may not be easily applicable. One could potentially formulate several effect estimations of interest (e.g., comparison of multiple group means to a control mean), construct simultaneous confidence intervals at an adjusted confidence level (e.g., 99% confidence level to adjust for five simultaneous confidence intervals), and perform sample size calculations that would guarantee that all confidence intervals were within the specified margin of error. However, sample size calculations become more complex and require more assumptions.

11.3.3 Example Power Calculations for a Two-Group Study

We consider the simplest design for repeated measures data, with one pre- and one post-treatment measure and two parallel groups (experimental and control). Our goal is to compare the mean improvements in the experimental group and the control group. Since we are focusing on change, we can perform power calculations as if this were a cross-sectional study with the change in the dependent measure as the outcome. We consider estimating sample size based on a t-test for two independent samples and based on a confidence interval for the difference in means.

11.3.3.1 Hypothesis Test for the Difference of Two Means

We first choose an outcome measure and evaluate prior data in order to figure out how large the standard deviation of this measure is. Suppose that it turns out to be about ten points. From previous studies, we anticipate that we will observe a change of about five points on the control treatment between baseline and endpoint, and that the correlation between repeated observations on that measure within the same individual is about 0.5. We will consider the experimental treatment to be better than the control treatment if it produces a change from baseline of at least ten points (five points more than the standard treatment produces). We plan to recruit equal numbers of individuals in the two groups. The planned analysis will be a t-test on differences in change from baseline to endpoint between the two groups. The question is, how many subjects do we need in order to detect the clinically meaningful difference with good power using a two-sided test? It is possible that up to 20% of the individuals could drop out during the study.

To estimate the required sample size we need to specify the other elements of the power calculation; namely, the significance level, the power level, and the effect size. Please note that we consider different combinations of these in order to evaluate the impact on our calculation. In particular, we consider 0.05 and 0.10 significance levels, power of 80% and 90%, and several effect sizes. To calculate the effect sizes based on the information available, we need to first calculate the standard deviation of the difference scores from the standard deviation of the outcome measure. The relationship between these two is as follows:

$$\sigma_{\text{diff}} = \sigma\sqrt{2(1-\rho)}$$

where:

- σ_{diff} is the standard deviation of the difference scores
- σ is the standard deviation of the measure

Since, from previous data, we know that σ is around ten, we consider values between eight and 12. Also, from previous data, we know that ρ is around 0.5, and hence, we consider correlations between 0.4 and 0.6. This gives the following range of values for σ_{diff}: $8\sqrt{2(1-0.6)} = 7.16$ to $12\sqrt{2(1-0.4)} = 13.15$. Note that the bigger the within-individual correlation, the smaller the standard deviation of the differences. If we have a direct measure of σ_{diff} from previous studies, then we do not need to go through this step, and can directly use the σ_{diff} value in the power calculations.

Since we want to be able to detect a minimum difference in change scores between the groups of $10-5=5$ points, this gives us the following range of values for the effect size d: $5/13.15 = 0.38$ (or approximately 0.40) to $5/7.16 = 0.70$. For the standard deviation and correlation equal to our prior estimate we obtain $d = 5/\left[10\sqrt{2(1-0.5)}\right] = 5/10 = 0.5$. Table 11.1 presents the required sample size per group for these combinations of values of the different parameters in the power calculation.

We see that the required sample size varies widely depending on what values we choose for the standard deviation, the within-individual correlation, and the required significance level and power. The bigger the effect size, the fewer individuals we need. The higher the power requirement and the lower the significance level, the more subjects we need. If we want to have sufficient power under all considered scenarios, we need 133 individuals per group.

TABLE 11.1

Sample Size Requirements for Two Independent Samples Comparison Using a t-test with Equal Variances

Effect Size d	Significance Level	Power	Required Sample Size Per Group
0.4	0.05	80%	100
0.4	0.05	90%	133
0.4	0.10	80%	78
0.4	0.10	90%	108
0.5	0.05	80%	64
0.5	0.05	90%	86
0.5	0.10	80%	51
0.5	0.10	90%	70
0.7	0.05	80%	34
0.7	0.05	90%	44
0.7	0.10	80%	26
0.7	0.10	90%	36

Note though, that if we expect to lose individuals because of drop out, we will not be able to calculate change scores for those individuals. Thus, the sample size should be increased further to account for dropout. The most conservative approach is to increase the required sample size in such a way as to have complete data on 133 individuals per group. Since we expect up to 20% drop out, we need to start with 167 individuals per group (80% of 167 is 133.6, truncated down to 133). A common mistake when accounting for drop out is to calculate 20% of the final number (20% of 133 = 26.6 or rounded up to 27) and add that to the target sample size for completers (133 + 27 = 160). However, this underestimates the total sample size. To obtain the required sample size prior to dropout, we divide the calculated sample size for completers by the expected completion rate (i.e., 133/0.8 = 166.25 rounded up to 167 per group).

As mentioned previously, this is a conservative approach to account for drop out. Since missing data could be handled using more sophisticated approaches (e.g., mixed models or multiple imputation, see Chapter 7), all available data on individuals could be used in the analysis and loss of power due to drop out may not be as extreme. We come back to this issue when we discuss power analysis methods for repeated measures studies in Section 11.4.

11.3.3.2 Confidence Interval for the Difference of Two Means

Suppose that the same parallel design with two groups of individuals with two repeated measures is chosen to compare the effects of experimental and control treatments. But, rather than performing a significance test, we are interested in estimating with good precision the difference in mean improvements on the two treatments. As before, the standard deviation of the outcome measure is about ten points and the expected within-individual correlation is 0.5. We would like to estimate the difference in mean improvement between groups with a confidence interval such that the half-width of the confidence interval is within a specified margin with high probability. To calculate the needed sample size (assumed equal in the two groups) we consider several possible values for the confidence level, the precision (half-width of the interval), the standard deviation, and the tolerance

TABLE 11.2

Sample Size Requirements for Two Independent Samples Comparison Using a Confidence Interval to Estimate Mean Differences

Confidence Level	Half-Width	Standard Deviation	Tolerance Probability	Required Sample Size Per Group
0.95	4	7	0.95	66
0.95	4	7	0.99	72
0.95	4	13	0.95	194
0.95	4	13	0.99	206
0.95	6	7	0.95	34
0.95	6	7	0.99	38
0.95	6	13	0.95	94
0.95	6	13	0.99	102
0.90	4	7	0.95	48
0.90	4	7	0.99	54
0.90	4	13	0.95	142
0.90	4	13	0.99	150
0.90	6	7	0.95	26
0.90	6	7	0.99	30
0.90	6	13	0.95	70
0.90	6	13	0.99	76

level (the probability that the half-width is smaller than the margin). Table 11.2 shows the needed sample size for the combination of values.

As in the previous power calculation, we see that the required sample size varies widely depending on what assumptions we make about the standard deviation of the change scores, the confidence level (which is equal to one minus the significance level), the tolerance probability, and the required precision (half-width of the confidence interval). We need more individuals when the standard deviation is higher, the confidence level is higher, the half-width is lower, and the tolerance probability is higher. If we want to have sufficient power under all considered scenarios, we need 206 individuals per group. If we are willing to use a lower tolerance probability (0.95 rather than 0.99) and lower confidence level (0.90 rather than 0.95), we can reach our goal with 142 individuals. Note that the highest impact on the power calculation comes from the width of the confidence interval and the standard deviation estimate. If we are way off the mark with these, we can get sample size estimates that are too high or too low. As in the power calculations for hypotheses testing, here we also need to increase the sample size if we anticipate subject dropout. The procedure for increasing the sample size is the same. We now turn our attention to more complicated designs with repeated measures.

11.4 Sample Size Calculations for Studies with Repeated Measures

The complexity of power calculations for studies with repeated measures stems from the need to account for correlations between repeated measures on the same individual (or within the same cluster) and the possibility of missing data (especially in longitudinal studies) and unequal variances over time. In the previous section, we presented an example with a simple pre–post comparison in which methods for cross-sectional data are applied to the change scores. We now extend our presentation by focusing on clustered data with an exchangeable correlation structure and then proceed by considering different correlation structures in longitudinal data. We consider power calculations for traditional methods for repeated measures analysis (rANOVA, rMANOVA), mixed-effects models, and GEE models. Our goal is to present the basic ideas only. A comprehensive reference on power analysis of repeated measures data is the book by Ahn et al. (2015).

11.4.1 Clustered Data

Let us consider the parallel two-group example from the previous section. Suppose that the treatments are administered in a group setting. Another instance when clustered data may arise is if we measure outcomes on students nested in classrooms (and perhaps schools) and we anticipate those outcomes to be correlated. In such scenarios, we expect observations on individual units to be equally correlated within clusters and uncorrelated across clusters. The intra-class correlation (ICC, which we denote by ρ) is given by the formula:

$$\rho = \frac{\sigma_b^2}{\sigma_b^2 + \sigma^2}$$

where:

σ_b^2 is the variance due to cluster
σ^2 is the residual variance (see Chapter 3)

If this correlation is ignored in statistical analysis, then type I error rate is usually increased. To prevent this inflation, analysis and power calculations need to take this correlation into account. This can happen if one uses rANOVA, mixed effects, or a GEE approach.

When data are equally correlated within clusters, sample size estimation proceeds as in cross-sectional data, with a simple adjustment for clustering. Specifically, one obtains a total number of individuals needed to detect a particular effect size with required power at a specified significance level. Then the resulting sample size is increased in order to take into account that some observations are equally correlated. Note there are two levels to the sample size: number of clusters and number of observations per cluster. The total sample size is the product of the two numbers when the data are balanced or the sum of individual observations across all clusters when the data are unbalanced.

Often, the number of individuals per cluster is fixed due to feasibility or practical constraints (e.g., class size is fixed, a provider treats a certain number of patients), and, in this case, one needs to calculate the number of clusters required. When it is possible to vary the number of individuals per cluster, one needs to decide on the optimal combination of number of clusters and number of individuals per cluster.

To illustrate how the sample size calculation is adjusted for within-cluster correlation, suppose that we have estimated that we need a total sample size of $T = n \cdot m$ individuals if the data both within and across clusters were independent. Here, n is the number of clusters, and m is the number of individuals in each cluster. The total sample size needed when there is positive ICC (equal to ρ) is then $nm[1 + (m-1)\rho]$.

The quantity $[1+(m-1)\rho]$ is the correction factor, also known as the *design effect* or the *variance inflation factor* (VIF). Note that the higher the ICC (ρ), the more we need to increase the sample size. If $\rho=0$, then no increase is necessary. If $\rho=1$, then we need to multiply the calculated sample size by the number of observations per cluster, m. For intermediate values of ρ, the inflation depends also on the cluster size. This increase is logical, since when there is dependence among the observations within clusters they provide less information than independent observations. We illustrate with a simple data example.

Suppose that we have calculated that for a two-group mean comparison we need a total of 200 individuals (100 per treatment group) assuming independence between observed values. We could divide these equally in 20 clusters per group (five individuals per cluster), or into ten clusters per group (ten individuals per cluster). Table 11.3 shows how the sample size increases under different assumptions for the ICC and cluster size. The first three columns of this table are fixed while the rest are calculated based on the information in the first three columns.

Note that the VIFs vary from 1 (when there is no within-cluster correlation) to 5.5 when the within-subject correlation is large and there are more observations within clusters. Thus, the required sample size could increase dramatically when the ICC is large. Fortunately, in most practical situations, the ICCs are not very large (we did not even consider values above 0.5) and hence the sample size requirements can be reined in.

The amount of independent information that is contained in a clustered sample (n^* clusters of size m) is reflected in the *effective sample size.* If all observations are perfectly correlated within a cluster, they provide as much information about the variance as a single observation. Thus, the *effective sample size* is equal to the number of clusters m. If observations are positively correlated, then the effective sample size is $n^*m/\left[1+(m-1)\rho\right]$ and is often considerably less than the total number of observations.

The effective sample size is interpreted as the sample size that is needed to detect the same effect size with the same power and at the same significance level as if the data were independent. In Table 11.3, the effective sample size is 200, while the actual sample sizes ranges between 200 and 1100 depending on the number of observations within clusters and the ICC.

Note that so far we have assumed that the data were balanced (i.e., number of units per cluster is the same). Modifications of the sample size formula are available for unbalanced data (see e.g., Ahn et al. [2015]). In addition, we did not specify what kinds of test we were using. This is because the general variance inflation formula applies whether we are

TABLE 11.3

Relationship between Sample Size Needed When Observations are Independent and When There Is Clustering with Positive Correlation among Some Observations

Sample Size for Independent Observations	Observations per Cluster	Intra-Class Correlation (ICC)	Variance-Inflation Factor (VIF)	Sample Size for Clustered Observations	Number of Clusters
200	5	0	1	200	40
200	5	0.10	1.4	280	56
200	5	0.25	2	400	80
200	5	0.50	3	600	120
200	10	0	1	200	20
200	10	0.10	1.9	380	38
200	10	0.25	3.25	650	65
200	10	0.50	5.5	1100	110

looking at comparisons of means or comparisons of other measures, such as proportions. Finally, if we anticipate that there will be missing data, we need to increase the sample size further in order to compensate for the loss of information. The sample size increase can be achieved by increasing the number of clusters and/or the number of individuals per cluster. Often, practical constraints dictate which option is more appropriate.

Note that, as with cross-sectional data, sample size calculations can be performed in reverse. That is, one could start with a feasible sample size and calculate power or detectable effect size. The only extra step that needs to be taken is to convert the feasible sample into an effective sample size before proceeding as indicated earlier in this chapter.

For example, practical restrictions might dictate that up to 500 individuals can be recruited in a study to compare two groups, clustered in groups of ten individuals (i.e., there are 50 clusters, ten individuals per cluster). The significance level for the test is 0.05. We want to calculate power to detect a particular effect size, or, conversely, we want to figure out what mean difference we can detect with 80% power. We expect from prior data a within-cluster correlation of around 0.2. To calculate the effective sample size, we first calculate the VIF, which is equal to $1+(10-1)(0.2)=2.8$. Thus, our effective sample size is $500/2.8=178.6$ (or close to 180 individuals). We round the number up in order to be able to distribute the individuals equally between groups. Now the problem reduces to performing reverse power calculations for a two independent samples t-test with 90 individuals per group.

Power calculations for confidence intervals are affected the same way as power calculations for hypotheses tests. Variance inflation adjustment is required. Models with more than one level of clustering require further adjustments of the sample size so that correlations within clusters at each level are taken into account. More information about the effects of clustering on power calculations can be found in Ahn et al. (2015).

11.4.2 Longitudinal Data

In order to perform power calculations for longitudinal data, several important decisions need to be made in addition to selecting the parameters of the calculation (i.e., power or tolerance level, significance level, effect size). The first is to decide what analysis will be performed, the second is what effect to power for, the third is to come up with reasonable values for the variances and covariances of repeated measures, and the fourth is to decide how to account for missing data.

The type of analysis is mainly a choice between mixed models and GEE models. Traditional rANOVA and rMANOVA methods could also be used in some scenarios, but are often not flexible enough, especially when it comes to dealing with missing data (see Chapter 2 for more detailed discussion of these approaches). Nevertheless, they might be useful for power calculations, as illustrated in Section 11.4.2.1. Non-parametric methods could also be used, but are usually not the first choice because they have less power and do not provide very meaningful effect size estimates (see Chapter 5).

Several possibilities for the effect of interest are commonly considered. The overall group by time effect is one option. However, there are many different ways in which one could achieve the same effect size for such a general test, with some of these potentially consistent with the study hypotheses and some not. Often, a more appropriate option to consider is a particular contrast of means over time (e.g., mean difference from baseline to endpoint, linear trend over time) either within or between groups. For example, one may be interested in assessing whether the average change from baseline to endpoint is greater in the experimental group than in the control group, or to estimate with good precision the rate of change over time (assuming that the trend is linear) and to assess whether it is significantly different from zero. A third option for the effect of interest may be the overall main effect of group; that is, whether post-baseline response in one group is consistently higher than in the other group on average. One could come up with other options depending on the goals of the study. Herein, we consider several basic options and present examples of how the study could be powered depending on the chosen method of analysis.

Prior data and substantive considerations can inform the choice of values for variances and covariances that are used in longitudinal data analysis. For example, previous studies may provide estimates for the variances of the outcome measure, indications of whether these variances are stable over time, and information about correlation structures that may fit the data well (e.g., autoregressive). Note that if a mixed-model approach with random effects is selected, then assumptions need to be made about the variances and covariances of the random effects in addition to assumptions about the errors. It often becomes a daunting task to specify the variance–covariance structure of the repeated measures before the study is initiated; hence, a range of values often need to be considered.

Missing data also affect the power of the study, sometimes considerably. Thus, it is important at the planning stage to establish what the expected rate and pattern of dropout is, and to decide how missing data will be handled. The latter is usually determined by the chosen method of analysis. For example, in mixed and GEE models, analyses are done following the intent-to-treat principle, with all available data on an individual used in the estimation. However, loss of some of the data usually leads to some loss of power, and hence the sample size should be adjusted so that sufficient power is available and effects are estimated with sufficient precision even after some dropout occurs.

We now consider sample size calculations for different methods of analysis of repeated measures data. We do not present general formulae as there is a wide variety of possibilities. Rather, we use data examples to explain what information we need to perform the power calculations and to emphasize interpretation of the results. SAS modules or freely available software programs are used to obtain the results. The code and output are available in the online materials.

11.4.2.1 Power Calculations for Summary Measures

One of the simplest approaches of performing power calculations for longitudinal data is to focus on summary measures for each individual and then perform power analysis for cross-sectional data on these summary measures as if they were the directly observed outcomes. Examples of summary measures are mean response over time, pre- to post-treatment change, area under the curve, and individual slope. We already illustrated how such power analysis is done on change scores from baseline to endpoint. However, this approach implies that the chosen analysis method is a two-stage analysis. At the first stage, the summary statistic is calculated for each individual, and at the second stage the summary measures are analyzed using traditional methods (e.g., t-test, ANOVA, ANCOVA) for cross-sectional data. As discussed in detail in Chapter 2, this analytic approach underestimates the variability in the data (e.g., slope uncertainties are ignored at the second stage) and missing data preclude calculation of the summary measures for some individuals. Although this may be offset by recruiting more individuals, a more appropriate approach is to consider analytic approaches and power calculations that take full advantage of the repeated measures nature of the data. Thus, we now focus on power calculations for traditional rANOVA and rMANOVA approaches, and then proceed to mixed and GEE models.

11.4.2.2 Power Calculations for Traditional Methods (rANOVA, rMANOVA)

When the main focus is on comparing groups and an exchangeable correlation structure is expected to fit the data well, the approach for clustered data from Section 11.4.1 could be used. That is, power calculations could be performed as if the data were cross-sectional and then the sample size could be increased according to the calculated variance inflation factor and dropout rate. The number of clusters is equal to the number of individuals and the number of observations per cluster is equal to the number of repeated measures on an individual. Different combinations of number of subjects and repeated measures could be considered. Missing data are taken into account by varying the cluster size according to the anticipated dropout rates.

When the correlation structure is not exchangeable and the design is balanced (i.e., individuals are measured at the same time points), power calculations could be based on the overall effect tests in rMANOVA. The effect sizes are determined based on the pattern of group means over time that we wish to detect and the values of the variances and correlations. More details and directions for the use of this method are provided in Castelloe (2014). Theoretical derivations and explanations are given in Muller and Peterson (1984) and in Muller et al. (1992). We show how power calculations could be performed for both the main effect of group and the overall interaction test between group and time using PROC GLMPOWER in SAS (see online materials for code).

In order to estimate the necessary sample size to detect clinically meaningful effects, we need to specify the design, the mean patterns over time by group, the variances by group and time point, the correlations among repeated observations within individuals, the power and significance levels, and the expected dropout rate. Power calculations could also be performed in reverse (i.e., we can fix the sample size and estimate the corresponding power at the levels of the other components of the calculation that are selected).

To illustrate sample size estimation in rMANOVA, we consider a hypothetical study with two parallel groups of individuals (equal number of individuals per group) with a normally distributed outcome measure evaluated at four equally spaced time points (e.g., month 1–4). The pattern of means is selected to represent clinically meaningful differences between groups that we do not want to miss, overall and by time point, and we consider the following mean values:

Group 1: 30, 25, 20, 15
Group 2: 30, 27, 24, 20

We assume two possible scenarios that describe the variability over time: a constant standard deviation of 4 for both groups at each time point, and increasing variances 3, 4, 5, and 6 at the first through fourth time points, respectively.

Several different variance–covariance structures are also considered: compound symmetry with a correlation of 0.5, autoregressive of first order with a correlation parameter 0.8, and unstructured with the following correlations:

$$\begin{pmatrix} 1 & 0.5 & 0.2 & 0.1 \\ 0.5 & 1 & 0.3 & 0.3 \\ 0.2 & 0.3 & 1 & 0.5 \\ 0.1 & 0.3 & 0.5 & 1 \end{pmatrix}$$

Performing power calculations under different assumptions for the variance–covariance structure is done because there may be uncertainty about the correct structure prior to analysis. We assume a 20% dropout during the study. Since rMANOVA excludes any individuals with missing data from the analysis, the analysis will be performed on 80% of the original sample; thus, we need to increase the sample size obtained from the power calculations so that even after dropping 20% of the individuals we still have sufficient power.

We are interested in testing the main effect of group, and the group by time interaction. The selected sample size should be sufficient so that for the mean and variance–covariance patterns already specified, we have 80% power at alpha levels of 0.05 for each test.

Table 11.4 shows the required total sample sizes under several different scenarios for the variance–covariance structure. The second-to-last column shows the estimated sample size using PROC GLMPOWER. The last column shows the final sample size that allows us to drop individuals with incomplete data from the analysis and still maintain 80% power. The numbers in the last column are obtained by dividing the corresponding numbers in the second-to-last column by 0.8 and rounding up to the nearest even number (since individuals need to be equally split between the two treatment groups).

Note that, in most cases, more individuals are needed to detect the group effect compared with the group by time effect, especially when the variances are unequal (increasing over time). The autoregressive structure is associated with larger sample size for the between-subject factor (group) than for the within-subject effect (group by time) when the correlation between neighboring observations is high. This is not surprising in view of our previous discussion of the effect of clustering, in that, when repeated observations are highly correlated, the effective sample size for between-group comparisons is much smaller than the total sample size. In contrast, for within-subject effects, the high correlation helps, as each individual serves as their own control. In general, compound symmetry needs the smallest sample sizes compared with the other structures.

As expected, dropout increases the sample size requirement, but unfortunately there is no guarantee that dropout will be uninformative, and it is quite possible that performing

TABLE 11.4

Required Sample Sizes to Detect Group and Group by Time Effects in rMANOVA under Different Correlation Structures

Effect	Variances	Correlation Structure	Required Number of Individuals with Complete Data	Required Number of Individuals Prior to Dropout
Group	Equal	CS	44	56
Group	Equal	AR(1)	54	68
Group	Equal	UN	36	46
Group	Unequal	CS	56	70
Group	Unequal	AR(1)	68	86
Group	Unequal	UN	58	74
Group×time	Equal	CS	28	36
Group×time	Equal	AR(1)	30	38
Group×time	Equal	UN	54	68
Group×time	Unequal	CS	38	48
Group×time	Unequal	AR(1)	40	50
Group×time	Unequal	UN	46	58

Note: Power Is Fixed at 80% and Significance Level at 0.05

the analysis on individuals with complete data leads to bias. This is one of the reasons why rANOVA and rMANOVA approaches are no longer widely used for longitudinal data analysis except in special cases (see Chapters 2 and 3 for more discussion on this issue).

Note that we did not specify the effect size directly in these calculations. Some programs (e.g., NCSS Statistical Software, 2014) calculate effects sizes in the form of ratios of the standard deviation of the means over the appropriate standard deviation of individual observations (which is a function of the variances and covariances). However, many different patterns of the means, standard deviations, and correlations could lead to the same effect size estimate, and not all of them reflect a pattern of the means consistent with the theoretical hypothesis. Thus, it is more meaningful to perform power calculations based on specific contrasts of the means. We illustrate this approach in the next two subsections in the context of mixed-effects models and GEE.

11.4.2.3 Power Calculations for Mixed-Effects Models

As described in Chapters 3 and 4, there is a wide variety of mixed models that can be considered. Mixed models can describe change over time using both fixed and random effects, and/or can assume different structures of the errors. Thus, it is important to decide *a priori* what model will be used for the analysis and to perform sample size calculations based on the chosen model. In many situations, a simulation approach is the only feasible option to obtain power estimates. That is, multiple simulated data sets are generated according to the chosen model and power is determined by the percent of samples for which the hypothesis test of interest rejects the null hypothesis.

One of the most meaningful comparisons in studies with longitudinal data is the difference in slopes between groups. Many other options are possible: overall main effects of group, time, group by time, user-specified mean contrasts including linear and quadratic effects over time, and particular mean differences by time point. Herein, we focus on the approach proposed by Hedeker et al. (1999), further developed by Roy et al. (2007) and Bhaumik et al. (2008) for linear mixed models, and used in the RMASS program (http://www.rmass.org/) for sample size calculations. It is focused on two-group repeated measures designs with attrition, allows for a variety of variance–covariance structures of the repeated measures, and for specification of either slope differences or mean differences by time point. Random effects may or may not be included. Attrition rates are specified by time point. Additional clustering can also be added (e.g., individuals clustered within centers). An example of a power calculation performed with the RMASS program follows.

Suppose we have a two-group design with four repeated measures and we anticipate linear trends over time with no difference between groups at baseline and a difference of 1.5 points by the end of the study (fourth time point). The model under the alternative hypothesis is:

$$Y_{ij} = 10 - 0.5\,t_{ij} - 0.5\,\text{Group}_i\,t_{ij} + \beta_{i0} + \beta_{i1}t_{ij} + \varepsilon_{ij},$$

where:

- i denotes individual
- j denotes observation within individual
- t_{ij} is observation time

Group_i is an indicator variable equal to 1 or 0 for the experimental and the control group, respectively.

There is no term in the linear predictor for group by itself because we assume that the groups' average responses are equal at baseline. The power calculation is based on the hypothesis test of the interaction between group and time and we would like to detect an absolute value for this coefficient of 0.5 or larger. This means that for one unit increase in time, the groups diverge from each other by 0.5 points. At the first time point (time 0) the groups have equal mean responses and by the fourth time point (time 3), the difference in outcome has become 1.5 points on average. Under the null hypothesis, the coefficient for the group by time effect is zero; that is, there is no difference in the rate of change over time.

The random intercept β_{i0} and slope β_{i1} are assumed to be correlated ($\rho = -0.2$) and normally distributed with variances of 0.25 and 0.09, respectively. The implied covariance (which is needed by the RMASS program in order to calculate the power) is then equal to $-0.2\sqrt{0.25}\sqrt{0.09} = -0.03$. The error variance is assumed to be equal to 0.5 and the errors are assumed to be uncorrelated with each other (i.e., all the correlations among the repeated observations within individuals are determined by the random effects). Power is set at 80% and the significance level is 0.05 (two-sided). Attrition is assumed to be 5% between consecutive time points.

Under these assumptions, the required sample size to detect the difference in slopes is calculated to be 27. Since this is an odd number and we plan to split the individuals evenly between groups, we need to recruit 28 individuals, 14 per group. As with the calculations for cross-sectional data, we should consider different values for the parameters of interest in order to investigate how the sample size changes. Table 11.5 shows how the estimated sample size depends on the effect size, on the assumptions about the variances and covariances of the random effects, and on the error variance value. In general, the greater the variability (i.e., larger variances of the random effects and/or the error), the more individuals we need, all other parameters of the calculation held equal. Also, the smaller the slope difference, the greater the sample size requirement.

Adjustment for attrition is integrated within the program so one does not need to inflate the sample size additionally. This approach results in a smaller sample size than if one

TABLE 11.5

Required Sample Size for Difference in Slopes in Linear Mixed Models under Different Assumptions for the Variances and Covariances of the Random Effects

Difference in Slopes	Intercept Variance	Slope Variance	Covariance between Intercept and Slope	Error Variance	Required Number of Individuals Prior to Dropout
0.5	0.25	0.09	−0.03	0.5	28
0.5	0.25	0.09	−0.03	0.2	18
0.5	0.25	0.09	−0.03	0.8	36
0.5	0.36	0.16	−0.06	0.5	36
0.5	0.36	0.16	−0.06	0.2	28
0.5	0.36	0.16	−0.06	0.8	46
0.4	0.25	0.09	−0.03	0.5	42
0.4	0.25	0.09	−0.03	0.2	30
0.4	0.25	0.09	−0.03	0.8	56
0.4	0.36	0.16	−0.06	0.5	58
0.4	0.36	0.16	−0.06	0.2	44
0.4	0.36	0.16	−0.06	0.8	70

Note: Power is fixed at 80% and significance level at 0.05. Attrition is fixed at 5% between consecutive time points.

calculates the needed sample size based on complete data, and then divides the resulting sample size by one minus the attrition rate as we did for traditional methods. This allows for a more efficient study.

Note that even in a simple scenario with just two groups and linear trends over time, there are many parameters that need to be fixed. This requires prior knowledge and good judgment, and gets even more complicated if we consider more groups, more complicated trends over time, and further levels of clustering.

Much research has been devoted in recent years to power calculations for mixed models (see e.g., Tu et al. (2004), Tu et al. (2007), Roy et al. (2007)), including non-linear growth models (Zhang and Wang, 2009) and methods for binary outcomes (Dang et al., 2008). In general, simulation methods are the only reasonable alternative for non-normal outcomes with complicated variance–covariance structures (see Chapter 16 in Stroup (2013)). More details about power calculations with or without simulations are provided in Chapter 12 of Littell (2006).

11.4.2.4 Power Calculations for GEE Models

Comparison of slopes between groups or other tests of interest can also be done in the context of GEE models. In GEE models, one only needs to specify the mean model correctly, and then even if the correlation structure of the repeated measures is miss-specified, estimates of the parameters describing the mean will be consistent. Nevertheless, if the working correlation structure is not well chosen, some loss of efficiency may occur. Like mixed models, GEE can be used for different types of data: continuous, binary, and count. To perform power calculations, one needs to specify the model (type of outcome, link, and predictors), the effect of interest (e.g., difference in slopes over time, overall group effect), mean patterns over time under the null and the alternative hypotheses, the working correlation structure that will be used (e.g., exchangeable, AR(1)), the significance level, and the required power level. To illustrate the process, we present a data example with binary data. We use the GEESize SAS macro (Version 3.1) based on the work of Rochon (1998) and Dahmen et al. (2004) (http://www.imbs-luebeck.de/imbs/node/30).

Our design is again a parallel group study with four repeated measures (at times 0, 1, 2, and 3). The underlying model under the alternative hypothesis is

$$\text{logit}\left(p_{ij}\right) = -1.0 + 0.2t_{ij} + 0.3\,Group_i\, t_{ij}$$

where p_{ij} is the probability of observing 1 for subject i at time j $Group_i$ is an indicator variable (1 for the active group and 1 for the control group)

Under the null hypothesis, the coefficient for the difference in slopes is 0 rather than 0.3. We are interested in the required sample size that would give us 80% power to detect an absolute difference in slopes as big as 0.3 or larger at a two-sided significance level of 0.05. We assume a 5% attrition rate between consecutive time points and an AR(1) working correlation structure. Table 11.6 shows the required sample sizes. We consider slope differences of 0.4 and 0.3.

From Table 11.6, we see that the magnitude of the slope difference and the correlation value affect the sample size calculation with a several-fold difference among the estimates. This illustrates how important it is to determine carefully what values are reasonable before the start of the study. Unlike normal data, where the identity link is used and hence it is easy translate slope differences into mean differences, in the case of binary data,

TABLE 11.6

Required Sample Size for Difference in Slopes in GEE Model for Binary Data with Logit Link under Different Assumptions

Difference in Slopes	Correlation	Required Number of Individuals
0.3	0.5	338
0.3	0.8	192
0.3	0.2	368
0.4	0.5	194
0.4	0.8	110
0.4	0.2	212

Note: Power is fixed at 80% and significance level is fixed at 0.05. Attrition is set at 5% between consecutive time points. AR(1) working correlation matrix is used.

one needs to apply non-linear transformation to the linear predictor (i.e., the inverse logit transformation) in order to see how intercept and slope values translate into probabilities. In the example that we considered we use the transformation:

$$p = \frac{\exp(lp)}{1+\exp(lp)}$$

where lp stands for linear predictor and p stands for probability.

Based on the values of the linear predictor at the four time points for the two groups (i.e., (−1, −0.5, 0, 0.5) in the active group and (−1, −0.8, −0.6, −0.4) in the placebo group when the slope difference is 0.3) we obtain the following probabilities (up to two digits after the decimal point): (0.27, 0.38, 0.50, 0.62) in the active group versus (0.27, 0.31, 0.35, 0.40) in the placebo group. This is a more meaningful metric in many applications and serves as a check on whether the effect sizes expressed as slope differences are reasonable when expressed as differences in proportions between treatment groups.

We chose to illustrate power calculations for GEE based on a slope difference for binary data, but there are many other options both for outcomes (e.g., count, ordinal, skewed continuous) and effects that one can power for (overall main effect, interactions, specific contrasts of the means). Different scenarios and theoretical justifications for power calculations for GEE data can be found in Chapter 4 of Ahn et al. (2015). Having illustrated a number of approaches for power calculations in longitudinal studies, we now turn our attention to another important aspect of study design; namely, consideration of different randomization methods.

11.5 Randomization Methods for Experimental Studies

In clinical trials and other experimental studies, causal inference can be performed because randomization ensures balance on potentially confounding variables. There are different methods of randomization that can be used, and some of them perform better in small samples than others. Herein, we present some of these methods at a non-technical level. The emphasis is again on basic concepts rather than on details. More information regarding issues of randomization can be found in Kalish and Begg (1985), Lachin (1988a),

Lachin (1988c), Chapter 5 of Altman (1991), and Suresh (2011). A sequence of papers in the journal *Controlled Clinical Trials* presents the most common procedures (Lachin, 1988b; Matts and Lachin, 1988; Wei and Lachin, 1988) and finishes with conclusions and recommendations for their use (Lachin et al., 1988).

To present the most common randomization methods, we consider a parallel group longitudinal study with two treatments (A and B). We focus on randomization at the individual level. This is in contrast to *cluster randomization* where randomization may be at the provider, clinician, or hospital level. The main randomization methods can be applied either at the individual or at the cluster level, but when randomization is carried out at the cluster level and outcomes are measured at the individual level, statistical analysis needs to take correlation of observations within clusters into account.

Simple randomization involves randomly assigning each individual to treatment A with a fixed probability p (often equal to 0.5) and to treatment B with probability $1-p$. The simplest way to execute such a randomization is by flipping a coin as each individual joins the study. As an example, consider that A corresponds to the "face" of the coin and B corresponds to the "tail." The following sequence is coded after flipping the coin 20 times:

AAABBABBAAABAAAABABA

In large samples, one can expect to get an approximately equal number of As and Bs in the sequence. However, in small samples, an imbalance may occur (in this particular sequence, which is random, there are 13 As and 7 Bs). Thus, there are several problems with this approach.

First, simple randomization can lead to a lack of balance in the number of individuals assigned to the two treatment groups and long sequences of A or B assignments could occur. Second, a flip of a coin cannot be reproduced, and hence no one could verify post-factum how the assignments were generated, whether the coin was indeed flipped 20 times, and whether the outcomes of the flips were as recorded. Third, in small samples, individuals assigned to treatment A could differ from individuals assigned to treatment B on a variety of other characteristics, some of which could potentially confound the association between treatment and the outcome.

To resolve these issues more sophisticated methods of randomization are used. The methods are categorized depending on whether they are *fixed* (i.e., randomization sequence is generated before individuals are recruited) or *adaptive* (information about treatment assignments, covariates, and, potentially, outcomes are used in order to inform future randomization assignments), and *completely unrestricted* (e.g., the simple randomization previously described) or *restricted* (e.g., the block randomization described in the following paragraph). Note that the goals of randomization are to ensure *balance of treatment assignments* (i.e., the proportion of individuals on each treatment is as according to the target), *covariate balance* (i.e., covariate distributions are similar in the different treatment groups), and in many cases to help keep individuals and/or providers *blinded to treatment assignment*. The latter is necessary so that systematic assessment bias is avoided.

The most common fixed randomization method that ensures balance of treatments even in small samples is *block randomization*. Rather than randomizing each individual separately, several consecutively recruited individuals form a block, and within this block, the treatment assignments are balanced. In the context of the earlier example with two treatments and equal probabilities of randomization to A or B, let us consider block randomization of block size four. There are six possible sequences of four treatments (two As and two Bs):

AABB, ABAB, ABBA, BAAB, BABA, BBAA

The randomization list consists of a sequence of such blocks. Thus, if, for example, 20 individuals are to be randomized, five blocks of four treatment assignments are randomly chosen with replacement. This randomization scheme guarantees that after each fourth patient, there is an equal number of individuals assigned to A and B. Note that the block size could be random (i.e., one can choose among blocks of size two, four, or six for example), which is often done in order to limit the possibility of individuals and/or providers guessing the treatment assignment. In addition, different randomization ratios can be used (e.g., twice as many individuals could be randomized to A, in which case the ratio of A to B assignments will be 2:1 within each block and overall). Block randomization guarantees balance of treatment assignments but does not ensure covariate balance in small samples.

When certain covariates are expected to be strong confounders of the relationship between treatment and outcome, it is advisable to *stratify the randomization* on these covariates. For example, if it is expected that gender may be a potentially confounding variable, separate randomization lists should be generated for each gender. Gender is a stratification variable, and if methods that achieve balance of treatment assignments are used within each stratum (e.g., block randomization), then we are also guaranteed to have balance on the stratification variable. Note that it is not necessary that the number of individuals be the same in each stratum. That is, we do not need to have the same number of male and female subjects in order to achieve balance on the covariate. Rather, stratified blocked randomization guarantees that the ratio of female to male subjects on each treatment is the same and thus there is balance of the covariate distribution across the two treatments.

Stratified blocked randomization is considered the gold standard for fixed randomization, and is especially useful in small clinical trials where stratification factors are prognostic of the outcome. However, it is limited in terms of the number of stratification variables that can be used. Additionally, since the list of participants is often not known at the onset of the study, it may be difficult to define the strata *a priori*. Finally, in large sample size studies, when the stratification factors are not substantially predictive of the outcome, stratified randomization does not provide clear advantages (see Kernan et al., 1999).

Note that fixed randomization schemes are usually generated by computer programs using pseudorandom numbers. The advantage of this approach over a coin toss is that it can be replicated.

Adaptive randomization schemes include *urn randomization*, *biased-coin randomization*, *covariate-adaptive randomization*, and *play-the-winner* randomization. The basic idea in all these methods is to update the assignment probabilities for future individuals enrolled in the clinical trial by using information about the current balance of treatment assignments, covariate distributions, and/or outcomes. In urn and biased-coin randomization, if there is lack of balance of treatment assignments (e.g., more individuals happen to be assigned to A than to B at some point in the study), then future assignment probabilities are adjusted so that the less commonly represented treatment is assigned more often. In play-the-winner randomization, more individuals are assigned to the treatment with the better outcome—this is often done for ethical reasons so that individuals are not assigned to an ineffective treatment as more evidence emerges. Perhaps the most widely used adaptive randomization procedure is *covariate-adaptive randomization*. This method can achieve balance on multiple potentially confounding variables. Assignment probabilities for future individuals enrolled in the clinical trial are updated based on information about the current balance of treatment assignments and covariate distributions across groups. For example, if at a certain recruitment point more older male individuals have been assigned to treatment A, then the probability of future treatment assignments to treatment A for older males is decreased. Rather than 0.5, the probability may be 0.4 or even lower. With a higher probability (0.6 or higher), individuals with such a combination of covariates are assigned to the alternative treatment B. Note that there is still an element of randomness; however, the idea is to gradually adjust for the lack of balance on covariates and treatments.

An alternative method to balance treatment assignments and covariates is the method of *minimization*. It assigns individuals to the treatment that leads to the least imbalance of treatments and covariates. However, because it is not random and allows the possibility of guessing the treatment assignments at some point in the study, this approach has not been extensively used. More information is provided in the review by Scott et al. (2002), who advise that minimization should be used more often.

In order to decide which randomization methods to use, one needs to consider the size of the trial, whether it is double-blind, single-blind, or not masked at all, and what the available resources are. Since randomization method needs to be taken into account in the analysis, fixed randomization schemes are often preferred, as they are simpler to analyze (e.g., stratification factor is included as a potential moderator in the analysis). Other procedures lead to more challenging statistical analyses. More information can be obtained in Kalish and Begg (1985), Wei and Lachin (1988), and Lachin et al. (1988).

11.6 Summary

In this chapter, we discussed study planning, presented the most commonly used designs for clustered and longitudinal studies, explained power calculations for cross-sectional and repeated measures data, and described different randomization options for experimental studies. Since serious mistakes at the study planning stage (e.g., confounding of the effects of treatment with the effects of time or other covariates) usually cannot be rectified at the analysis stage, it is crucially important to make the right decisions at the design stage. This includes clearly defining the goals of the study, carefully selecting the target population and clarifying inclusion and exclusion criteria, choosing an appropriate sampling method, outcome measure(s), and study design, calculating a sample size that gives a high probability that the goals of the study will be achieved, developing a plan for randomization, and an appropriate analysis approach. It also involves decisions about data collection, management, monitoring, and approaches to handling missing data.

The main advantages of studies with repeated measures compared with cross-sectional studies is that individuals serve as their own controls and thus it is possible to evaluate the effect of treatment or exposure within individuals. However, when repeated measures are collected over time, the effects of treatment or exposure need to be disentangled from the effects of time. Furthermore, dropout needs to be carefully planned for and controlled if possible. Thus, studies with longitudinal data present unique challenges and opportunities.

Some general recommendations at the planning stage of studies with repeated measures and future topics are as follows:

- Choose randomized study designs (such as parallel group clinical trials) whenever possible. Randomization is the only reliable method to achieve balance on measured and unmeasured covariates and thus allow for causal inference. Although methods for causal inference can also be used in observational studies, they rely on assumptions that are often not satisfied.

- Perform power calculations based on clinically meaningful effects before the study is initiated. Post hoc power calculations do not serve any useful purpose. Also, it is not appropriate to directly use the effect size from a small pilot study as the target effect in power calculations (see e.g., Leon et al. (2011)). Such estimates are usually imprecise and do not necessarily provide information about clinically meaningful differences. Previous studies could be used to provide information about the expected variability in the planned investigation (although this is also imprecise, it is often the best we have available) and the response in the control group. The effect size should be based on clinically meaningful effects (i.e., differences that one does not want to miss because of subject-matter considerations).
- Although power calculations are traditionally based on hypotheses tests, it is possible and often preferable to select the sample size so that the effect of interest can be estimated with good precision. Thus, power calculations based on confidence intervals could and should be used more often.
- Every power calculation should take into account the effects of missing data. Missing data can both bias estimates and lead to a decrease in power. Thus, sample size usually needs to be adjusted upward and sensitivity analyses need to be planned to examine the effects of missing data.
- Although sample size is determined at the onset of the study, one can plan an interim analysis at the design stage and define rigorous criteria for stopping the study for reasons of efficacy or futility at the interim time point. It is possible that a new treatment may be more effective than anticipated, and that this can be shown when only a fraction of the planned sample has been enrolled. On the other hand, it is also possible that, based on the outcomes observed up to the time of interim analysis, there is no possibility of demonstrating superiority of the new treatment by the end of the study. Thus, it may be futile to continue the study. In both cases, stopping the study early is indicated. Rigorous criteria for such decisions are described in O'Brien and Fleming (1979). More recent discussion and an overview of methods are available in Pocock (2006) and Chow (2014).
- Herein, we did not consider studies with more than one design stage. However, a sequence of treatments is often necessary to achieve an optimal response. In recent years, sequential study designs have increasingly been used, and much research is devoted to dynamic treatment regimes (e.g., Chakraborty and Murphy (2014)). In these types of studies, a sequence of decisions are made for each patient based on treatment and covariate histories. The ultimate goal is to personalize treatment assignments for the individual patients in order to achieve the best possible outcome.

In conclusion, study planning is a crucially important stage in any data investigation, involving careful consideration of many aspects. There are unique challenges to consider when clustered or longitudinal data are collected. One needs to select a proper design, an analysis method that allows correlated data to be handled, and to decide how to handle dropout and other missingness. Sample size calculations are more complicated for correlated data than for cross-sectional data and require many more assumptions. There is a wide variety of study designs to choose from, which makes this both a very challenging and exciting process involving close collaboration between subject-matter researchers and statisticians.

12

Summary and Further Readings

This book has focused on advanced statistical methods for the analysis of correlated data in clinical trials and observational studies with emphasis on applications in psychiatry and related fields. Data collected in psychiatric longitudinal studies are complex because outcomes are rarely directly observed, there are multiple correlated repeated measures within individuals, and there is natural heterogeneity in treatment responses and other characteristics in the populations. Simple statistical methods do not work well with such data as described in Chapter 2. More advanced statistical methods capture the complexity of psychiatric data better but are difficult to apply appropriately and correctly by investigators who do not have advanced training in statistics.

To facilitate understanding and increase appreciation of the versatility of these methods, we presented, at a non-technical level, several approaches for the analysis of correlated data, namely, mixed-effects and generalized estimating equation (GEE) models (Chapters 3 and 4), mixture models for longitudinal data (Chapter 10), and non-parametric methods for repeated measures studies (Chapter 5). These methods have revolutionized our ability to analyze data from clinical trials and epidemiological studies. In particular, mixed models use all data on subjects without the need for imputation, properly account for correlations of the repeated measures within individuals, minimize bias in estimates, and are appropriate for a wide range of applications from longitudinal to brain imaging data. GEE have similar advantages but require careful consideration of missing data. Mixture models allow for data-driven estimation of underlying latent classes of subjects with particular characteristics or trajectories over time. Non-parametric methods are useful when data exhibit floor and ceiling effects or when distributions vary wildly across time points and are otherwise unwieldy.

By presenting these methods at a non-technical level, focusing on the assumptions of the methods, applicability, and interpretation, and providing online resources for their use, we aimed to increase understanding of the advantages and potential caveats of these methods and to contribute to their more extensive and appropriate use. The examples provided from published studies in psychiatry, neuroscience, and mental health throughout the book were meant to illustrate the methods and to provide guidelines as to how commonly encountered data should be analyzed and interpreted.

We also focused on several important topics in the analysis of longitudinal and clustered data that deserve special attention. In particular, we presented methods of adjustment for multiple testing (Chapter 6), which are essential when one analyzes multiple outcome measures or needs to adjust for multiple post hoc tests. We also devoted a chapter (Chapter 7) to methods for dealing with missing data including gold standard approaches such as multiple imputation and full information maximum likelihood. Proper methods of adjustment for potentially confounding variables in experimental and observational studies were also presented and discussed (Chapter 8). We also covered assessment of moderator effects that allow us to determine for whom or under what circumstances a particular treatment works, and of mediator effects that allow us to evaluate how (i.e., via what potential mechanism) a treatment exerts its effect. We also briefly covered design considerations for planning studies with clustered and longitudinal data (Chapter 11), including sample size estimation, randomization, and most commonly used longitudinal designs. References to relevant publications in both the statistical literature and the subject-matter literature were provided throughout the book. Further reading suggestions with applications in psychiatry and related fields are as follows. The textbook of Hedeker and Gibbons (2006) is an excellent but more technical reference for longitudinal data analysis. The book edited by Jones et al. (2012) covers a wide range of topics with applications in aging. The book by Long (2011) focuses on applications in the behavioral sciences and shows how R software could be used for longitudinal modeling. The book of Dunn (2000) is focused specifically on psychiatry, but emphasizes issues of measurement, agreement, and factor analysis rather than methods for clustered and longitudinal data.

There are a number of topics that we considered beyond the scope of this book and hence did not cover. Sections 12.1 through 12.9 introduce some of these and include references for further reading.

12.1 Models for Multiple Outcomes

Mixed-effects and GEE models have been extended in the statistical literature to situations when multiple outcome measures are repeatedly collected. For example, multiple measures of disease severity could be recorded over time, or one might be interested in a simultaneous analysis of efficacy and safety outcomes. If the outcomes are analyzed separately, one does not obtain information about their correlation and either needs to adjust the significance level for performing separate analyses, thus potentially decreasing power, or risk inflating the familywise type I error rate, thus increasing the risk of false positive findings. Joint analysis of the outcome variables allows us to make inferences about the correlation of the different measures and allows us to test or estimate an overall treatment effect on all outcomes, thus reducing the need to correct for multiple testing. In addition, if the outcomes are highly correlated, then one could potentially gain efficiency in the estimates for an outcome by borrowing information from the other outcomes. This is especially attractive if some of the outcome measures are more precise but not measured as frequently, and other measures are less precise but are collected more frequently.

Joint analysis also comes with the disadvantage that models become more complex, more difficult to formulate and estimate, and there is an increased probability of convergence issues or other computational problems. This is especially relevant when the outcomes are of different types (e.g., continuous and categorical).

There are multiple methodological publications on this topic in recent years in the statistical literature. The recent review by Verbeke et al. (2014) and Verbeke and Davidian (2009) are good starting points and cite many other relevant publications.

12.2 Non-linear and Spline Modeling of Time Effects

In all models for longitudinal data presented so far, we modeled the time effect using a simple categorical predictor for balanced designs or polynomial trends to describe change over time parsimoniously. However, the categorical time approach is only applicable for balanced designs when individuals are measured at the same time points, and works only when the number of repeated assessments is not large. It also does not allow prediction of the outcome at intermediate time points. Modeling time with polynomials (i.e., linear, quadratic, cubic, and other trends) is rather limited in describing different patterns of change. Very often, the response is not described well by a straight line or by part of a parabola, and this lack of fit may lead to bias in parameter estimates and invalid conclusions. There are several alternative approaches that one could consider if more flexibility in modeling time effects is needed.

In particular, *non-linear models for longitudinal data,* where a non-linear function in the parameters is used to describe the pattern of change over time, are discussed in the book of Davidian and Giltinan (1995) and in Davidian (2009). Such models are routinely used in pharmacokinetics and pharmacodynamics and less often in other areas. The form of the model (e.g., S-shaped curve, exponential curve) is often suggested by mechanistic theoretical considerations and describes phenomena at the individual level. Thus, non-linear models are most commonly used in a random effects framework but marginal (GEE-type) models are also available and can be fit. A fairly non-technical review of these approaches is provided by Serroyen et al. (2009).

Another possibility is to describe the time effect using models based on *splines.* Splines are piecewise polynomials that are tied together at different time points so that there is a seamless (smooth) transition from one polynomial to the other. One can think of such models as having the time range divided into different windows, within each of which we fit a polynomial model, and force these individual polynomials to join hands with polynomials from neighboring windows at the borders. This approach allows us to fit virtually any pattern of change over time but of course comes with an added complexity level, especially in the context of longitudinal data, where correlations among repeated observations on the same individual over time also need to be taken into account. There are different types of spline models that can be used for longitudinal data, such as *regression splines, smoothing splines,* and *penalized splines.* A gentle introduction to the spline approach for longitudinal data is provided in Chapter 7 of Weiss (2005) and in Chapter 19 of Fitzmaurice et al. (2011). Theoretical details of the methods can be found in Chapters 8 through 12 of Fitzmaurice et al. (2009).

12.3 Transition Models

In this book, we focused on two major types of models for longitudinal data based on the generalized linear model: subject-specific models with random effects and marginal models with structured variances and covariances (GEE). There is a third type of models that extends the generalized linear models for longitudinal data, in which previous outcomes are included in the linear predictor. Thus, one can estimate the effect of past outcomes on current and future outcomes with the added advantage of seamlessly taking into account serial correlations among the repeated measures. These models are called *transition (or Markov) models* and are also sometimes referred to as *conditional models* because they express the conditional distribution of each response as a function of previous responses and covariates. One of the simplest transition models is the first-order autoregressive generalized linear model, in which the previous outcome affects the current outcome. Markov models of order k are achieved when the previous k outcomes are affecting the current outcome. When the outcome is categorical, these models are known as *Markov chains*. More details about transition models for longitudinal data can be obtained in Chapter 10 of Diggle et al. (2002).

A further extension of this approach are *latent Markov models* for longitudinal data, where one assumes that there are unobserved latent classes, and individuals stay in the same class over time or transition from one latent class to another with certain probabilities. Both the number of latent classes and the parameters describing the effect of covariates and potentially previous outcomes on the transition probabilities are estimated from the data. A good reference on such models is the book of Bartolucci et al. (2012).

12.4 Survival Analysis

Another topic that we did not cover in this book is *survival analysis*. In survival analysis, the outcome is time until an event of interest occurs. The event may be death, treatment response, remission, or any other outcome that could be reliably ascertained to have happened. Typically, the event occurs once during the study for an individual (and hence we do not have multiple repeated measures within the individual on this outcome); however, there are situations when the event could be recurring. For example, an alcohol-dependent individual who has achieved abstinence could relapse to heavy drinking repeatedly.

The goal in survival analysis could be to estimate the distribution of time-to-event, to compare groups in terms of their survival times, or assess the effects of covariates on the time-to-event. A complicating factor with survival data is that for some individuals the event of interest does not occur during the observation time. Such individuals are said to have been *censored* since we do not know whether they had or did not have the event. Censoring necessitates the use of special methods for survival analysis. Some of the most recognized approaches are *Kaplan-Meier estimates* of the survival function, *log-rank* tests to compare survival times of groups of individuals, and the *Cox proportional hazards model* for evaluating the impact of predictors on survival times. Good references for survival analysis are the classical text of Sir David Cox (Cox et al., 1984), the introduction to survival analysis in a medical context by Collett (2003), and the comprehensive and more technical book of Kalbfleisch and Prentice (2002).

12.5 Joint Analysis of Survival Outcomes and Repeated Measures

In many studies, there is an interest in both repeatedly measured outcomes and survival outcomes. For example, one might measure disease severity repeatedly, and also time to treatment discontinuation, time to treatment response, or time to dropout. Methods for joint analysis of repeated measures and survival outcomes have received much attention in the statistics literature in recent years. The goals of such analyses can be to simultaneously assess influences of predictors on the longitudinal and survival outcomes (if both outcomes are considered to be equally important and are substantially correlated), to perform inference for the repeatedly measured outcome by accounting for the survival outcome (this is especially useful if the survival outcome is dropout and accounting for that outcome allows us to correct for bias in the estimates of the repeatedly measured outcome), or to perform inference for the survival outcome while accounting for the repeatedly measured outcome (this might be useful if the survival outcome is not frequently observed and we borrow information from the repeatedly measured outcome to improve estimates of the survival outcome).

Models for joint analysis are necessarily complex, as they require joining together models for different types of outcomes. They typically combine linear mixed-effects models for repeated measurements and Cox models for censored survival outcomes, although other combinations are possible. Due to model complexity, joint models could have convergence problems and issues with identifiability. While describing such methods is beyond the scope of our book, we refer the interested reader to a gentle introduction by Asar et al. (2015), or the more technical and comprehensive manuscripts of Henderson et al. (2000) and Diggle et al. (2008).

12.6 Models for Intensive Longitudinal Data

All examples presented in this book had a relatively low number of repeated observations per individual (less than 10). With the increased ease of collecting, storing, and analyzing data, studies that record information much more intensively (e.g., several times per day) are quite common. For example, *ecological momentary assessment* (EMA) studies collect data on feelings or actions (Shiffman and Stone, 1998) in groups of individuals often using smartphones and other hand-held devices. Although mixed-effects and GEE models could be used to analyze such data, the problem is not only the intensity of the data collection, but also that there are unique aspects of EMA data that are not well captured with the classical formulations of these models. In particular, the variety of individual trajectories with possible daily or weekly oscillations are not well captured by simple polynomial trends. Additionally, interest in EMA studies often centers not so much on the mean trends over time, but on fluctuations in individuals' responses. Individuals who show more variability may be inherently more unstable and more prone to adverse outcomes. Furthermore, how the response or variation in response affects what happens next may be of interest. In order to tackle the additional challenges that intensive longitudinal data present, special methods often need to be adopted. These include *functional data analysis, state-space models, dynamic systems modeling,* and *point process models.* An excellent reference on these approaches with illustrative examples and many references from the behavioral sciences is the book edited by Walls and Schafer (2006).

12.7 Models for Spatial Data

Although we provided some examples with clustering, including an analysis of region of interest data from an fMRI study, we did not focus specifically on situations in which we model the spatial associations among the data points. Such data are encountered in structural and functional imaging studies, in disease mapping applications, and in geographic information systems. Data can be intensively collected (e.g., one might have data on thousands of voxels within individuals or hundreds of locations on a map). Both spatial and time components are present when one is interested in modeling how the response of the spatial network of points changes over time. In such applications, it is critically important to take into account the interrelationships among the observed responses in space and time. When modeling disease spread or brain connectivity, the strength of associations varies not only by proximity but also by the connections that exist among different observation units in space and time. Therefore, although some simple spatial applications can be handled with the methods described in this book by using the spatial power variance–covariance structure of the repeated measures (Chapter 3), specialized methods are needed for more complex data. The book by Diggle (2003) is an excellent reference for analyzing spatial point patterns. Geostatistical modeling is described at a fairly non-technical level by Diggle and Ribeiro (2007). Temporal trend modeling in geographic information systems is presented from an applied perspective by Ott and Swiaczny (2001). The book of Gelfand (2010) is a general reference on spatial statistics. An overview of brain imaging analysis and statistical methods is provided by Bowman (2014).

12.8 Bayesian Methods

We presented the material in this book from a frequentist perspective. That is, we regard the parameters of the models as unobserved fixed quantities that are estimated from the information in the sample. Alternatively, one could adopt a Bayesian perspective and treat parameters as random quantities with some prior distribution (whether informative or non-informative). We update our belief about the distribution of these parameters based on the observed data and thus construct posterior distributions. The posterior modes are used as point estimates of the parameters, and 95% credible intervals provide information about the likely range in which the parameters vary. In addition to the conceptual differences regarding parameter interpretation, Bayesian models have potential computational advantages over their frequentist counterparts in small samples and when the number of random effects increases. However, they require more sophistication to use and software is not as widespread as for frequentist models. We refer readers interested in the Bayesian approach and inference methods to the books of Carlin and Louis (2009) and Gelman et al. (2014).

12.9 Software

We used SAS STAT software for illustration throughout the book. More information and a variety of examples for the analysis of longitudinal and clustered data using SAS can be found in Littell (2006). SAS Institute has a related software program (*JMP*) that has excellent graphical capabilities and a friendly user interface that still allows to use the powerful SAS machinery behind the scenes. Sall et al. (2014) provide an introduction on the use of JMP.

There are a number of other software programs that could be used for analysis of longitudinal and clustered data. Of particular note is the free programming environment *R*, which provides great flexibility, is open source, and is accessible all around the world. A good reference for R is the book of Crawley (2007), whereas Li and Baron (2012) focus on applications from the behavioral sciences and show how models for longitudinal and clustered data could be fit in R. Another programming environment that has modules for longitudinal and clustered data analysis is MATLAB® (see e.g., Gilat (2011) for an introduction).

Stata is a flexible and powerful software program for statistical analysis that can also handle the models covered in this book. A gentle introduction to data analysis with Stata is provided in Kohler and Kreuter (2005). A more comprehensive reference on models for repeatedly measured outcomes is the book of Rabe-Hesketh and Skrondal (2008).

Software commonly used by applied researchers for data analysis is the *Statistical Package for the Social Sciences* (SPSS). It does have a user-friendly interface and capabilities to fit mixed models, but is not as flexible as the other software options mentioned. An introduction to SPSS is provided by Argyrous (2005).

A number of more specialized programs for the analysis of different models for repeated measures are available. For example, MLWin (http://www.bristol.ac.uk/cmm/software/mlwin/) and HLM (http://www.ssicentral.com/hlm/) are well suited for multilevel models, Supermix fits mixed models for continuous and categorical data (http://www.ssicentral.com/supermix/), LISREL is focused on structural equation models (http://www.ssicentral.com/lisrel/), and MPlus has wide-ranging capabilities for the analysis of correlated data (https://www.statmodel.com/).

12.10 Concluding Remarks

While some novel statistical methods have been used to plan studies and analyze data in psychiatry and related fields, progress toward bridging the gap between methodological developments in statistics and analyses of psychiatric clinical trials and epidemiological studies has been slow. This is partly due to difficulties in "translating" statistical methods so that their assumptions, applicability, model fitting, and interpretation are understandable to quantitatively oriented applied researchers. Statistical methodological papers are often full of statistical notation and jargon that makes them hard to follow by less mathematically inclined readers. There are multiple other publications that aim to explain statistical methods to non statistical audiences but they are spread over many different subject-matter journals and often focus on just a particular aspect of statistical methods or only on a particular area of application. The current book summarizes recent statistical developments to a non statistical audience of quantitatively oriented researchers in psychiatry and mental health, and will hopefully be a valuable resource promoting the use of appropriate statistical methods for analysis of complex psychiatric data sets.

References

Agresti, A. (2002). *Categorical Data Analysis* (2nd edn). New York: Wiley.

Agresti, A. (2007). *An Introduction to Categorical Data Analysis* (2nd edn). Hoboken, NJ: Wiley.

Agresti, A. (2015). *Foundations of Linear and Generalized Linear Models*. Hoboken, NJ: Wiley.

Ahn, C., Heo, M., and Zhang, S. (2015). *Sample Size Calculations for Clustered and Longitudinal Outcomes in Clinical Research*. Boca Raton, FL: CRC Press.

Allison, P. D. (2000). Multiple imputation for missing data: A cautionary tale. *Sociological Methods and Research*, 28(3), 301–309.

Allison, P. D. (2002). *Missing Data*. Thousand Oaks, CA: Sage Publications.

Altman, D. G. (1991). *Practical Statistics for Medical Research* (1st edn). New York: Chapman and Hall.

Altman, D. G., and Simera, I. (2016). A history of the evolution of guidelines for reporting medical research: The long road to the EQUATOR Network. *Journal of the Royal Society of Medicine*, 109(2), 67–77.

Altman, D. G. (1982). How large a sample? In S. M. Gore, & D. G. Altman (Eds.), *Statistics in practice. London: British Medical Association.*

Angrist, J. D., Imbens, G. W., and Rubin, D. B. (1996). Identification of causal effects using instrumental variables. *Journal of the American Statistical Association*, 91(434), 444–455.

Anton, R. F., O'Malley, S. S., Ciraulo, D. A., Cisler, R. A., Couper, D., Donovan, D. M., ... and Longabaugh, R. (2006). Combined pharmacotherapies and behavioral interventions for alcohol dependence: The COMBINE study: A randomized controlled trial. *JAMA*, 295(17), 2003–2017.

Argyrous, G. (2005). *Statistics for Research: With A Guide to SPSS* (2nd edn). Thousand Oaks, CA: SAGE Publications.

Asar, O., Ritchie, J., Kalra, P. A., and Diggle, P. J. (2015). Joint modelling of repeated measurement and time-to-event data: An introductory tutorial. *International Journal of Epidemiology*, 44(1), 334–344.

Austin, P. C. (2008). A critical appraisal of propensity-score matching in the medical literature between 1996 and 2003. *Statistics in Medicine*, 27(12), 2037–2049.

Bailar, J. C., and Mosteller, F. (1992). *Medical Uses of Statistics* (2nd edn). Boston, MA: NEJM Books.

Baiocchi, M., Cheng, J., and Small, D. S. (2014). Instrumental variable methods for causal inference. *Statistics in Medicine*, 33(13), 2297–2340.

Baron, R. M., and Kenny, D. A. (1986). The moderator mediator variable distinction in social psychological-research: Conceptual, strategic, and statistical considerations. *Journal of Personality and Social Psychology*, 51(6), 1173–1182.

Bartolucci, F., Farcomeni, A., and Pennoni, F. (2012). *Latent Markov Models for Longitudinal Data*. Boca Raton, FL: CRC Press.

Bauer, D. J., and Curran, P. J. (2003). Distributional assumptions of growth mixture models: Implications for overextraction of latent trajectory classes. *Psychological Methods*, 8(3), 338–363.

Bauer, D. J., and Reyes, H. L. M. (2010). Modeling variability in individual development: Differences of degree or kind? *Child Development Perspectives*, 4(2), 114–122.

Bauer, D. J., Preacher, K. J., and Gil, K. M. (2006). Conceptualizing and testing random indirect effects and moderated mediation in multilevel models: New procedures and recommendations. *Psychological Methods*, 11(2), 142–163.

Bauer, P., Bretz, F., Dragalin, V., Konig, F., and Wassmer, G. (2016). Twenty-five years of confirmatory adaptive designs: Opportunities and pitfalls. *Statistics in Medicine*, 35(3), 325–347.

Benjamini, Y. (2010a). Discovering the false discovery rate. *Journal of the Royal Statistical Society Series B—Statistical Methodology*, 72, 405–416.

Benjamini, Y. (2010b). Simultaneous and selective inference: Current successes and future challenges. *Biometrical Journal*, 52(6), 708–721.

Benjamini, Y., and Hochberg, Y. (1995). Controlling the false discovery rate: A practical and powerful approach to multiple testing. *Journal of the Royal Statistical Society Series B—Methodological*, 57(1), 289–300.

Benjamini, Y., and Yekutieli, D. (2001). The control of the false discovery rate in multiple testing under dependency. *Annals of Statistics*, 29(4), 1165–1188.

Benjamini, Y., and Yekutieli, D. (2005). False discovery rate-adjusted multiple confidence intervals for selected parameters. *Journal of the American Statistical Association*, 100(469), 71–81.

Benjamini, Y., Krieger, A. M., and Yekutieli, D. (2006). Adaptive linear step-up procedures that control the false discovery rate. *Biometrika*, 93(3), 491–507.

Berlin, K. S., Parra, G. R., and Williams, N. A. (2014). An introduction to latent variable mixture modeling (part 2): Longitudinal latent class growth analysis and growth mixture models. *Journal of Pediatric Psychology*, 39(2), 188–203.

Bhaumik, D. K., Roy, A., Aryal, S., Hur, K., Duan, N. H., Normand, S. L. T., … and Gibbons, R. D. (2008). Sample size determination for studies with repeated continuous outcomes. *Psychiatric Annals*, 38(12), 765–771.

Bind, M. A. C., Vanderweele, T. J., Coull, B. A., and Schwartz, J. D. (2016). Causal mediation analysis for longitudinal data with exogenous exposure. *Biostatistics*, 17(1), 122–134.

Blankers, M., Smit, E. S., van der Pol, P., de Vries, H., Hoving, C., and van Laar, M. (2016). The missing = smoking assumption: A fallacy in internet-based smoking cessation trials? *Nicotine Tob Res*, 18(1), 25–33.

Bolker, B. M., Brooks, M. E., Clark, C. J., Geange, S. W., Poulsen, J. R., Stevens, M. H. H., and White, J. S. S. (2009). Generalized linear mixed models: A practical guide for ecology and evolution. *Trends in Ecology and Evolution*, 24(3), 127–135.

Bollen, K. A., and Curran, P. J. (2004). Autoregressive latent trajectory (ALT) models a synthesis of two traditions. *Sociological Methods and Research*, 32(3), 336–383.

Borenstein, M. (1997). Hypothesis testing and effect size estimation in clinical trials. *Annals of Allergy, Asthma and Immunology*, 78(1), 5–11.

Bowden, R. J., and Turkington, D. A. (1984). *Instrumental Variables*. Cambridge: Cambridge University Press.

Bowman, F. D. (2014). Brain imaging analysis. *Annual Review of Statistics and Its Application*, 1, 61–85.

Box, G. E. P. (1950). Problems in the analysis of growth and wear curves. *Biometrics*, 6(4), 362–389.

Brown, C. H., Wang, W., Kellam, S. G., Muthen, B. O., Petras, H., Toyinbo, P., … and Sloboda, Z. (2008). Methods for testing theory and evaluating impact in randomized field trials: Intent-to-treat analyses for integrating the perspectives of person, place, and time. *Drug and Alcohol Dependence*, 95, S74–S104.

Brown, H., and Prescott, R. (2006). *Applied Mixed Models in Medicine* (2nd edn). Hoboken, NJ: Wiley.

Brunner, E., and Puri, M. L. (2001). Nonparametric methods in factorial designs. *Statistical Papers*, 42(1), 1–52.

Brunner, E., Domhof, S., and Langer, F. (2002). *Nonparametric Analysis of Longitudinal Data in Factorial Experiments*. New York: Wiley.

Brunner, E., Munzel, U., and Puri, M. L. (1999). Rank-score tests in factorial designs with repeated measures. *Journal of Multivariate Analysis*, 70(2), 286–317.

Bryk, A. S., and Raudenbush, S. W. (1987). Application of hierarchical linear-models to assessing change. *Psychological Bulletin*, 101(1), 147–158.

Carey, V., Zeger, S. L., and Diggle, P. (1993). Modeling multivariate binary data with alternating logistic regressions. *Biometrika*, 80(3), 517–526.

Carlin, B. P., and Louis, T. A. (2009). *Bayesian Methods for Data Analysis* (3rd edn). Boca Raton, FL: CRC Press.

Carpenter, J. R., and Kenward, M. G. (2013). *Multiple Imputation and Its Application* (1st edn). Chichester: Wiley.

Casella, G. (1985). An introduction to empirical Bayes data-analysis. *American Statistician*, 39(2), 83–87.

Castelloe, J. (2014). Power and sample size for MANOVA and repeated measures with the GLMPOWER procedure. SAS Global Forum Proceedings. Paper SA030-2014. http://support.sas.com/resources/papers/proceedings14/SAS030-2014.pdf

Chakraborty, B., and Murphy, S. A. (2014). Dynamic treatment regimes. *Annual Review of Statistics and Its Application*, 1, 447–464.

Chekroud, A. M., Gueorguieva, R., Krumholz, H. M., Trivedi, M. H., Krystal, J. H., and McCarthy, G. (2017). Reevaluating the efficacy and predictability of antidepressant treatments: A symptom clustering approach. *JAMA Psychiatry*, 74(4), 370–378.

Chekroud, A. M., Zotti, R. J., Shehzad, Z., Gueorguieva, R., Johnson, M. K., Trivedi, M. H., ... Corlett, P. R. (2016). Cross-trial prediction of treatment outcome in depression: A machine learning approach. *Lancet Psychiatry*, 3(3), 243–250.

Chow, S. C. (2014). Adaptive clinical trial design. *Annual Review of Medicine*, 65, 405–415.

Chow, S. C., and Liu, J. P. (2013). *Design and Analysis of Clinical Trials: Concepts and Methodologies. Wiley Series in Probability and Statistics*. Hoboken, NJ: Wiley.

Chung, M. K. (2014). *Statistical and Computational Methods in Brain Image Analysis*. Boca Raton, FL: CRC Press.

Claeskens, G., and Hjort, N. L. (2008). *Model Selection and Model Averaging*. Cambridge: Cambridge University Press.

Clayton, D. (1992). Generalized linear mixed models in biostatistics. *Statistician*, 41(3), 327–328.

Coffey, C. S., and Kairalla, J. A. (2008). Adaptive clinical trials: Progress and challenges. *Drugs in R&D*, 9(4), 229–242.

Cohen, J. (1988). *Statistical Power Analysis for the Behavioral Sciences* (2nd edn). Hillsdale, NJ : L. Erlbaum Associates.

Cole, D. A., and Maxwell, S. E. (2003). Testing mediational models with longitudinal data: Questions and tips in the use of structural equation modeling. *Journal of Abnormal Psychology*, 112(4), 558–577.

Collett, D. (2003). *Modelling Survival Data in Medical Research* (2nd edn). Boca Raton, FL: Chapman and Hall/CRC.

Cox, D. R., Oakes, D., and Oakes, D. (1984). *Analysis of Survival Data*. New York: Chapman and Hall.

Crawley, M. J. (2007). The R book (pp. 1 online resource (viii, 942 p.)) Retrieved from http://onlinelibrary.wiley.com/book/10.1002/9780470515075.

D'Agostino, R. B. (1998). Propensity score methods for bias reduction in the comparison of a treatment to a non-randomized control group. *Statistics in Medicine*, 17(19), 2265–2281.

Dahmen, G., Rochon, J., Konig, I. R., and Ziegler, A. (2004). Sample size calculations for controlled clinical trials using generalized estimating equations (GEE). *Methods of Information in Medicine*, 43(5), 451–456.

Dang, Q. Y., Mazumdar, S., and Houck, P. R. (2008). Sample size and power calculations based on generalized linear mixed models with correlated binary outcomes. *Comput Methods Programs Biomed*, 91(2), 122–127.

Davidian, M., and Giltinan, D. M. (1995). *Nonlinear Models for Repeated Measurement Data* (1st edn). New York: Chapman and Hall.

Davidian, M. (2009). Non-linear mixed-effects models. In G. Fitzmaurice, M. Davidian, G. Verbeke, and G. Molenberghs (Eds.), *Longitudinal Data Analysis*, Boca Raton, FL: CRC Press, 107–142.

Dawson, K. S., Gennings, C., and Carter, W. H. (1997). Two graphical techniques useful in detecting correlation structure in repeated measures data. *American Statistician*, 51(3), 275–283.

Delucchi, K. L. (1994). Methods for the analysis of binary outcome results in the presence of missing data. *Journal of Consulting and Clinical Psychology*, 62(3), 569–575.

Diggle, P. J. (2003). *Statistical Analysis of Spatial Point Patterns* (2nd edn). London: Arnold.

Diggle, P. J., Sousa, I., and Chetwynd, A. G. (2008). Joint modelling of repeated measurements and time-to-event outcomes: The fourth Armitage lecture. *Statistics in Medicine*, 27(16), 2981–2998.

Diggle, P., and Ribeiro, P. J. (2007). *Model-Based Geostatistics*. New York: Springer.

Diggle, P., Liang, K.-Y., and Zeger, S. L. (2002). *Analysis of Longitudinal Data* (2nd edn). Oxford: Oxford University Press.

Dmitrienko, A., Tamhane, A. C., and Bretz, F. (2010). *Multiple Testing Problems in Pharmaceutical Statistics* Boca Raton, FL: Chapman and Hall/CRC.

Driesen, N. R., Leung, H. C., Calhoun, V. D., Constable, R. T., Gueorguieva, R., Hoffman, R., ... and Krystal, J. H. (2008). Impairment of working memory maintenance and response in schizophrenia: Functional magnetic resonance imaging evidence. *Biological Psychiatry*, 64(12), 1026–1034.

Dudoit, S., and van der Laan, M. J. (2008). *Multiple Testing Procedures with Applications to Genomics*. New York: Springer.

Duncan, D. B. (1955). Multiple range and multiple F tests. *Biometrics*, 11(1), 1–42.

Dunn, G. (2000). *Statistics in Psychiatry*. London: Oxford University Press.

Dunn, O. J. (1961). Multiple comparisons among means. *Journal of the American Statistical Association*, 56(293), 52–64.

Dunnett, C. W. (1955). A multiple comparison procedure for comparing several treatments with a control. *Journal of the American Statistical Association*, 50(272), 1096–1121.

Edwards, D., and Berry, J. J. (1987). The efficiency of simulation-based multiple comparisons. *Biometrics*, 43(4), 913–928.

Efron, B. (1994). Missing data, imputation, and the bootstrap. *Journal of the American Statistical Association*, 89(426), 463–475.

Egbewale, B. E., Lewis, M., and Sim, J. (2014). Bias, precision and statistical power of analysis of covariance in the analysis of randomized trials with baseline imbalance: A simulation study. *BMC Medical Research Methodology*, 14, 49.

Enders, C. K. (2010). *Applied Missing Data Analysis*. New York: Guilford Press.

Enders, C. K. (2011). Analyzing longitudinal data with missing values. *Rehabilitation Psychology*, 56(4), 267–288.

Epperson, N., Czarkowski, K. A., Ward-O'Brien, D., Weiss, E., Gueorguieva, R., Jatlow, P., and Anderson, G. M. (2001). Maternal sertraline treatment and serotonin transport in breast-feeding mother-infant pairs. *American Journal of Psychiatry*, 158(10), 1631–1637.

Ertefaie, A., and Stephens, D. A. (2010). Comparing approaches to causal inference for longitudinal data: Inverse probability weighting versus propensity scores. *International Journal of Biostatistics*, 6(2), 1–24.

Fava, M., Evins, A. E., Dorer, D. J., and Schoenfeld, D. A. (2003). The problem of the placebo response in clinical trials for psychiatric disorders: Culprits, possible remedies, and a novel study design approach. *Psychotherapy and Psychosomatics*, 72(3), 115–127.

Ferrer, E., and McArdle, J. J. (2003). Alternative structural models for multivariate longitudinal data analysis. *Structural Equation Modeling—a Multidisciplinary Journal*, 10(4), 493–524.

Fisher, R. A. (1925). *Statistical Methods for Research Workers*. London: Oliver and Boyd.

Fitzmaurice, G. M., Davidian, M., Verbeke, G., and Molenberghs, G. (2009). (Eds). *Longitudinal Data Analysis*. Boca Raton, FL: CRC Press.

Fitzmaurice, G. M., Laird, N. M., and Ware, J. H. (2011). *Applied Longitudinal Analysis* (2nd edn). Hoboken, NJ: Wiley.

Fleiss, J. L. (1986). *The Design and Analysis of Clinical Experiments*. New York: Wiley.

Frankfurt, S., Frazier, P., Syed, M., and Jung, K. R. (2016). Using group-based trajectory and growth mixture modeling to identify classes of change trajectories. *Counseling Psychologist*, 44(5), 622–660.

Frazier, P. A., Tix, A. P., and Barron, K. E. (2004). Testing moderator and mediator effects in counseling psychology research. *Journal of Counseling Psychology*, 51(1), 115–134.

Friedman, L. M., Furberg, C., and DeMets, D. L. (2010). *Fundamentals of Clinical Trials*. New York: Springer.

Friston, K. J. (2007). *Statistical Parametric Mapping: The Analysis of Functional Brain Images* (1st edn). London: Elsevier/Academic Press.

Fuller, W. A. (1987). *Measurement Error Models*. New York: Wiley.

Gaynes, B. N., Rush, A. J., Trivedi, M. H., Wisniewski, S. R., Spencer, D., and Fava, M. (2008). The STAR*D study: Treating depression in the real world. *Cleveland Clinic Journal of Medicine*, 75(1), 57–66.

Gelfand, A. E. (2010). *Handbook of Spatial Statistics*. Boca Raton, FL: CRC Press.

Gelman, A., Carlin, J. B., Stern, H. S., Dunson, D. B., Vehtari, A., Rubin, D. B., and Ebooks Corporation. (2014). *Bayesian Data Analysis*. Boca Raton, FL: Chapman and Hall/CRC.

Genovese, C., and Wasserman, L. (2004). A stochastic process approach to false discovery control. *Annals of Statistics*, 32(3), 1035–1061.

Gibbons, R. D., Hedeker, D., Elkin, I., Waternaux, C., Kraemer, H. C., Greenhouse, J. B., ... and Watkins, J. T. (1993). Some conceptual and statistical issues in analysis of longitudinal psychiatric data. Application to the NIMH treatment of Depression Collaborative Research Program dataset. *Arch Gen Psychiatry*, 50(9), 739–750.

Gilat, A. (2011). *MATLAB: An Introduction with Applications* (4th edn). Hoboken, NJ: Wiley.

Ginexi, E. M., Howe, G. W., and Caplan, R. D. (2000). Depression and control beliefs in relation to reemployment: What are the directions of effect? *Journal of Occupational Health Psychology*, 5, 323–336.

Goldstein, H. (1987). *Multilevel Models in Educational and Social Research*. London: Griffin.

Graham, J. W. (2009). Missing data analysis: Making it work in the real world. *Annual Review of Psychology*, 60, 549–576.

Greenhouse, S. W., and Geisser, S. (1959). On methods in the analysis of profile data. *Psychometrika*, 24(2), 95–112.

Gueorguieva, R., and Krystal, J. H. (2004). Move over ANOVA: Progress in analyzing repeated-measures data and its reflection in papers published in the Archives of General Psychiatry. *Archives of General Psychiatry*, 61(3), 310–317.

Gueorguieva, R., Wu, R., Couper, D., Donovan, D., Rounsanville, B., Krystal, J., and O'Malley, S. (2011). Baseline trajectories of drinking moderate acamprosate effects on drinking in the COMBINE study. *Alcoholism—Clinical and Experimental Research*, 35(3), 523–531.

Gueorguieva, R., Wu, R., Donovan, D., Rounsaville, B. J., Couper, D., Krystal, J. H., and O'Malley, S. S. (2010). Naltrexone and combined behavioral intervention effects on trajectories of drinking in the COMBINE study. *Drug and Alcohol Dependence*, 107, 221–229.

Gueorguieva, R., Wu, R., Donovan, D., Rounsaville, B. J., Couper, D., Krystal, J. H., and O'Malley, S. S. (2012). Baseline trajectories of heavy drinking and their effects on postrandomization drinking in the COMBINE Study: Empirically derived predictors of drinking outcomes during treatment. *Alcohol*, 46(2), 121–131.

Gueorguieva, R., Wu, R., Krystal, J. H., Donovan, D., and O'Malley, S. S. (2013). Temporal patterns of adherence to medications and behavioral treatment and their relationship to patient characteristics and treatment response. *Addictive Behaviors*, 38(5), 2119–2127.

Gueorguieva, R., Wu, R., O'Connor, P. G., Weisner, C., Fucito, L. M., Hoffmann, S., ... and O'Malley, S. S. (2014). Predictors of abstinence from heavy drinking during treatment in COMBINE and external validation in PREDICT. *Alcoholism—Clinical and Experimental Research*, 38(10), 2647–2656.

Gueorguieva, R., Wu, R., Pittman, B., Cramer, J., Rosenheck, R. A., O'Malley, S. S., and Krystal, J. H. (2007). New insights into the efficacy of naltrexone based on trajectory-based reanalyses of two negative clinical trials. *Biological Psychiatry*, 61(11), 1290–1295.

Hanley, J. A., Negassa, A., Edwardes, M. D. D., and Forrester, J. E. (2003). Statistical analysis of correlated data using generalized estimating equations: An orientation. *The American Journal of Epidemiology*, 157(4), 364–375.

Harder, V. S., Stuart, E. A., and Anthony, J. C. (2010). Propensity score techniques and the assessment of measured covariate balance to test causal associations in psychological research. *Psychological Methods*, 15(3), 234–249.

Hardin, J. W., and Hilbe, J. (2013). *Generalized Estimating Equations* (2nd edn). Berlin: Springer Science+Business Media.

Harville, D. A. (1977). Maximum likelihood approaches to variance component estimation and to related problems. *Journal of the American Statistical Association*, 72(358), 320–338.

Hastie, T., and Tibshirani, R. (1987). Generalized additive models: Some applications. *Journal of the American Statistical Association*, 82(398), 371–386.

Hastie, T., Tibshirani, R. J., and Tibshirani, R. (1990). *Generalized Additive Models* (1st edn). New York: Chapman and Hall.

Have, T. R., Joffe, M. M., Lynch, K. G., Brown, G. K., Maisto, S. A., and Beck, A. T. (2007). Causal mediation analyses with rank preserving models. *Biometrics*, 63(3), 926–934.

Haviland, A. M., and Nagin, D. S. (2005). Causal inferences with group based trajectory models. *Psychometrika*, 70(3), 557–578.

Haviland, A. M., Jones, B. L., and Nagin, D. S. (2011). Group-based trajectory modeling extended to account for nonrandom participant attrition. *Sociological Methods and Research*, 40(2), 367–390.

Hayes, A. F. (2013). *Introduction to Mediation, Moderation, and Conditional Process Analysis: A Regression-Based Approach*. New York: Guilford Press.

Heagerty, P. J., and Zeger, S. L. (1996). Marginal regression models for clustered ordinal measurements. *Journal of the American Statistical Association*, 91(435), 1024–1036.

Hedeker, D. R., and Gibbons, R. D. (2006). *Longitudinal Data Analysis*. Hoboken, NJ: Wiley.

Hedeker, D., Gibbons, R. D., and Waternaux, C. (1999). Sample size estimation for longitudinal designs with attrition: Comparing time-related contrasts between two groups. *Journal of Educational and Behavioral Statistics*, 24(1), 70–93.

Hedeker, D., Mermelstein, R. J., and Demirtas, H. (2007). Analysis of binary outcomes with missing data: Missing = smoking, last observation carried forward, and a little multiple imputation. *Addiction*, 102(10), 1564–1573.

Heilbron, D. C. (1994). Zero-altered and other regression models for count data with added zeros. *Biometrical Journal*, 36(5), 531–547.

Hemming, K., Haines, T. P., Chilton, P. J., Girling, A. J., and Lilford, R. J. (2015). The stepped wedge cluster randomised trial: Rationale, design, analysis, and reporting. *British Medical Journal*, 350:h391.

Henderson, R., Diggle, P., and Dobson, A. (2000). Joint modelling of longitudinal measurements and event time data. *Biostatistics*, 1(4), 465–480.

Hernan, M. A., and Robins, J. M. (2006). Instruments for causal inference: An epidemiologist's dream? *Epidemiology*, 17(4), 360–372.

Hipp, J. R., and Bauer, D. J. (2006). Local solutions in the estimation of growth mixture models. *Psychological Methods*, 11(1), 36–53.

Hochberg, Y. (1988). A sharper Bonferroni procedure for multiple tests of significance. *Biometrika*, 75(4), 800–802.

Hochberg, Y., and Benjamini, Y. (1990). More powerful procedures for multiple significance testing. *Statistics in Medicine*, 9(7), 811–818.

Hochberg, Y., and Tamhane, A. C. (1983). Multiple comparisons in a mixed model. *American Statistician*, 37(4), 305–307.

Hochberg, Y., and Tamhane, A. C. (1987). *Multiple Comparison Procedures*. New York: Wiley.

Hoenig, J. M., and Heisey, D. M. (2001). The abuse of power: The pervasive fallacy of power calculations for data analysis. *American Statistician*, 55(1), 19–24.

Hogan, J. W., and Lancaster, T. (2004). Instrumental variables and inverse probability weighting for causal inference from longitudinal observational studies. *Statistical Methods in Medical Research*, 13(1), 17–48.

Hogan, J. W., Roy, J., and Korkontzelou, C. (2004). Tutorial in biostatistics: Handling drop-out in longitudinal studies. *Statistics in Medicine*, 23(9), 1455–1497.

Hollander, M., and Wolfe, D. A. (1999). *Nonparametric Statistical Methods* (2nd edn). New York: Wiley.

Holm, S. (1979). A simple sequentially rejective multiple test procedure. *Scandinavian Journal of Statistics*, 6(2), 65–70.

Hommel, G. (1988). A stagewise rejective multiple test procedure based on a modified Bonferroni test. *Biometrika*, 75(2), 383–386.

Hong, G. (2015). *Causality in a Social World: Moderation, Mediation and Spill-Over*. Chichester, UK: Wiley.

Hosmer, D. W., and Lemeshow, S. (1989). *Applied Logistic Regression*. New York: Wiley.

Hsu, J. C. (1981). Simultaneous confidence intervals for all distances from the best. *Annals of Statistics*, 9(5), 1026–1034.

Hsu, J. C. (1996). *Multiple Comparisons: Theory and Methods* (1st edn). London: Chapman and Hall.

Hu, M. C., Pavlicova, M., and Nunes, E. V. (2011). Zero-inflated and hurdle models of count data with extra zeros: Examples from an HIV-risk reduction intervention trial. *American Journal of Drug and Alcohol Abuse*, 37(5), 367–375.

Huitema, B. (2011). *Analysis of Covariance and Alternatives: Statistical Methods for Experiments, Quasi-Experiments, and Single-Case Studies*. Hoboken, NJ: Wiley.

Huynh, H., and Feldt, L. S. (1976). Estimation of the box correction for degrees of freedom from sample data in randomized block and split-plot designs. *Journal of Educational Statistics*, 1(1), 69–82.

Ibrahim, J. G., and Molenberghs, G. (2009). Missing data methods in longitudinal studies: A review. *Test*, 18(1), 1–43.

Imai, K., and van Dyk, D. A. (2004). Causal inference with general treatment regimes: Generalizing the propensity score. *Journal of the American Statistical Association*, 99(467), 854–866.

Imai, K., Keele, L., and Tingley, D. (2010). A general approach to causal mediation analysis. *Psychological Methods*, 15(4), 309–334.

Imai, K., Keele, L., and Yamamoto, T. (2010). Identification, inference and sensitivity analysis for causal mediation effects. *Statistical Science*, 25(1), 51–71.

Imbens, G. W. (2000). The role of the propensity score in estimating dose-response functions. *Biometrika*, 87(3), 706–710.

Imbens, G. W. (2014). Instrumental variables: An econometrician's perspective. *Statistical Science*, 29(3), 323–358.

Jiang, J. (2007). *Linear and Generalized Linear Mixed Models and their Applications*. New York, NY: Science + Business Media.

Joffe, M. M., and Rosenbaum, P. R. (1999). Invited commentary: Propensity scores. *The American Journal of Epidemiology*, 150(4), 327–333.

Jones, B. L., and Nagin, D. S. (2007). Advances in group-based trajectory modeling and an SAS procedure for estimating them. *Sociological Methods and Research*, 35(4), 542–571.

Jones, B. L., Nagin, D. S., and Roeder, K. (2001). A SAS procedure based on mixture models for estimating developmental trajectories. *Sociological Methods and Research*, 29(3), 374–393.

Jones, R. N., Newsom, J. T., and Hofer, S. M. (2012). *Longitudinal Data Analysis: A Practical Guide for Researchers in Aging, Health, and Social Sciences*. New York: Routledge.

Jose, P. E. (2013). *Doing Statistical Mediation and Moderation*. New York: Guilford Press.

Judd, C. M., and Kenny, D. A. (1981). Process analysis: Estimating mediation in treatment evaluations. *Evaluation Review*, 5(5), 602–619.

Jung, T., and Wickrama, K. A. S. (2008). An introduction to latent class growth analysis and growth mixture modeling. *Social and Personality Psychology Compass*, 2(1), 302–317.

Kalbfleisch, J. D., and Prentice, R. L. (2002). *The Statistical Analysis of Failure Time Data* (2nd edn). Hoboken, NJ: Wiley.

Kalish, L. A., and Begg, C. B. (1985). Treatment allocation methods in clinical trials: A review. *Statistics in Medicine*, 4(2), 129–144.

Katz, M. H. (2006). *Study Design and Statistical Analysis: A Practical Guide for Clinicians*. Cambridge: Cambridge University Press.

Kenny, D. A., Korchmaros, J. D., and Bolger, N. (2003). Lower level mediation in multilevel models. *Psychological Methods*, 8(2), 115–128.

Kernan, W. N., Viscoli, C. M., Makuch, R. W., Brass, L. M., and Horwitz, R. I. (1999). Stratified randomization for clinical trials. *Journal of Clinical Epidemiology*, 52(1), 19–26.

Kohler, U., and Kreuter, F. (2005). *Data Analysis Using Stata*. College Station, TX: Stata Press.

Kong, M. Y., Xu, S., Levy, S. M., and Datta, S. (2015). GEE type inference for clustered zero-inflated negative binomial regression with application to dental caries. *Computational Statistics and Data Analysis*, 85, 54–66.

Kraemer, H. C. (2011). Moderators and mediators: The MacArthur updated view. In *Handbook of Behavioral Medicine: Methods and Applications*, 869–880. New York: Springer.

Kraemer, H. C., and Blasey, C. (1987). *How Many Subjects?: Statistical Power Analysis in Research* (2nd edn). Thousand Oaks, CA: Sage Publications.

Kraemer, H. C., Stice, E., Kazdin, A., Offord, D., and Kupfer, D. (2001). How do risk factors work together? Mediators, moderators, and independent, overlapping, and proxy risk factors. *American Journal of Psychiatry*, 158(6), 848–856.

Kraemer, H. C., Wilson, G. T., Fairburn, C. G., and Agras, W. S. (2002). Mediators and moderators of treatment effects in randomized clinical trials. *Archives of General Psychiatry*, 59(10), 877–883.

Krull, J. L., and MacKinnon, D. P. (1999). Multilevel mediation modeling in group-based intervention studies. *Evaluation Review*, 23(4), 418–444.

Kutner, N. N., Nachtsheim, C. J., Neter, J., and Li, W. (2005). *Applied Linear Statistical Models*, 5th edn. New York, NY: McGraw-Hill.

Lachin, J. M. (1981). Introduction to sample-size determination and power analysis for clinical trials. *Controlled Clinical Trials*, 2(2), 93–113.

Lachin, J. M. (1988a). Properties of randomization in clinical-trials: Foreword. *Controlled Clinical Trials*, 9(4), 287–288.

Lachin, J. M. (1988b). Properties of simple randomization in clinical trials. *Controlled Clinical Trials*, 9(4), 312–326.

Lachin, J. M. (1988c). Statistical properties of randomization in clinical trials. *Controlled Clinical Trials*, 9(4), 289–311.

Lachin, J. M., Matts, J. P., and Wei, L. J. (1988). Randomization in clinical trials: Conclusions and recommendations. *Controlled Clinical Trials*, 9(4), 365–374.

Laird, N. M., and Ware, J. H. (1982). Random effects models for longitudinal data. *Biometrics*, 38(4), 963–974.

Lambert, D. (1992). Zero-inflated poisson regression, with an application to defects in manufacturing. *Technometrics*, 34(1), 1–14.

Lenth, R. V. (2001). Some practical guidelines for effective sample size determination. *American Statistician*, 55(3), 187–193.

Leon, A. C., Davis, L. L., and Kraemer, H. C. (2011). The role and interpretation of pilot studies in clinical research. *Journal of Psychiatric Research*, 45(5), 626–629.

Leon, A. C., Hedeker, D., Li, C., and Demirtas, H. (2012). Performance of a propensity score adjustment in longitudinal studies with covariate-dependent representation. *Statistics in Medicine*, 31(20), 2262–2274.

Levy, P. S., and Lemeshow, S. (1999). *Sampling of Populations: Methods and Applications* (3rd edn). New York: Wiley.

Li, L. L., Shen, C. Y., Li, X. C., and Robins, J. M. (2013). On weighting approaches for missing data. *Statistical Methods in Medical Research*, 22(1), 14–30.

Li, Y., and Baron, J. (2012). Behavioral research data analysis with R Use R! New York, NY: Springer Science+Business Media.

Lin, H. Z., and Pan, J. X. (2013). Nonparametric estimation of mean and covariance structures for longitudinal data. *Canadian Journal of Statistics—Revue Canadienne De Statistique*, 41(4), 557–574.

Lin, X. H., and Carroll, R. J. (2009). Non-parametric and semi-parametric regression methods for longitudinal data. In G. Fitzmaurice, M. Davidian, G. Verbeke, and G. Molenberghs (Eds.), *Longitudinal Data Analysis*, Boca Raton, FL: CRC Press, 199–221.

Lindsey, J. K. (1999). *Models for Repeated Measurements* (2nd edn). Oxford: Oxford University Press.

Littell, R. C. (2006). *SAS for Mixed Models* (2nd edn). Cary, NC: SAS Institute.

Littell, R. C., Pendergast, J., and Natarajan, R. (2000). Modelling covariance structure in the analysis of repeated measures data. *Statistics in Medicine*, 19(13), 1793–1819.

Little, R. J., and Rubin, D. B. (2000). Causal effects in clinical and epidemiological studies via potential outcomes: Concepts and analytical approaches. *Annual Review of Public Health*, 21, 121–145.

Little, R. J., D'Agostino, R., Cohen, M. L., Dickersin, K., Emerson, S. S., Farrar, J. T., ... and Stern, H. (2012). The prevention and treatment of missing data in clinical trials. *New England Journal of Medicine*, 367(14), 1355–1360.

Little, R. J. A. (1988). A test of missing completely at random for multivariate data with missing values. *Journal of the American Statistical Association*, 83(404), 1198–1202.

Little, R. J. A., and Rubin, D. B. (2014). *Statistical Analysis with Missing Data*. New York: Wiley.

Liu, L., Ma, J. Z., and Johnson, B. A. (2008). A multi-level two-part random effects model, with application to an alcohol-dependence study. *Statistics in Medicine*, 27(18), 3528–3539.

Liu, L., Strawderman, R. L., Johnson, B. A., and O'Quigley, J. M. (2012). Analyzing repeated measures semi-continuous data, with application to an alcohol dependence study. *Statistical Methods in Medical Research*, 25(1), 133–152.

Lo, Y. T., Mendell, N. R., and Rubin, D. B. (2001). Testing the number of components in a normal mixture. *Biometrika*, 88(3), 767–778.

Long, J. D. (2011). *Longitudinal Data Analysis for the Behavioral Sciences Using R*. Thousand Oaks, CA: SAGE Publications.

Longford, N. T. (1993). *Random Coefficient Models*. Oxford; New York: Clarendon Press; Oxford University Press.

Lu, B. (2005). Propensity score matching with time-dependent covariates. *Biometrics*, 61(3), 721–728.

MacKinnon, D. P. (2008). *Introduction to Statistical Mediation Analysis*. Abingdon, United Kingdom: Routledge.

MacKinnon, D. P., and Luecken, L. J. (2008). How and for whom? Mediation and moderation in health psychology. *Health Psychology*, 27(2), S99–S100.

MacKinnon, D. P., Fairchild, A. J., and Fritz, M. S. (2007). Mediation analysis. *Annual Review of Psychology*, 58, 593–614.

MacKinnon, D. P., Lockwood, C. M., Brown, C. H., Wang, W., and Hoffman, J. M. (2007). The intermediate endpoint effect in logistic and probit regression. *Clinical Trials*, 4(5), 499–513.

Mallinckrodt, C., Roger, J., Chuang-Stein, C., Molenberghs, G., Lane, P. W., Kelly, M. O., ... and Thijs, H. (2013). Missing data: Turning guidance into action. *Statistics in Biopharmaceutical Research*, 5(4), 369–382.

Mallinckrodt, C., Roger, J., Chuang-Stein, C., Molenberghs, G., O'Kelly, M., Ratitch, B., ... and Bunouf, P. (2014). Recent developments in the prevention and treatment of missing data. *Therapeutic Innovation and Regulatory Science*, 48(1), 68–80.

Marcus, R., Peritz, E., and Gabriel, K. R. (1976). Closed testing procedures with special reference to ordered analysis of variance. *Biometrika*, 63(3), 655–660.

Matts, J. P., and Lachin, J. M. (1988). Properties of permuted-block randomization in clinical trials. *Controlled Clinical Trials*, 9(4), 327–344.

McArdle, J. J. (2009). Latent variable modeling of differences and changes with longitudinal data. *Annual Review of Psychology*, 60, 577–605.

McCullagh, P., and Nelder, J. A. (1989). *Generalized Linear Models* (2nd edn). New York: Chapman and Hall.

McCulloch, C. E., and Searle, S. R. (2001). *Generalized, Linear, and Mixed Models*. New York: Wiley.

Miller, G. A., and Chapman, J. P. (2001). Misunderstanding analysis of covariance. *Journal of Abnormal Psychology*, 110(1), 40–48.

Milliken, G. A., and Johnson, D. E. (1984). *Analysis of Messy Data*. Belmont, CA: Lifetime Learning Publications.

Milliken, G. A., and Johnson, D. E. (2008). *Analysis of Messy Data*, 2nd edn. Boca Raton, FL: CRC Press.

Min, Y. Y., and Agresti, A. (2005). Random effect models for repeated measures of zero-inflated count data. *Statistical Modelling*, 5(1), 1–19.

Moher, D., Hopewell, S., Schulz, K. F., Montori, V., Gotzsche, P. C., Devereaux, P. J., ... and Altman, D. G. (2012). CONSORT 2010 explanation and elaboration: Updated guidelines for reporting parallel group randomised trials. *Journal of Clinical Epidemiology*, 65(3), 351–351.

Molenberghs, G., and Kenward, M. G. (2007). *Missing Data in Clinical Studies*. Hoboken, NJ: Wiley.

Molenberghs, G., Fitzmaurice, G., Kenward, M. G., Tsiatis, A., and Verbeke, G. (Eds.) (2014). *Handbook of Missing Data Methodology*: Boca Raton, FL: Chapman and Hall/CRC.

Molenberghs, G., Verbeke, G., and Kenward, M. G. (2009a). Sensitivity analysis for incomplete data. *Longitudinal Data Analysis*, 501–551.

Molenberghs, G., Verbeke, G., and Kenward, M. G. (2009b). *Sensitivity Analysis for Incomplete Data*. Boca Raton, FL: CRC Press-Taylor & Francis Group.

Montgomery, D. C. (2013). *Design and Analysis of Experiments* (8th edn). Hoboken, NJ: Wiley.

Moodie, E. E. M., and Stephens, D. A. (2011). Marginal structural models: Unbiased estimation for longitudinal studies. *International Journal of Public Health*, 56(1), 117–119.

Morgan, P. T., Angarita, G. A., Canavana, S., Pittman, B., Oberleitner, L., Malison, R. T., ... and Forselius, E. (2016). Modafinil and sleep architecture in an inpatient-outpatient treatment study of cocaine dependence. *Drug and Alcohol Dependence*, 160, 49–56.

Morgan, S. L., and Winship, C. (2015). *Counterfactuals and Causal Inference: Methods and Principles for Social Research*, 2nd edn. Cambridge: Cambridge University Press.

Morgan-Lopez, A. A., and MacKinnon, D. P. (2006). Demonstration and evaluation of a method for assessing mediated moderation. *Behavior Research Methods*, 38(1), 77–87.

Muller, D., Judd, C. M., and Yzerbyt, V. Y. (2005). When moderation is mediated and mediation is moderated. *Journal of Personality and Social Psychology*, 89(6), 852–863.

Muller, K. E., and Peterson, B. L. (1984). Practical methods for computing power in testing the multivariate general linear hypothesis. *Computational Statistics and Data Analysis*, 2(2), 143–158.

Muller, K. E., Lavange, L. M., Ramey, S. L., and Ramey, C. T. (1992). Power calculations for general linear multivariate models including repeated measures applications. *Journal of the American Statistical Association*, 87(420), 1209–1226.

Muller, R., and Buttner, P. (1994). A critical discussion of intraclass correlation coefficients. *Statistics in Medicine*, 13(23–24), 2465–2476.

Muthén, B., and Asparouhov, T. (2015). Causal effects in mediation modeling: An introduction with applications to latent variables. *Structural Equation Modeling—a Multidisciplinary Journal*, 22(1), 12–23.

Muthén, B., and Asparouhov, T. (2015). Growth mixture modeling with non-normal distributions. *Statistics in Medicine*, 34(6), 1041–1058.

Muthén, B., and Muthén, L. (1998–2015). *MPlus User's Guide*, 7th edn. Los Angeles, CA: Muthen and Muthen.

Muthén, B., and Muthén, L. K. (2000). Integrating person-centered and variable-centered analyses: Growth mixture modeling with latent trajectory classes. *Alcoholism—Clinical and Experimental Research*, 24(6), 882–891.

Muthén, B., and Shedden, K. (1999). Finite mixture modeling with mixture outcomes using the EM algorithm. *Biometrics*, 55(2), 463–469.

Muthén, B., Asparouhov, T., Hunter, A. M., and Leuchter, A. F. (2011). Growth modeling with non-ignorable dropout: Alternative analyses of the STAR*D antidepressant trial. *Psychological Methods*, 16(1), 17–33.

Muthén, B., Brown, C. H., Masyn, K., Jo, B., Khoo, S. T., Yang, C. C., ... and Liao, J. (2002). General growth mixture modeling for randomized preventive interventions. *Biostatistics*, 3(4), 459–475.

Nagin, D. S. (1999). Analyzing developmental trajectories: A semiparametric, group-based approach. *Psychological Methods*, 4(2), 139–157.

Nagin, D. S. (2014). Group-based trajectory modeling: An overview. *Annals of Nutrition and Metabolism*, 65(2–3), 205–210.

Nagin, D. S., and Odgers, C. L. (2010). Group-based trajectory modeling in clinical research. *Annual Review of Clinical Psychology*, 6, 109–138.

Nagin, D. S., and Tremblay, R. E. (2001). Analyzing developmental trajectories of distinct but related behaviors: A group-based method. *Psychological Methods*, 6(1), 18–34.

Nagin, D. S., and Tremblay, R. E. (2005). Developmental trajectory groups: Fact or a useful statistical fiction? *Criminology*, 43(4), 873–904.

NCSS Statistical Software. (2014). PASS 13 Power Analysis and Sample Size Software. Kaysville, UT: NCSS. http://ncss.com/software/pass.

Nelder, J. A., and Wedderburn, R. W. M. (1972). Generalized linear models. *Journal of the Royal Statistical Society Series A—General*, 135(3), 370–384.

Nelson, D. B., Partin, M. R., Fu, S. S., Joseph, A. M., and An, L. C. (2009). Why assigning ongoing tobacco use is not necessarily a conservative approach to handling missing tobacco cessation outcomes. *Nicotine Tob Res*, 11(1), 77–83.

Newman, D. (1939). The distribution of range in samples from a normal population, expressed in terms of an independent estimate of standard deviation. *Biometrika*, 31, 20–30.

Nobre, J. S., and da Motta Singer, J. (2007). Residual analysis for linear mixed models. *Biometrical Journal*, 49(6), 863–875.

Normand, S. L. T. (1999). Meta-analysis: Formulating, evaluating, combining, and reporting. *Statistics in Medicine*, 18(3), 321–359.

Nylund, K. L., Asparouhov, T., and Muthén, B. O. (2007) Deciding on the number of classes in latent class analysis and growth mixture modeling: A Monte Carlo simulation study. *Structural Equation Modeling—a Multidisciplinary Journal*, 14, 535–569.

O'Brien, P. C., and Fleming, T. R. (1979). A multiple testing procedure for clinical trials. *Biometrics*, 35(3), 549–556.

Ott, T., and Swiaczny, F. (2001). *Time-Integrative Geographic Information Systems: Management and Analysis of Spatio-Temporal Data*. Berlin: Springer Science+Business Media.

Paik, M. C. (1997). The generalized estimating equation approach when data are not missing completely at random. *Journal of the American Statistical Association*, 92(440), 1320–1329.

Pan, W. (2001). Akaike's information criterion in generalized estimating equations. *Biometrics*, 57(1), 120–125.

Parfrey, P. S., and Barrett, B. (2009). *Clinical Epidemiology: Practice and Methods*. New York: Springer.

Pearl, J. (2003). Statistics and causal inference: A review. *Test*, 12(2), 281–318.

Pearl, J. (2010). An introduction to causal inference. *International Journal of Biostatistics*, 6(2), 1–62.

Pickles, A., and Croudace, T. (2010). Latent mixture models for multivariate and longitudinal outcomes. *Statistical Methods in Medical Research*, 19(3), 271–289.

Pirlott, A. G., and MacKinnon, D. P. (2016). Design approaches to experimental mediation. *Journal of Experimental Social Psychology*, 66, 29–38.

Pocock, S. J. (2006). Current controversies in data monitoring for clinical trials. *Clinical Trials*, 3(6), 513–521.

Preacher, K. J. (2015). Advances in mediation analysis: A survey and synthesis of new developments. *Annual Review of Psychology*, 66, 825–852.

Preacher, K. J., and Hayes, A. F. (2008). Asymptotic and resampling strategies for assessing and comparing indirect effects in multiple mediator models. *Behavior Research Methods*, 40(3), 879–891.

Preacher, K. J., Rucker, D. D., and Hayes, A. F. (2007). Addressing moderated mediation hypotheses: Theory, methods, and prescriptions. *Multivariate Behavioral Research*, 42(1), 185–227.

Rabe-Hesketh, S., and Skrondal, A. (2008). *Multilevel and Longitudinal Modeling Using Stata*, 2nd edn. College Station, TX: Stata Press.

Ram, N., and Grimm, K. J. (2009). Growth mixture modeling: A method for identifying differences in longitudinal change among unobserved groups. *International Journal of Behavioral Development*, 33(6), 565–576.

Robins, J. M., and Greenland, S. (1992). Identifiability and exchangeability for direct and indirect effects. *Epidemiology*, 3(2), 143–155.

Robins, J. M., and Hernan, M. A. (2009). Estimation of the causal effects of time-varying exposures. In G. Fitzmaurice, M. Davidian, G. Verbeke, and G. Molenberghs (Eds.), *Longitudinal Data Analysis*, Boca Raton, FL: CRC Press, 553–599.

Robins, J. M., Hernan, M. A., and Brumback, B. (2000). Marginal structural models and causal inference in epidemiology. *Epidemiology*, 11(5), 550–560.

Rochon, J. (1998). Application of GEE procedures for sample size calculations in repeated measures experiments. *Statistics in Medicine*, 17(14), 1643–1658.

Rosenbaum, P. R. (2002). *Observational Studies* (2nd edn). New York: Springer.

Rosenbaum, P. R. (2010). *Design of Observational Studies*. New York: Springer.

Rosenbaum, P. R., and Rubin, D. B. (1983). The central role of the propensity score in observational studies for causal effects. *Biometrika*, 70(1), 41–55.

Rosenbaum, P. R., and Rubin, D. B. (1984). Reducing bias in observational studies using subclassification on the propensity score. *Journal of the American Statistical Association*, 79(387), 516–524.

Rosenbaum, P. R., and Rubin, D. B. (1985). Constructing a control group using multivariate matched sampling methods that incorporate the propensity score. *American Statistician*, 39(1), 33–38.

Rosenblum, M., and van der Laan, M. J. (2010). Targeted maximum likelihood estimation of the parameter of a marginal structural model. *International Journal of Biostatistics*, 6(2). doi: Artn 19 10.2202/1557-4679.1238.

Rothman, K. J., Greenland, S., and Lash, T. L. (2008). *Modern Epidemiology* (3rd edn). Philadelphia, PA: Wolters Kluwer Health/Lippincott Williams & Wilkins.

Rotnitzky, A. (2009). Inverse probability weighted methods. In Fitzmaurice, G., Davidian, M., Verbeke, G., Molenberghs, G. (Eds.), *Longitudinal Data Analysis*, 453–476. Boca Raton, FL: CRC Press.

Rotnitzky, A., and Robins, J. (1997). Analysis of semi-parametric regression models with non-ignorable non-response. *Statistics in Medicine*, 16(1–3), 81–102.

Rotnitzky, A., Lei, Q. H., Sued, M., and Robins, J. M. (2012). Improved double-robust estimation in missing data and causal inference models. *Biometrika*, 99(2), 439–456.

Roy, A., Bhaumik, D. K., Aryal, S., and Gibbons, R. D. (2007). Sample size determination for hierarchical longitudinal designs with differential attrition rates. *Biometrics*, 63(3), 699–707.

Rubin, D. B. (1976). Inference and missing data. *Biometrika*, 63(3), 581–590.

Rubin, D. B. (1996). Multiple imputation after 18+ years. *Journal of the American Statistical Association*, 91(434), 473–489.

Rubin, D. B. (2005). Causal inference using potential outcomes: Design, modeling, decisions. *Journal of the American Statistical Association*, 100(469), 322–331.

Rush, A. J., Bernstein, I. H., Trivedi, M. H., Carmody, T. J., Wisniewski, S., Mundt, J. C., ... Fava, M. (2006). An evaluation of the quick inventory of depressive symptomatology and the Hamilton rating scale for depression: A sequenced treatment alternatives to relieve depression trial report. *Biological Psychiatry*, 59(6), 493–501.

Rutherford, A. (2012). *ANOVA and ANCOVA: A GLM Approach (2)*. Hoboken, NJ: Wiley.

Sall, J., Lehman, A., Stephens, M., and Creighton, W. L. (2014). JMP start statistics: A guide to statistics and data analysis using JMP, 5th edn. Cary, NC: SAS Institute.

Sanacora, G., Berman, R. M., Cappiello, A., Oren, D. A., Kugaya, A., Liu, N. J., … and Charney, D. S. (2004). Addition of the alpha 2-antagonist yohimbine to fluoxetine: Effects on rate of antidepressant response. *Neuropsychopharmacology*, 29(6), 1166–1171.

Schaefer, H., Timmesfeld, N., and Muller, H. H. (2006). An overview of statistical approaches for adaptive designs and design modifications. *Biometrical Journal*, 48(4), 507–520.

Schafer, J. L. (1997). *Analysis of Incomplete Multivariate Data*. New York: Chapman and Hall.

Schafer, J. L. (1999). Multiple imputation: A primer. *Statistical Methods in Medical Research*, 8(1), 3–15.

Scharfstein, D. O., Rotnitzky, A., and Robins, J. M. (1999). Adjusting for nonignorable drop-out using semiparametric nonresponse models. *Journal of the American Statistical Association*, 94(448), 1096–1120.

Scheffé, H. (1952). An analysis of variance for paired comparisons. *Journal of the American Statistical Association*, 47(259), 381–400.

Scheffé, H. (1953). A method for judging all contrasts in the analysis of variance. *Biometrika*, 40(1–2), 87–104.

Scheffé, H. (1999). *The Analysis of Variance* (Wiley Classics library edn). New York: Wiley.

Schlomer, G. L., Bauman, S., and Card, N. A. (2010). Best practices for missing data management in counseling psychology. *Journal of Counseling Psychology*, 57(1), 1–10.

Schweder, T., and Spjøtvoll, E. (1982). Plots of p-values to evaluate many tests simultaneously. *Biometrika*, 69(3), 493–502.

Scott, N. W., McPherson, G. C., Ramsay, C. R., and Campbell, M. K. (2002). The method of minimization for allocation to clinical trials: A review. *Controlled Clinical Trials*, 23(6), 662–674.

Senn, S. (2006). Change from baseline and analysis of covariance revisited. *Statistics in Medicine*, 25(24), 4334–4344.

Serroyen, J., Molenberghs, G., Verbeke, G., and Davidian, M. (2009). Nonlinear models for longitudinal data. *American Statistician*, 63(4), 378–388.

Sher, K. J., Jackson, K. M., and Steinley, D. (2011). Alcohol use trajectories and the ubiquitous cat's cradle: Cause for concern? *Journal of Abnormal Psychology*, 120(2), 322–335.

Shiffman, S., and Stone, A. A. (1998). Ecological momentary assessment: A new tool for behavioral medicine research. In Krantz, D.S. and Baum, A.S. (Eds.), *Technology and Methods in Behavioral Medicine*, Lawrence Erlbaum Associates, 117–131.

Shults, J., and Hilbe, J. M. (2014). *Quasi-least Squares Regression*. Boca Raton, FL: CRC Press.

Sidak, Z. (1967). Rectangular confidence regions for means of multivariate normal distributions. *Journal of the American Statistical Association*, 62(318), 626–633.

Simera, I., Moher, D., Hirst, A., Hoey, J., Schulz, K. F., and Altman, D. G. (2010). Transparent and accurate reporting increases reliability, utility, and impact of your research: Reporting guidelines and the EQUATOR Network. *BMC Medicine*, 8(1), Article 24.

Simes, R. J. (1986). An improved Bonferroni procedure for multiple tests of significance. *Biometrika*, 73(3), 751–754.

Singer, J. D., and Willett, J. B. (2003). *Applied Longitudinal Data Analysis: Modeling Change and Event Occurrence*. Oxford: Oxford University Press.

Skardhamar, T. (2010). Distinguishing facts and artifacts in group-based modeling. *Criminology*, 48(1), 295–320.

Snijders, T. A. B., and Bosker, R. J. (2012). *Multilevel Analysis: An Introduction to Basic and Advanced Multilevel Modeling* (2nd edn). Los Angeles, CA: Sage.

Soric, B. (1989). Statistical "discoveries" and effect-size estimation. *Journal of the American Statistical Association*, 84(406), 608–610.

Spratt, M., Carpenter, J., Sterne, J. A. C., Carlin, J. B., Heron, J., Henderson, J., and Tilling, K. (2010). Strategies for multiple imputation in longitudinal studies. *The American Journal of Epidemiology*, 172(4), 478–487.

Storey, J. D. (2003). The positive false discovery rate: A Bayesian interpretation and the q-value. *Annals of Statistics*, 31(6), 2013–2035.

Stroup, W. W. (2012). Generalized linear mixed models: Modern concepts, methods and applications. Boca Raton, FL: CRC Press.

Suresh, K. (2011). An overview of randomization techniques: An unbiased assessment of outcome in clinical research. *J Hum Reprod Sci*, 4(1), 8–11.

Sutradhar, B. C., and Das, K. (2000). On the accuracy of efficiency of estimating equation approach. *Biometrics*, 56(2), 622–625.

Ten Have, T. R., and Joffe, M. M. (2012). A review of causal estimation of effects in mediation analyses. *Statistical Methods in Medical Research*, 21(1), 77–107.

Tleyjeh, I. M., Ghomrawi, H. M. K., Steckelberg, J. A., Montori, V. M., Hoskin, T. L., Enders, F., … and Baddour, L. M. (2010). Propensity score analysis with a time-dependent intervention is an acceptable although not an optimal analytical approach when treatment selection bias and survivor bias coexist. *Journal of Clinical Epidemiology*, 63(2), 139–140.

Tofighi D., Enders C. K. (2008). Identifying the correct number of classes in a growth mixture model. In Hancock, G. R., and Samuelsen, K. M. (Eds.), *Advances in latent variable mixture models*. Charlotte, NC: Information Age, 317–341.

Tofighi, D., West, S. G., and MacKinnon, D. P. (2013). Multilevel mediation analysis: The effects of omitted variables in the 1–1–1 model. *British Journal of Mathematical and Statistical Psychology*, 66(2), 290–307.

Trivedi, M. H., Rush, A. J., Wisniewski, S. R., Nierenberg, A. A., Warden, D., Ritz, L., … and Shores-Wilson, K. (2006). Evaluation of outcomes with citalopram for depression using measurement-based care in STAR*D: Implications for clinical practice. *American Journal of Psychiatry*, 163(1), 28–40.

Tu, X. M., Kowalski, J., Zhang, J., Lynch, K. G., and Crits-Christoph, P. (2004). Power analyses for longitudinal trials and other clustered designs. *Statistics in Medicine*, 23(18), 2799–2815.

Tu, X. M., Zhang, J., Kowalski, J., Shults, J., Feng, C., Sun, W., and Tang, W. (2007). Power analyses for longitudinal study designs with missing data. *Statistics in Medicine*, 26(15), 2958–2981.

Tukey, J. (1953). Multiple comparisons. *Journal of the American Statistical Association*, 48(263), 624–625.

Tukey, J. W. (1949). Comparing individual means in the analysis of variance. *Biometrics*, 5(2), 99–114.

Twisk, J. W. (2013a). *Applied Longitudinal Data Analysis for Epidemiology: A Practical Guide*. Cambridge: Cambridge University Press.

Twisk, J. W. R. (2013b). *Applied Multilevel Analysis: A Practical Guide*. Cambridge: Cambridge University Press.

Valentine, G. W., DeVito, E. E., Jatlow, P., Gueorguieva, R., and Sofuoglu, M. Acute effects of inhaled menthol on the rewarding effects of intravenous nicotine in smokers. *Journal of Psychopharmacology*, under review.

Valeri, L., and VanderWeele, T. J. (2013). Mediation analysis allowing for exposure-mediator interactions and causal interpretation: Theoretical assumptions and implementation with SAS and SPSS macros. *Psychological Methods*, 18(2), 137–150.

Van Breukelen, G. J. P. (2006). ANCOVA versus change from baseline had more power in randomized studies and more bias in nonrandomized studies. *Journal of Clinical Epidemiology*, 59(9), 920–925.

Van Buuren, S. (2012). Longitudinal data. In *Flexible Imputation of Missing Data* (pp. 221–245). Boca Raton, FL: Chapman and Hall/CRC.

Van Buuren, S., Brand, J. P. L., Groothuis-Oudshoorn, C. G. M., and Rubin, D. B. (2006). Fully conditional specification in multivariate imputation. *Journal of Statistical Computation and Simulation*, 76(12), 1049–1064.

van de Schoot, R. (2015). Latent trajectory studies: The basics, how to interpret the results, and what to report. *European Journal of Psychotraumatology*, 6(1), 27514.

van der Wal, W. M., Prins, M., Lumbreras, B., and Geskus, R. B. (2009). A simple G-computation algorithm to quantify the causal effect of a secondary illness on the progression of a chronic disease. *Statistics in Medicine*, 28(18), 2325–2337.

VanderWeele, T. (2015). *Explanation in Causal Inference: Methods for Mediation and Interaction*. Oxford: Oxford University Press.

VanderWeele, T. J. (2010). Direct and indirect effects for neighborhood-based clustered and longitudinal data. *Sociological Methods and Research*, 38(4), 515–544.

VanderWeele, T. J. (2013). A three-way decomposition of a total effect into direct, indirect, and interactive effects. *Epidemiology*, 24(2), 224–232.

VanderWeele, T. J. (2016). Mediation analysis: A practitioner's guide. *Annual Review of Public Health*, 37, 17–32.

VanderWeele, T. J., and Tchetgen, E. J. T. (2016). Mediation analysis with matched case-control study designs. *The American Journal of Epidemiology*, 183(9), 869–870.

VanderWeele, T. J., and Vansteelandt, S. (2009). Conceptual issues concerning mediation, interventions and composition. *Statistics and Its Interface*, 2(4), 457–468.

VanderWeele, T. J., Vansteelandt, S., and Robins, J. M. (2014). Effect decomposition in the presence of an exposure-induced mediator-outcome confounder. *Epidemiology*, 25(2), 300–306.

VanderWeele, T., and Vansteelandt, S. (2014). Mediation analysis with multiple mediators *Epidemiologic Methods*. 2(1), 95-115.

Verbeke, G., and Davidian, G. (2009). Joint models for longitudinal data: Introduction and overview. In G. Fitzmaurice, M. Davidian, G. Verbeke, and G. Molenberghs (Eds.), *Longitudinal Data Analysis*, Boca Raton, FL: CRC Press.

Verbeke, G., and Lesaffre, E. (1996). A linear mixed-effects model with heterogeneity in the random-effects population. *Journal of the American Statistical Association*, 91(433), 217–221.

Verbeke, G., Fieuws, S., Molenberghs, G., and Davidian, M. (2014). The analysis of multivariate longitudinal data: A review. *Statistical Methods in Medical Research*, 23(1), 42–59.

Vermunt, J. K. (2010). Longitudinal research using mixture models. In K. van Mentfort, A. Satorra and J.H.L. Oud. (Eds.), *Longitudinal Research with Latent Variables*, Berlin: Springer-Verlag, 119–152.

Vickers, A. J. (2001). The use of percentage change from baseline as an outcome in a controlled trial is statistically inefficient: A simulation study. *BMC Medical Research Methodology*, 1(1), 6.

Vonesh, E. F., and Chinchilli, V. M. (1997). *Linear and Nonlinear Models for the Analysis of Repeated Measurements*. New York: M. Dekker.

Walls, T. A., and Schafer, J. L. (2006) (Eds). *Models for Intensive Longitudinal Data*. Oxford: Oxford University Press.
Wang, C. P., Brown, C. H., and Bandeen-Roche, K. (2005). Residual diagnostics for growth mixture models: Examining the impact of a preventive intervention on multiple trajectories of aggressive behavior. *Journal of the American Statistical Association*, 100(471), 1054–1076.
Wang, H., Shao, J., and Chow, S.-C. (2008). *Sample Size Calculations in Clinical Research* (2nd edn). Boca Raton, FL: Chapman and Hall/CRC.
Wang, R., and Ware, J. H. (2013). Detecting moderator effects using subgroup analyses. *Prevention Science*, 14(2), 111–120.
Ware, J. H. (1985). Linear models for the analysis of longitudinal studies. *American Statistician*, 39(2), 95–101.
Wei, L. J., and Lachin, J. M. (1988). Properties of the urn randomization in clinical trials. *Controlled Clinical Trials*, 9(4), 345–364.
Weiss, R. E. (2005). *Modeling Longitudinal Data*. New York: Springer.
Westfall, P. H., and Young, S. S. (1993). *Resampling-Based Multiple Testing: Examples and Methods for P-Value Adjustment*. New York: Wiley.
Westfall, P. H., Tobias, R. D., and Wolfinger, R. D. (2011). *Multiple Comparisons and Multiple Tests Using SAS*, 2nd edn. Cary, NC: SAS Institute.
White, I. R., Royston, P., and Wood, A. M. (2011). Multiple imputation using chained equations: Issues and guidance for practice. *Statistics in Medicine*, 30(4), 377–399.
Widaman, K. F. (2006). III. Missing data: What to do with or without them. *Monographs of the Society for Research in Child Development*, 71(3), 42–64.
Williamson, E. J., and Forbes, A. (2014). Introduction to propensity scores. *Respirology*, 19(5), 625–635.
Winship, C., and Morgan, S. L. (1999). The estimation of causal effects from observational data. *Annual Review of Sociology*, 25, 659–706.
Woods, S. W., Gueorguieva, R. V., Baker, C. B., and Makuch, R. W. (2005). Control group bias in randomized atypical antipsychotic medication trials for schizophrenia. *Archives of General Psychiatry*, 62(9), 961–970.
Woodward, M. (1999). *Epidemiology: Study Design and Data Analysis*. Boca Raton, FL: Chapman and Hall/CRC Press.
Wu, H., and Zhang, J.-T. (2006). *Nonparametric Regression Methods for Longitudinal Data Analysis*. Hoboken, NJ: Wiley.
Zeger, S. L., Liang, K. Y., and Albert, P. S. (1988). Models for longitudinal data: A generalized estimating equation approach. *Biometrics*, 44(4), 1049–1060.
Zhang, X., Huang, S. P., Sun, W., and Wang, W. (2012). Rapid and robust resampling-based multiple-testing correction with application in a genome-wide expression quantitative trait loci study. *Genetics*, 190(4), 1511–1520.
Zhang, Z. Y., and Wang, L. J. (2009). Statistical power analysis for growth curve models using SAS. *Behavior Research Methods*, 41(4), 1083–1094.
Ziegler, A. (2011). *Generalized Estimating Equations*. New York, NY: Springer Science + Business Media.

Index

M

S